MENTAL HEALTH AND CANADIAN SOCIETY

MCGILL-QUEEN'S ASSOCIATED MEDICAL SERVICES
Studies in the History of Medicine, Health, and Society

Series Editors: S.O. Freedman and J.H. Connor

Volumes in this series have financial support from Associated Medical Services, Inc. (AMS). Associated Medical Services Inc. was established in 1936 by Dr Jason Hannah as a pioneer not-for-profit health care organization in Ontario. With the advent of medicare, AMS became a charitable organization supporting innovations in academic medicine and health services, specifically the history of medicine and health care, as well as innovations in health professional education and bioethics.

Contents

Tables, Figures, and Map

Acknowledgments

The editors are greatly indebted to the participants in the conference from whence this edited volume arose – the 2001 Hannah International Conference on the History of Mental Disorders – and to those institutions that financially supported the meeting: Associated Medical Services, Inc. (Toronto), McMaster University, and the University of Toronto. Associated Medical Services provided an additional subvention in support of this publication, as did the Aid to Scholarly Publications Programme of the Social Sciences and Humanities Research Council of Canada. Many thanks in particular to Dr Bill Seidelman, the president of Associated Medical Services, for his personal encouragement in the publication of the book.

The construction of the volume was made possible through the generous and unfailing administrative assistance of Barbara-Ann Bartlett of the History of Medicine Unit, McMaster University. Erika Dyck provided further editorial input and word-processing expertise. The French-language and legal-language translation was assisted respectively by Don Fyson of the Université Laval and Ian Wright of Scott, Petrie, Brander, Walters & Wright, LLP (London). We are very grateful for the excellent editorial team at McGill-Queen's University Press and, in particular, for the support and patience of Jonathan Crago, Joan McGilvray, and John Zucchi. Elizabeth Hulse's meticulous copy-editing smoothed over a few rough edges, added additional clarity to the text, and provided consistency between chapters of disparate disciplinary lineage. Thanks also to two anonymous referees for their detailed and constructive criticism. A final word of thanks to our colleagues for their excellent contributions.

Contributors

ANDRÉ CELLARD is professor in the Criminology and History departments at the University of Ottawa. He has published numerous articles and books on the history of madness and criminality, including *l'Histoire de le folie au Québec, 1600–1850* (Québec: Boréal, 1991), *Punishment, Imprisonment and Reform in Canada: From New France to the Present* (Ottawa: Canadian Historical Association, Historical Booklet no. 60, 2000), and (with Gérald Pelletier) "Le Code criminel canadien, 1892–1927: Étude des acteurs sociaux," *Canadian Historical Review.* 79, no. 2 (June 1998).

IAN DOWBIGGIN is professor of history at the University of Prince Edward Island. He is the author of *Inheriting Madness: Professionalization and Psychiatric Knowledge in Nineteenth-Century France* (Berkeley: University of California Press, 1991), *Keeping America Sane: Eugenics and Psychiatry in the United States and Canada, 1880–1940* (Ithaca: Cornell University Press, 1997), *Suspicious Minds: The Triumph of Paranoia in Everyday Life* (Toronto: McFarlane Walter and Ross, 1999), and *A Merciful End: The Euthanasia Movement in Modern America* (New York: Oxford University Press, 2002). He is currently researching a book on the history of sterilization.

ERIKA DYCK is assistant professor in the history of medicine at the University of Alberta. Her recently-completed doctoral dissertation from McMaster University explores the history of psychiatric experimentation in post-war Canada. In particular, she is researching the role of two Saskatchewan psychiatrists, Abram Hoffer and Humphrey Osmond, and their contribution to LSD experimentation in the 1950s and 1960s.

JUDITH FINGARD was a member of the Department of History at Dalhousie University from 1967 until her retirement in 1998. Among her many publications are *Jack in Port: Sailortowns of Eastern Canada* (1982), *The Dark Side of Life in Victorian Halifax* (1989), and, with others, *Mothers of the Municipality: Women, Work, and Social Policy in Post-1945 Halifax* (2005). She has been examining, with John Rutherford, the development of public policy, professionalization of health care workers, evolution of treatment, and delivery of services in the mental health care field in the twentieth century.

ALLISON KIRK-MONTGOMERY is an independent historian and has been a social worker and a member of the Ontario Parole Board. Her article is drawn from her doctoral dissertation, which was completed at the University of Toronto in 2001 and entitled, "'Courting Madness': Insanity and Testimony in the Criminal Justice System of Victorian Ontario."

ROBERT MENZIES is the J.S. Woodsworth Resident Scholar in the Humanities at Simon Fraser University. He is co-editor, with Wendy Chan and Dorothy E. Chunn, of the recently published *Women, Madness and the Law: A Feminist Reader* (London and Portland, OR: Glasshouse Press, 2005) and has published numerous articles on the history of crime and madness.

JANET MIRON completed her PhD in the History Department at York University, in 2004. Her chapter derives from her dissertation, entitled "'As in a Menagerie': The Custodial Institution as Spectacle in Nineteenth-Century North America." It explores the popular pastime of "institutional visiting," which saw thousands of people tour the growing number of prisons and asylums in Canada and the United States.

JAMES E. MORAN is assistant professor, Department of History, University of Prince Edward Island. He has published widely in the history of mental health, including *Committed to the State Asylum: Insanity and Society in Nineteenth-Century Quebec and Ontario* (Montreal and Kingston: McGill-Queen's University Press, 2000), and with co-editors Leslie Topp and Jonathan Andrews, *Madness, Space and the Built Envi-*

ronment: Psychiatric Spaces in International Context, 1600–2000 (London: Routledge, 2006).

THIERRY NOOTENS completed a doctorate in history in 2003 at the Université du Québec à Montréal. His dissertation examined the nature of interactions between the many actors (families, justice officials, doctors, and institutions) involved in the care and control of some types of devi-ance (mental illness, alcoholism, and spendthrift attitudes) in nineteenth-century Montreal. As a post-doctoral fellow, he has worked on the problem of sons of the bourgeoisie who were seen as "failures" by their social circles. He is now a lecturer at the University of Sherbrooke.

TED PALYS is professor in the School of Criminology at Simon Fraser University. His book on research methods and sociology of science, entitled *Research Decisions: Qualitative and Quantitative Perspectives* (3rd ed., Scarborough, ON: Thomson Nelson,2003) is used in a variety of disciplines in universities and colleges across the country. He is currently collaborating on a book regarding the law and ethics of research confidentiality. In addition to his methodological interests, Professor Palys does research and engages policy issues regarding Aboriginal justice in Canada and the international community.

GEOFFREY REAUME is assistant professor in the Critical Disability Studies MA program at York University, Toronto, where he teaches "Mad People's History." He is the author of *Remembrance of Patients Past: Patient Life at the Toronto Hospital for the Insane, 1870–1940* (Toronto: Oxford University Press Canada, 2000) and is also involved in establishing the Psychiatric Survivor Archives, Toronto.

JOHN RUTHERFORD is professor in the Department of Anatomy and Neurobiology, Dalhousie University. Along with Judith Fingard, he has been examining the history of mental health care in post-war Atlantic Canada. This study considers the development of public policy, professionalization of health care workers, evolution of treatment, and delivery of services.

MARIE-CLAUDE THIFAULT received her PhD in history from the University of Ottawa in 2003. Her thesis was entitled "Citoyennes de St-Jean-de-Dieu: L'enfermement asilaire des femmes au Québec: 1873–1921." She is now teaching history at the University of Hearst, Ontario.

DAVID WRIGHT is Hannah Chair in the History of Medicine and an asso-
ciate professor in the Department of Psychiatry and Behavioural Neuro-
sciences and the Department of History, McMaster University. His publi-
cations include, with Anne Digby as co-editor, *From Idiocy to Mental
Deficiency: Historical Perspectives on People with Learning Disabilities*
(London: Routledge, 1996); with Peter Bartlett as co-editor, *Outside the
Walls of the Asylum: The History of Care in the Community* (London:
Athlone, 1999); *Mental Disability in Victorian England: The Earlswood
Asylum, 1847–1901* (Oxford University Press, 2001); and with Roy Porter
as co-editor, *The Confinement of the Insane, 1800–1965: International
Perspectives* (Cambridge University Press, 2003).

MENTAL HEALTH AND CANADIAN SOCIETY

Introduction

DAVID WRIGHT AND JAMES E. MORAN

Public stereotypes and private myths about mental disorders run deep in Canadian society. We feel a revulsion and sympathy towards mental illness and its treatment in equal measure. From the Victorian backdrop to Margaret Atwood's *Alias Grace*[1] to Timothy Findlay's post-war *Headhunter*,[2] the mental hospital and the practice of psychiatry act as a fictional repository for our darkest fears. Such ambivalent and contradictory attitudes are further shaped by and reflected in popular representations in visual media, such as the gothic depiction of schizophrenia in David Cronenberg's thriller *Spider* or the more sympathetic portrayal of psychosis in the 2001 American Oscar winner, *A Beautiful Mind*. Empowered with guarding against the descent into madness is the profession of psychiatry, which is met with fascination and mistrust, adulation and mockery. Some of the most successful North American television comedies of all time have been about psychological and psychiatric treatment, from the group counselling of the 1970s *Bob Newhart Show* to the psychoanalytically inclined 1990s radio therapy program *Fraser*. Both popular shows reawaken old tropes of the satire of inversion, giving the audience an opportunity to turn the tables (or couch) and psychoanalyze the psychoanalyzer. "Who is more mad," we ask ourselves, "the insane or those who treat them?"

The fascination with "madness" and the "mad-doctor" is not limited to popular culture; mental health topics remain one of the most actively researched areas in the more rarefied milieu of academe. Indeed, it is noteworthy how often relatively esoteric mental health research often has had wider intellectual appeal and impact. Erving Goffman's *Asylums* (1961)[3] remains a classic of sociology, as well a stinging commentary on the state of post-war American psychiatric institutions, providing some of the inspiration for Ken Kesey's 1962 novel *One Flew over the Cuckoo's Nest*.[4] Phyllis Chesler's *Women and Madness*[5] not only was an indictment of what she saw as the psychiatrisation of women's behaviour by the (male) medical profession, but it also became an important contribution to the emerging "second wave" of feminism that would profoundly change Western society in the 1970s. Michel Foucault's *Folie et déraison: Histoire de la folie à l'âge classique*[6] was not just a major treatise challenging the triumphalist account of the mental hospital (though it was in part that); but it also revolutionized intellectual theorizing about the way power and knowledge(s) were created, shaped, and contested in modern society. Some consider it one of the first major works of poststructuralism.

Considering this rare intersection of societal fascination and scholarly frisson, it is perhaps not surprising that the *history* of "madness" or, to use a more neutral turn of phrase, the historical relationship between mental ill health and society has proved very popular within and without Canada. In the last quarter of the century, there have been no fewer than a dozen English-language edited volumes published on the history of mental health and psychiatry, mostly focused on British and, to a lesser degree, American sources and topics.[7] What is new is the way in which, in the just the last few years, the Anglo-American dominance in the English-language literature has been complemented by rich subcultures of the history of psychiatry in other countries, as witnessed in edited volumes on mental health and society in Holland,[8] Australia,[9] and Argentina.[10] So popular has been the topic that an edited volume was published in New Zealand made up entirely of undergraduate and master's theses on the history of mental health.[11] Prominent themes in these new works include the ways in which dominant Western European psychiatric ideas and mental institutions were transplanted, resisted, and adapted to colonial or quasi-colonial environments and the ways in which Native approaches to madness and mental healing persisted alongside Western "scientific" approaches. A recent edited volume of international perspectives on the confinement of the insane sampled only a small fraction of this emerging literature, but included chapters on countries as disparate as Japan, Switzerland, and colonial India.[12] Recent research monographs on the history of mental health in North Wales[13] and East Anglian England[14] and on non-European asylums in India[15] show that the excitement in this contentious field continues unabated. These new, original contributions are now added to major monographs published in the 1990s on British India,[16] Nigeria,[17] and early nineteenth-century Germany.[18] The literature on the history of mental health now is truly global in scope and activity, as evidenced by the extraordinary range of papers now being published in the journal *History of Psychiatry* and the appearance of sweeping international histories of psychiatry and of mental symptoms.[19]

It thus seems an appropriate time to provide a collection of leading scholarship on the history of mental health and society in Canada. Articles have been published in historical periodicals for the last two decades on various aspects of mental health in this country (see below), but there has yet been no edited volume looking back on the contribution of Canadian researchers to this field and forward to the exciting work yet to be addressed. Consequently, the following collection of essays focuses on the relationship between mental disorder and Canadian society over the past two centuries. They are, in part, a product of a Hannah International Conference on the History of Mental Disorders held at the University of Toronto and McMaster University in April 2001.[20]

TRENDS IN THE HISTORY OF MENTAL HEALTH
IN CANADA

A peculiar characteristic of mental health historiography in Canada is that there have been very few attempts at national synthesis, or at least the integration of regional perspectives into a single volume. It is also significant that a full century separates the only two published efforts to achieve something of a national history. T.J.W. Burgess's *Historical Sketch of Our Canadian Institutions for the Insane* (1898), written as a presidential address to the Royal Society of Canada, is the pioneering work in this respect that includes information on the nineteenth-century changes in the care of the insane in all provinces and territories of Canada. Burgess argued that, while "Canada has yet no reason to be proud of her early treatment of this unfortunate class ... the care of the insane has shown a gradual process of evolution" leading up to "the present epoch of progress," in which patients "are cared for in special governmental institutions."[21] Over one hundred years later, Quentin Rae-Grant's introduction to an edited volume of articles commemorating the founding of the Canadian Psychiatric Association offers a similar prognosis of psychiatric progress as it lauds the shift from the late nineteenth-century psychiatric paradigm of institutional care to the late twentieth-century paradigm of community-based outpatient biological psychiatry. In *Psychiatry in Canada: 50 Years, 1951–2001*, Rae-Grant confidently asserts, "We may not have found the penicillin or streptomycin for mental illnesses, but we are rapidly getting closer."[22]

Sandwiched between these optimistic histories is Harvey Stalwick's 1969 doctoral dissertation on asylum administration in Canada prior to Confederation, which offered a more sombre interpretation of psychiatry's legacy.[23] In Stalwick's view, the asylum's potential as an institutional solution to mental illness was thwarted from the start by social conditions and political priorities beyond the control of pioneering alienists (psychiatrists). His sympathetic assessment of psychiatry and its successes and shortcomings was thematically consistent with works produced by Gerald Grob in the United States and by Kathleen Jones in Britain.[24] Their work continues to attract considerable support from researchers in Canada. For example, Peter Keating has argued that the "moral treatment" of insanity that inspired the first generation of asylums is best understood as a hopeful new breakthrough in medical practice. Keating explains the failure of asylum treatment and the rise of late nineteenth-century degeneration theory in Quebec as the result of social and political factors outside the power of the early asylum promoters.[25] More recently still, Danielle Terbenche's account of moral therapy and female patients at the Kingston Asylum claims that many historians remain caught in the custodial/curative debates which inevitably equate custodial asylums with "failed" institutions. Terbenche concludes not only that the Kingston Asylum was curative for a certain number of short-term female patients, but that it also served a "benevolent" custodial function for the one-quarter of female patients who were among its long-term residents.[26]

If the lack of a national narrative is one peculiar characteristic of our historiography, another is surely that the literature on the history of madness in Canada bypassed what is often referred to as the "revisionist" phase of the 1970s, a phase that, as historians of madness know too well, witnessed an unprecedented scholarly attack on the traditional view of the rise of mental hospitals and the consolidation of Anglo-American psychiatry. Revisionist historians such as David Rothman and Andrew Scull offered more cynical views of the rise of the asylum (in the United States and Britain respectively), situating the mental hospital within a new range of institutional solutions designed to incarcerate the "deviant" of industrial society. Following closely on the work of Michel Foucault, whose *Histoire de la folie* was first translated into English in 1965, these scholars rejected the views of Gerald Grob and Kathleen Jones, which had placed the establishment of asylums within the perspective of enlightened humanitarianism. In contrast, revisionist scholars viewed the asylum and the psychiatric profession that emerged within it as thinly veiled attempts to control the marginal, anti-social, and violent in an urbanizing society. However, these authors differed in their explanations for this rapid institution-based social-control response. Rothman emphasized the power and influence of new urban elites eager to find a replacement for the diminishing moral authority of traditional institutions such as the church. Scull, by contrast, highlighted the emerging capitalist work ethic, which devalued those who could not contribute to their own subsistence, and newly conceived productive relations that made it impossible for next of kin to care for the unproductive. He also directed his scathing critique at the "entrepreneurial" ambitions of asylum doctors, who, he suggests, had no real claim to expertise regarding the treatment of the insane.[27] By definition, therefore, revisionist interpretations of the history of psychiatry questioned both the inevitability of medicine's control over the treatment of madness and whether the history of psychiatry can be seen as a narrative of gradual progress.

The absence of a body of complementary revisionist histories of the asylum and the psychiatric profession in Canada is curious, but it may be in part explained by the country's own historical development. The colonial configuration of British North America in the nineteenth century and the subsequent decentralized nature of Canadian confederation (in which health care became a provincial jurisdiction) have steered historians in this country towards histories of mental health services at the provincial or institutional level.[28] Thus, although some regional studies incorporated aspects of Rothman's and Scull's critique of the emergence of modern psychiatry and the social-control uses of the asylum, no overarching revisionist monograph appeared in Canada during this important period in psychiatric historiography. One can perceive, however, an articulation of this revisionist perspective in André Cellard's *Histoire de la folie au Québec,* which placed asylum development in the wider volatile social, cultural, and political contexts of early nineteenth-century French Canadian society. Cellard identifies a broadening of the definition of and a narrowing of tolerance for insanity among eighteenth- and early nineteenth-century francophones leading up to the creation of the Montreal and Beauport asylums. In the tradition of Foucault, Rothman, and Scull, Cellard places the meaning, social constitution, and medical classification of behaviours labelled "insane" in critical perspective.[29]

Of greater importance to Canadian medical historiography in the last two decades has been the emergence of a new approach that emphasizes doing medical history "from below,"[30] or rewriting the history of health by bringing patients' perspectives to the fore. A plethora of recent monographs and journal articles has reflected these new perspectives, particularly an interest in the social history of patient populations. Like their British and American counterparts, these works have been skeptical of the earlier traditional approaches at the same time as they critically engaged with (though did not fully embrace) the revisionist accounts. The seminal Canadian publications of the last two decades remain S.E.D. Shortt's book on the London, Ontario, asylum and Cheryl Warsh's monograph on the private Homewood Retreat. In Shortt's book, renowned alienist Richard Maurice Bucke and his intellectual work on madness and evolution are considered in relation to the social and intellectual milieu of nineteenth-century psychiatry. Shortt also employed statistical analysis to place the patient population of the London Asylum in a broader social and economic context.[31] It is not coincidental that his important book was published almost simultaneously with the two other outstanding English-language institutional studies of the time period – Anne Digby's book on the Tukes and the Quaker York Retreat and Nancy Tomes's study of Thomas Kirkbride and the Pennsylvania state asylum.[32] For her part, Warsh examined how the changing nature of the middle-class Victorian family affected the definition of insanity, asylum committal practices, and the diagnostic and treatment strategies of Homewood's medical directors. Warsh was the first Canadian author to offer a sophisticated, sustained analysis of the gendered nature of middle-class responses to madness. The trend in institutional histories towards those that incorporate the patients' world has been taken to a provocative new level with Geoffrey Reaume's history of the Toronto Asylum, a book directed almost entirely to patients' perspectives.[33]

Recent scholarship by Canadian medical historians has reflected other major themes in the Anglo-American historiography of madness during the past two decades. For example, Wendy Mitchinson's feminist analysis of admissions to the Toronto and London asylums echoes the famous work of Elaine Showalter[34] by emphasizing "the way the medical profession treated women as patients" when they "suffered from problems that were or could be related to their being female." According to Mitchinson, at issue was the use of the male body as the norm against which women's health – including mental health – was gauged.[35] Rainer Baehre has contributed to the growing interest in the interconnexion between legal history and the history of madness by putting forth a complex meta-analysis of penal and lunacy reform in early nineteenth-century Canada. He argues that lunacy reform in early Victorian Upper Canada preceded the major political unrest of the late 1830s, reflecting more a consensus of political culture among Tory and Reform politicians than the outcome of any classic form of class conflict.[36] Allison Kirk-Montgomery and Robert Menzies have explored aspects of the relationship between criminality and lunacy through their studies, respectively, of the insanity plea in Victorian Ontario and asylums for the criminally insane in early twentieth-century British Columbia.[37]

The recent intensity of focus upon the asylum and upon patient populations has led, perhaps inevitably, to a questioning of the centrality of the asylum itself within social responses to mad behaviour. Reflecting the growing interest in the history of care and control of the insane outside the asylum on both sides of the Atlantic, James Moran has highlighted the importance in understanding traditional responses to madness as practised by local familial, legal, medical, and social authorities in New Jersey, Quebec, and Ontario.[38] His work reflects a new interest in extramural care and a slow decentring of the asylum as the locus of historical inquiry. Along with scholars such as Mark Jackson, he challenges the broader and overused notion of medicalization of madness as a top-down process.[39] Recent and forthcoming research by Thierry Nootens and André Cellard investigates similar patterns of care and control in the community in the context of nineteenth-century Quebec.[40]

The work on the care and control of insane individuals outside lunatic asylums has refocused an older debate over the reasons for asylum committal. Clearly, just as not every person confined in an asylum was "insane," historians also now appreciate the many thousands of individuals who, although they were recognized as insane by family members and local community members, were never institutionalized in the formal sense of the word.[41] So what combination of medical, behavioural, and socioeconomic factors combined to create a situation whereby a family would seek an institutional solution? And did these factors change over time? Interest in the context of asylum committal and in the strategic use of mental hospitals by families and communities dates back to the late 1970s. At that time, Richard Fox, John Walton, and Mark Finnane examined the background of patients admitted to the California state (United States), Lancaster county (England), and Omagh county (Ireland) asylums respectively, in order to determine the social and economic factors influencing the arrival of patients at the mental hospital. All three agreed that the process of confinement was more complex than the standard revisionist claim that the state (or middle classes) used the asylum as a means of social control. Each pointed to migration as an important factor, though in very different ways. Fox identified isolated unmarried and newly arrived immigrants in California as particularly vulnerable to confinement.[42] John Walton, by contrast, argued that the dislocating process of urbanization placed strains on family and kin resources of those who had left the countryside for work in the developing industrial city of Lancaster.[43] For his part, Finnane suggested that the emigration of fit young men and women from Ireland (following the Famine) robbed households of caring resources, thus making affected families vulnerable to seeking institutional solutions should crises of caring arise.[44] Building on this work, Cheryl Warsh identified the isolation of young immigrants as she directed her attention to the characteristics of patients admitted to the London, Ontario, asylum.[45] These studies of sample populations looked for factors that may have made certain individuals vulnerable to being confined. In addition to migration (emigration, immigration, and in-migration), they also analyzed the behaviour of patients, gender, marital status, and the availability of beds.

Another central theme emanating from the sustained focus on the complexities of asylum committal was the active and determining role of the family in the confinement of their insane kin. In her analysis of admissions to the Toronto Asylum, Wendy Mitchinson argued that the asylum was used by families to deal with those social excesses of insanity that they thought warranted institutionalization.[46] Mary-Ellen Kelm's work on the British Columbia Provincial Hospital for the Insane pushed the historiography further by detailing the influence of families *after* the patient had been admitted.[47] Other Canadian researchers have focused on particular patient groups. Edward-André Montigny, for instance, has explored the confinement of the elderly to the Rockwood (Kingston) Asylum in the latter part of the nineteenth century. He argues that asylum superintendents exaggerated the numbers of aged in their institutions as a means of exculpating themselves for low cure rates. Far from being flooded with elderly admissions, the Kingston asylum, according to this author, saw a moderate, if slightly increasing, representation of admissions over the age of sixty. Montigny, like many of the other historians just cited, was struck by the distance families went to try to accommodate insane family members within the community, before turning to the asylum as a measure of last resort.[48]

NEW DIRECTIONS IN MENTAL HEALTH HISTORY

While several of the contributors to this volume clearly bear the stamp of this "history from below" approach, they take advantage of the growing general body of research and writing on mental health history in Canada to nuance and augment the debate. Janet Miron employs the tools of the cultural historian to explore the phenomenon of "asylum tourism" in greater detail than this important subject usually receives. Miron breaks new ground by placing the very popular public visits to the asylum in the wider cultural context of custodial tourism, modern spectacle, and social reform. She indicates that the study of asylum visiting puts to rest two assertions frequently made by previous historians – that nineteenth-century psychiatric institutions were closed or "total" institutions, and that such institutional tourism was merely a mean form of voyeurism. In Miron's view, the reasons for visiting the asylums were multiple, reflecting not merely the Victorian zeal for public spectacle but also various agendas for moral and educational uplift and the public's quest for identity in an urbanizing environment. In studying the debate among psychiatrists about the merits of visitations to their asylums, Miron also highlights the anxieties among superintendents about how their institutions were being perceived by the public.

In his chapter, Thierry Nootens takes the family as his focus, but his interest lies in an in-depth sociological consideration of nineteenth-century families and their dynamic relationship to "the mad among them." Nootens combines a materialist analysis of the imperatives of family reproduction in industrializing Montreal with a consideration of the culturally constructed familial responses to madness, in order to better appreciate the complex relationships of sane and insane family members in the Victorian period. Drawing on the rich body of evidence on legal "interdictions" (decisions of incapacity), he reveals the balancing act of family decisions about the insane driven by socio-economic necessity, with those that were the product of more enduring familial concerns about interdependence, social status, and honour. It is his effort to penetrate the dynamics of industrializing families facing the spectre of madness that sends Nootens' work in challenging new historiographical directions.

In a hard-hitting analysis characteristic of his work on psychiatric patient perspectives, Geoffrey Reaume focuses on the relationship between the principles of moral therapy and the reality of patient work. Reaume charts the dramatic increase in patient labour in Ontario asylums over the course of the nineteenth century, work that became central to the institutional lives of most patients. He argues that asylum and government officials articulated a rationale for this work that utilized therapeutic paradigms to justify involuntary labour. Patient labour, they claimed, was of great benefit in the recovery of patients, though it simultaneously helped to reduce the costs of an ever-expanding asylum system. Reaume exposes the inconsistencies in this rationale, pointing out that officials maximized free work and talked up its cost-effectiveness in some contexts, while in other situations they underplayed its value in order to duck the thorny question of compensation (compensation that was, by contrast, paid to ordinary criminal inmates at the same time). He concludes that moral therapy was by the late nineteenth century merely "a public works program" run on "free" labour. In one of the most poignant passages of recent scholarship, Reaume illustrates how patients were forced to build the stone walls that enclosed them from society.

André Cellard and Marie-Claude Thifault reconsider the ever-increasing tendency to commit the insane to institutional care in Quebec, a trend consistent with many regions and nation-states in the nineteenth-century Western world. Cellard and Thifault argue that the family played a central but complex role in this process. While acknowledging the arguments of revisionist academics about the efforts (and potential influence) of asylum superintendents, social reformers, and government officials to make the asylum a more acceptable place for the insane, they remind us that the decision to commit ultimately rested in most cases with families. Drawing on both an impressive database of patient admission statistics and qualitative evidence, they argue that in Quebec this crucial transformation in the locus of care of the mad from the household to the asylum played itself out in identifiable phases. These included an initial phase of resistance by families to the asylum, a phase of class-ethnic division in the institutionalization of the insane early in the century, and a later period of asylum acceptance after a complex process of institutional reappropriation. This perspective challenges earlier historical accounts that lay more emphasis on the role of the state and the psychiatric profession in the "great confinement" in the second half of the nineteenth century.[49] It also appreciates that the influence of families has its own history, which reflects the changing relationship between the family unit and the asylum.

Allison Kirk-Montgomery's contribution considers the complex historical relationship between criminality and insanity. Focusing on the development of forensic psychiatry, Kirk-Montgomery argues that the leading psychiatrists of the nineteenth century held a "conservative view" of the insanity plea, which made its use an increasingly dangerous option for the accused. Although this conservatism decreased psychiatrists' direct involvement in criminal trials, their position nevertheless had an important effect on the way that the courts and Victorian society responded to the relationship between insanity and criminal responsibility. According to Kirk-Montgomery, psychiatrists all but eliminated the concept of "not guilty by reason of insanity" for the great majority of those from less-privileged backgrounds accused of major crime, while preserving the concept of "diminished responsibility" for the socially and economically respectable. She concludes that, in so far as their participation in criminal courts was concerned, psychiatrists served as powerful moral regulators, not by becoming a dominant voice, but by being selective about their decreasing involvement.

Robert Menzies's and Ted Palys's work highlights a central category of social historical analysis, race, which has been little studied by historians of madness. In a welcome contribution to both the national and international literature, Menzies and Palys explore the relationship between Aboriginality and state institutional responses to mental illness between 1870 and 1950. Drawing on superb records pertaining to a hundred First Nations psychiatric patients in British Columbia, they put Aboriginal treatment in the mental health system into the wider context of Native-white relations in order to explain the "racialized" response to those mentally troubled Aboriginals who came into the ambit of institutional (Western) psychiatry. They also examine the negative effects of that response on Aboriginal peoples, and they consider Aboriginal agency in the face of trying experiences.

Three of the contributions to this book offer refreshing histories of psychiatry and mental illness in the twentieth century. While the authors' research interests are distinct, all three chapters chart the history of very prominent Canadian psychiatric developments and show the importance of the international contexts out of which these developments emerged. Ian Dowbiggin leads off this trio by examining Canada's most internationally famous psychiatrist, Brock Chisholm. Dowbiggin's focus is Chisholm's gravitation towards the psychiatry of reproduction, population control, and ultimately the social-hygiene and sterilization movements, for which he became a vociferous proponent in his influential capacity as deputy minister of health and later as the first director-general of the World Health Organization. Dowbiggin draws out the early professional relationships that contributed to Chisholm's views on population control and the influence that he wielded in the Canadian, American, and international theatres of public health reform on this subject. For Dowbiggin, Chisholm's concerns about population were very much the product of the prevailing elite professional views on eugenics. Chisholm was part of the influential mainstream of this important chapter in psychiatry – a lightning rod for the psychiatrization of overlapping eugenicist intellectual currents – but he was not, as others have argued, a medical maverick.

Judith Fingard and John Rutherford tackle the rise to national and international prominence of psychiatric research in Nova Scotia in the 1940s and 1950s. They carefully explicate the myriad local, regional, national, and international factors leading to the creation of a research milieu that was very conducive to the growth of psychiatric research in Nova Scotia. Fingard and Rutherford argue that professional interests, the experiences of World War II, post-war societal anxieties, the funding proclivities of national and international organizations, and the growing faith in scientific research all intersected with local circumstance in Nova Scotia to fuel three case studies of psychiatric research. One of these projects under scrutiny, the Stirling County Study, would prove to be one of the most famous, and long-lasting, explorations of the epidemiology of community-based mental illnesses in the post-war Western world.

If large epidemiological studies were the modus operandi of professional psychiatry in Nova Scotia, Erika Dyck reminds us that an equally significant but radically different form of psychiatric research was being developed during the same period in the Canadian west. In "Prairie Psychedelics," Dyck examines how influential regional context can be in the development of specific directions in psychiatric research. In the case of Saskatchewan in the 1950s and 1960s, the energetic reform agenda of the post-war social progressive Co-operative Commonwealth Federation (CCF), under the leadership of Tommy Douglas, created a very receptive environment to experimentation and innovation when it came to mental health research and delivery. Two psychiatrists in particular, Humphry Osmond and Abram Hoffer, established themselves in Saskatchewan. These men shared a penchant for unorthodox theories and critical views of their profession, a profession which, they contended, constrained rather than expanded scientific and therapeutic horizons. They were able to take advantage of Saskatchewan's sunny psychiatric climate, implementing what would become internationally debated experiments in the therapeutic uses of LSD.

Despite the geographical and temporal coverage of this volume, it need hardly be said that collections such as this are, by nature, selective in their composition and tentative in their conclusions. However, they do serve a useful function by forcing scholars to pause, reflect, reconsider old arguments, and map out new directions of professional research. The complex and dynamic relationship between mental ill health and society over the course of Canadian history will no doubt continue to evolve, addressing new problems of interpretation, uncovering new historical sources, and applying new theoretical perspectives. Taken together, the following chapters present a history which is geographically and temporally comprehensive, but which also demonstrates that Canadian scholarship has been and is at the forefront of historiographical innovation in a field that has not lost its vitality and resonance since the period of transformation introduced by Michel Foucault.

NOTES

1 Margaret Atwood, *Alias Grace* (Toronto: Doubleday, 1997).
2 Timothy Findlay, *Headhunter* (Toronto: Harper Collins, 1987).
3 Erving Goffman, *Asylums: Essays on the Social Situation of Mental Patients and Other Inmates* (New York: Anchor Books, 1961). For an commentary on the influence of Goffman's treatise on 1970s sociology and the emergence of anti-psychiatry, see Peter Sedgwick, *Psycho politics: Laing, Foucault, Goffman, Szasz, and the Future of Mass Psychiatry* (New York: Harper and Row, 1982), 5 and chapter 1.
4 Ken Kesey, *One Flew Over the Cuckoo's Nest* (New York: New American Library, 1962).
5 Phyllis Chesler, *Women and Madness* (New York: Avon Books, 1973).
6 Michel Foucault, *Folie et déraison: Histoire de la folie à l'âge classique* (Paris: Plon, 1961) first translated into English by Richard Howard as *Madness and Civilization: A History of Insanity in the Age of Reason* (New York: Pantheon, 1965).
7 The literature on the history of mental health and psychiatry in Britain and the United States is vast. For edited volumes largely devoted to Britain, see Andrew Scull, ed., *Mad-Houses, Mad-Doctors and Madmen: The Social History of Psychiatry in the Victorian Era* (London: University of Pennsylvania Press, 1981); W.F. Bynum, Roy Porter, and Michael Shepherd, eds., *The Anatomy of Madness: Essays in the History of Psychiatry* (3 vols.; London: Tavistock, 1985–7); Scull, ed., *Social Order/Mental Disorder: Anglo-American Psychiatry in Historical Perspective* (Berkeley: University of California Press, 1989); German Berrios and Hugh Freeman, eds., *150 Years of British Psychiatry, 1841–1991* (London: Gaskell, 1991); Mark Micale and Roy Porter, eds., *Discovering the History of Psychiatry* (Oxford: Oxford University Press, 1994); German Berrios and Roy Porter, eds., *A History of Clinical Psychiatry: The Origin and History of Psychiatric Disorders* (London: The Athlone Press, 1996); Hugh Freeman and German Berrios, eds., *150 Years of British Psychiatry, 1841–1991*, Vol. 2, *The Aftermath* (London: Athlone, 1996); David Wright and Anne Digby, eds., *From Idiocy to Mental Deficiency: Historical Perspectives on People with Learning Disabilities* (London: Routledge, 1996); Dorothy Atkinson, Mark Jackson and Jan Walmsley, eds., *Forgotten Lives: Exploring the History of Learning Disability* (Kidderminster: British Institute of Learning Disabilities, 1997); Joseph Melling and Bill Forsythe, eds., *Insanity, Institutions and Society: A Social History of Madness in Comparative Perspective* (London: Routledge, 1999); Peter Bartlett and David Wright, eds., *Outside the Walls of the Asylum: The History of Care in the Community, 1750–2000* (London: Athlone Press, 1999); Jonathan Andrews and Anne Digby, eds., *Sex and Seclusion, Class and Custody: Perspectives on Class and Gender in the History of British and Irish Psychiatry* (Amsterdam: Rodolpi, 2004).

8 Marijke Gijswijt-Hofstra and Roy Porter, eds., *Cultures of Psychiatry and Mental Health Care in Postwar Britain and the Netherlands* (Amsterdam: Rodolpi, 1998).

9 Catharine Coleborne and Dolly MacKinnon, eds., *'Madness' in Australia: Histories, Heritage and the Asylum* (St Lucia: University of Queensland Press, 2003).

10 Mariano Plotkin, ed., *Argentina on the Couch: Psychiatry, State, and Society, 1880 to Present* (Albuquerque: University of New Mexico Press, 2003).

11 Barbara Brookes and Jane Thomson, ed., *"Unfortunate Folk": Essays on the History of Mental Health Treatment, 1863–1992* (Dunedin, NZ: University of Otago Press, 2001).

12 See chapters in Roy Porter and David Wright, eds., *The Confinement of the Insane: International Perspectives, 1800–1965* (Cambridge: Cambridge University Press, 2003).

13 Pamela Michael, *Care and Treatment of the Mentally Ill in North Wales, 1800–2000* (Cardiff: University of Wales Press, 2003).

14 Steven Cherry, *Mental Health Care in Modern England: The Norfolk Lunatic Asylum, St Andrew's Hospital, 1810–1998* (London: Boydell & Brewer, 2003).

15 James H. Mills, *Madness, Cannabis and Colonialism: The "Native Only" Lunatic Asylums of British India, 1857–1900* (London: Palgrave MacMillan, 2000).

16 Waltraud Ernst, *Mad Tales from the Raj: The European Insane in British India, 1800–1858* (London: Routledge, 1991).

17 Jonathan Sadowsky, *Imperial Bedlam: Institutions of Madness in Southwest Nigeria* (Berkeley: University of California Press, 1999).

18 Ann Goldberg, *Sex, Religion and the Making of Modern Madness* (Oxford: Oxford University Press, 1999).

19 German Berrios, *A History of Mental Symptoms: Descriptive Psychopathology since the Nineteenth Century* (Cambridge: Cambridge University Press, 1996); Edward Shorter, *A History of Psychiatry: From the Era of the Asylum to the Age of Prozac* (New York: John Wiley and Sons, 1997); Roy Porter, *Madness: A Brief History* (Oxford: Oxford University Press, 2003).

20 The "international" papers arising from this conference appeared partly in an edited volume and partly in a special issue of the interdisciplinary journal, *History of Psychiatry* 14 (Sept. 2003).

21 T.J.W. Burgess, "A Historical Sketch of Our Canadian Institutions for the Insane," *Transactions of the Royal Society of Canada* 4, 18 (1898): 4.

22 Quentin Rae-Grant, ed., *Psychiatry in Canada: 50 Years, 1951–2001* (Ottawa: Canadian Psychiatric Association, 2001), xii–xiii.

23 Henry Stalwick, "A History of Asylum Administration in Pre-Confederation Canada" (PhD thesis, University of London, 1969).

24 *Kathleen Jones, A History of the Mental Health Services* (London: Routledge and Kegan Paul, 1972), and Gerald N. Grob, *Mental Institutions in America: Social*

Policy to 1875 (New York: Free Press, 1973). For revisions of these influential monographs, see Jones, *Asylums and After: A Revised History of the Mental Health Services* (London: Athlone Press, 1993), and Grob, *The Mad among Us: A History of the Care of America's Mentally Ill* (Cambridge: Harvard University Press, 1994).

25 Peter Keating, *La science du mal: L'institution de la psychiatrie au Québec, 1800–1914* (Québec: Boréal, 1993).

26 Danielle Terbenche, "'Curative' and 'Custodial': Benefits of Patient Treatment at the Asylum for the Insane, Kingston, 1878–1906," *Canadian Historical Review* 86, 1 (2005): 29–52.

27 David Rothman, *The Discovery of the Asylum: Social Order and Disorder in the New Republic* (Boston: Little Brown, 1971); Andrew Scull, *Museums of Madness: The Social Organization of Insanity in Nineteenth-Century England* (London: Allen Lane, 1979).

28 See, for example, Thomas Brown, "'Living with God's Afflicted': A History of the Provincial Lunatic Asylum at Toronto, 1830–1911" (PhD thesis, Queen's University, 1980), 43–51.

29 André Cellard, *Histoire de la folie au Québec, de 1600 à 1850: Le désordre* (Québec: Boréal, 1991).

30 Roy Porter, "The Patient's View: Doing Medical History from Below," *Theory and Society* 14 (1985): 175–98.

31 S.E.D. Shortt, *Victorian Lunacy: Richard M. Bucke and the Practice of Late Nineteenth-Century Psychiatry* (Cambridge: Cambridge University Press, 1986).

32 Anne Digby, *Madness, Morality and Medicine: A Study of the York Retreat, 1792–1914* (Cambridge: Cambridge University Press, 1985); Nancy Tomes, *A Generous Confidence: Thomas Story Kirkbride and the Art of Asylum Keeping, 1840–1883* (Cambridge: Cambridge University Press, 1985).

33 Cheryl Warsh, *Moments of Unreason: The Practice of Canadian Psychiatry and the Homewood Retreat* (Montreal-Kingston: McGill-Queen's University Press, 1989); Geoffrey Reaume, *Remembrance of Patients Past: Patient Life at the Toronto Hospital for the Insane, 1870–1940* (Toronto: Oxford University Press, 2000).

34 Elaine Showalter, *The Female Malady: Women, Madness and English Culture, 1830–1980* (New York: Pantheon, 1985).

35 Wendy Mitchinson, *The Nature of Their Bodies: Women and Their Doctors in Victorian Canada* (Toronto: University of Toronto Press, 1991).

36 Rainer Baehre, "Imperial Authority and Colonial Officialdom of Upper Canada in the 1830s: The State, Crime, Lunacy and Everyday Social Order," in Louis Knafla and Susan Binnie, eds., *Law, Society and the State: Essays in Modern Legal History* (Toronto: University of Toronto Press, 1995).

37 Allison Kirk-Montgomery, "Courting Madness: Insanity and Testimony in the Criminal Justice System in Victorian Ontario" (PhD thesis, University of Toronto, 2001); Robert Menzies, "'I Do Not Care for a Lunatic's Role': Modes of Regula-

tion and Resistance inside the Colquitz Mental Home, British Columbia, 1919–33," *Canadian Bulletin of Medical History* 16 (1999): 181–214; Peter Bartlett, "Structures of Confinement in 19th-Century Asylums: A Comparative Study Using England and Ontario," *International Journal of Law and Psychiatry* 23 (2000): 1–13.

38 James E. Moran, *Committed to the State Asylum: Insanity and Society in Nineteenth-Century Quebec and Ontario* (Montreal-Kingston: McGill-Queen's University Press, 2000); Moran, "Asylum in the Community: Managing the Insane in Antebellum America," *History of Psychiatry* 9, 2 (1998): 217–40.

39 Mark Jackson, "'It Begins with the Goose and Ends with the Goose': Medical, Legal, and Lay Understandings of Imbecility in *Ingram v Wyatt*, 1824–1832," *Social History of Medicine* 11 (1998): 361–80.

40 Thierry Nootens, "Fous, prodigues et ivrognes: Internormativité et déviance à Montréal au 19e siècle" (PhD thesis, Université du Québec à Montréal, 2003); André Cellard, "Folie, internment et érosion des solidarités familiales au Québec: Un analyse quantitative" (conference paper, Folie et société au Québec: 19e–20e siécles, Centre d'histoire des régulations sociales, Université du Québec à Montréal, 10 March 1999).

41 David Wright, "Getting Out of the Asylum: Understanding the Confinement of the Insane in the Nineteenth Century," *Social History of Medicine* 10 (1997): 137–55.

42 Richard Fox, *So Far Disordered in Mind: Insanity in California, 1870–1930* (Berkeley: University of California Press, 1978).

43 John Walton, "Lunacy in the Industrial Revolution: A Study of Asylum Admissions in Lancashire, 1848–1850," *Journal of Social History* 13 (1979): 1–22.

44 Mark Finnane, *Insanity and the Insane in Post-Famine Ireland* (London: Croom Helm, 1981), chapter 4.

45 Cheryl Warsh, "'In Charge of the Loons': A Portrait of the London, Ontario Asylum for the Insane in the Nineteenth Century," *Ontario History* 74 (1982): 138–84.

46 Wendy Mitchinson, "Reasons for Committal to a Mid-Nineteenth-Century Ontario Insane Asylum: The Case of Toronto," in Wendy Mitchinson and Janice Dickin McGinnis, eds., *Essays in the History of Canadian Medicine* (Toronto: McClelland and Stewart, 1988); Warsh, *Moments of Unreason.*

47 Mary-Ellen Kelm, "Women, Families and the Provincial Hospital for the Insane, British Columbia, 1905–1915," *Journal of Family History* 19 (1994): 177–93.

48 Edward-André Montigny, "'Foisted upon the Government': Institutions and the Impact of Public Policy upon the Aged: The Elderly Patients of Rockwood Asylum, 1866–1906," *Journal of Social History* (1995): 819–36.

49 See note 27.

"Open to the Public"

Touring Ontario Asylums in the Nineteenth Century

JANET MIRON

In the 1880s E. Katharine Bates embarked on a transatlantic tour of North America, visiting such cities as Montreal, New York, Boston, Philadelphia, and Washington. While in Toronto for a few days, she included in her sightseeing itinerary the law courts of Osgoode Hall, the University of Toronto, Rosedale Park, and the insane asylum on Queen Street.[1] A few years earlier, Thomas Dick, a young farmer living outside the city, came to Toronto for a visit on the occasion of the national exhibition and chose to spend his time seeing not only the Central Prison but the asylum grounds as well.[2] The visits by Bates and Dick to Toronto's asylum were part of an extremely popular pastime in Ontario in the nineteenth century, whereby large numbers of people poured into the asylums hoping to inspect both the buildings and the people confined within them.[3]

Historians have tended to dismiss visitors such as Bates and Dick as cruel voyeurs who were drawn to mental institutions in search of cheap thrills and excitement, and as irritating intruders who greatly vexed institutional officials.[4] However, when the aims of these visitors, their experiences on their tours, and the attitudes of asylum employees towards them are critically analyzed, institutional tourism becomes a complex phenomenon that represented more than a mere "shameful" or "degrading spectacle."[5] Indeed, the practice embodies invaluable information for the historian and helps to illuminate both the relationship between asylums and their broader community and popular attitudes towards the insane. In particular, the discourse surrounding visitors demonstrates that many asylum superintendents and government inspectors believed the public had the potential to influence both the success of the asylum and the treatment of mental illness. Moreover, it suggests that an array of motives lay behind people's decision to visit a hospital for the mentally ill. While not all alienists shared the views of visitors and not all visitors were propelled by the same considerations, the debates that arose and the records left behind by officials and visitors provide important insight into the role these institutions served in the nineteenth century, the influence the public had upon their functionings, and the relationships that were forged with the communities beyond the asylum's walls.

Thousands of tourists such as Bates and Dick strolled across the grounds and walked through the wards of Ontario's mental hospitals in the nineteenth century, and traces of their steps have been left behind in a wide variety of sources, including institutional records, travel narratives, memoirs, and newspapers. Frequently conceived of by historians as existing in isolation from broader society, the tours taken by casual visitors and the responses of institutional officials to them challenge the assumption that insanity became hidden or privatized simply with the construction of edifices to house those labelled "mad." Further, these tours reveal the fact that the public played an essential role in determining the place these institutions would hold within the nineteenth-century social and cultural landscape. In this regard, visiting shows that asylums were closely connected to the communities around them and were familiar sights to local citizens and tourists alike.

Although their interpretations differ in many fundamental ways, pioneering scholars such as Michel Foucault, Erving Goffman, David J. Rothman, and Andrew Scull tended to portray the asylum as a dumping ground for undesirables that existed in isolation from "normal" society. For example, Goffman's idea of the "total institution" depicted asylum inmates as completely barricaded from the wider world, a separation that "lasts around the clock." Similarly, Rothman argued that "the new institutions were in every sense apart from society, bounded by sturdy walls and by administrative regulations that self-consciously and successfully separated inmate from outsider."[6] However, the practice of visiting suggests that these institutions were not simply sites of confinement but, within the context of the Victorian culture of looking, important loci of social activity that fostered popular understandings of and insight into mental illness.

Recently, scholars have begun to explore the history of asylums from the viewpoint of patients, as well as the relationship between asylums and the communities surrounding them. For example, S.E.D. Shortt, Ellen Dwyer,

Peter McCandless, James E. Moran, and Geoffrey Reaume have examined asylums beyond the perspective of the medical profession, documenting the subcultures that existed amongst patients and attendants and the roles played by families in the committal process.[7] Moreover, an emerging body of literature has challenged the idea that the asylum superseded other methods of dealing with the mentally ill and instead has argued that community or familial care remained the primary response. In particular, Peter Bartlett and David Wright, editors of the book *Outside the Walls of the Asylum*, criticized historians for their narrow focus on the asylum and institutionalization, claiming that this approach has eclipsed other responses to mental illness, even though "mental hospitals never *replaced* community care."[8] While still focusing on asylums, this study continues in this vein by situating these institutions within their broader communities and exploring the visits to asylums by ordinary people – local residents and tourists from other communities – and the responses of institutional officials to the general public.

This chapter focuses on the asylums located in southern Ontario (in particular, those established in London, Hamilton, and Toronto), examining the attitudes of officials towards asylum visiting and the relationships they tried to construct between their institutions and broader society. It then explores the incentives behind visiting and the experiences of people such as Bates and Dick as they toured Ontario's asylums. Although "professional" visitors, prominent reformers, and family members or friends of patients could also be found in the asylum, it is the thousands of casual observers with which this chapter primarily is concerned. When we explore asylums through the eyes of such individuals, it becomes clear that nineteenth-century Canadians and tourists from abroad were not mere passive receptacles of the ideologies espoused by those in the medical profession but, instead, were active participants in the effort to understand and study what was deemed to be aberrant behaviour.

INSTITUTIONAL POLICIES AND ATTITUDES OF ASYLUM OFFICIALS

Throughout the nineteenth century, tens of thousands of tourists passed through the growing number of asylums in Ontario. From their very establishment, the province's asylums attracted tourists from the surrounding countryside and from abroad as well. The public displayed an insatiable appetite for inspecting institutions for the mentally ill, compelling John Scott, the first superintendent of the permanent Provincial Lunatic Asylum in Toronto, to remark in the early 1850s that "the desire of the public seems unabated, to examine the arrangements and learn the state of the inmates."[9] Nevertheless, in spite of society's fascination with these new institutions, for many of those who were intimately or professionally connected to asylums, institutional tourism represented an ideological conundrum: should patients be exposed to the public gaze, or should they be completely isolated from the outside world? The question was not easily resolved, and as a result, the increasingly popular pastime of visiting led to lengthy and often heated discussions over whether or not the public should have access to asylums at all.

While official policies and statements did not always reflect what was actually being practised, institutional documents nevertheless help us to understand attitudes towards custodial tourism and the place employees envisioned for their institutions within nineteenth-century society. The debates that arose and the ensuing efforts of officials to determine the relationships these institutions would have with the greater society illuminate administrators' perceptions of their institutions and those under their care, the intellectual currents informing their practices, and the pressures they faced in their efforts to develop effectively managed institutions. The writings of institutional and government employees included defences of or attacks on the idea of visiting, an informal record of the annual number of visitors, and the reactions of visitors and patients. There was no consensus as to whether or not visiting should be practised in Ontario's asylums, yet all agreed upon the fact that members of the public were interested in seeing the interiors of asylums and that they had the potential to greatly influence the workings of these institutions and the lives of those within them.

PROPONENTS OF VISITING

Most superintendents and government inspectors did not believe that asylums could be easily isolated from greater society; nor did many of them actually desire complete segregation. Instead, a number of administrators strove to foster close ties with the communities beyond their walls, arguing that such relationships were beneficial for a variety of reasons. Moreover, many recognized that the public was crucial to these institutions in a number of ways and that perceptions of and attitudes towards asylums were as dependent on "official" discourse as they were on the laity's experiences while passing through them. As state-run institutions relied on government funding, public approval was essential for asylums, and inevitably, this dependence led asylum officials to embark on campaigns to bolster popular support through the practice of visiting.

Many officials perceived visiting as an important part of the process of social legitimization and believed that the practice was the best means by which public confidence could be gained. These officials were aware of the public's growing fascination with asylums, evinced by the fact that the reports of superintendents, government inspectors, and commissioners were regularly reprinted in the popular press and that the recommendations, criticisms, and impressions of "professional" visitors or prominent reformers commonly appeared in newspapers as well. However, officials were also cognizant of the prejudice towards asylums that pervaded society and undermined the view of their institutions as curative. Indeed, much of the printed information available to the general populace painted a grim picture of institutions for the mentally ill. In the nineteenth century, "shocking" tales of conditions inside asylums appeared regularly in newspapers, sparking concern over the treatment of the institutionalized and fostering suspicion about the buildings that housed them. Until the latter half of the nineteenth century, medical practitioners affiliated with either hospitals or asylums were treated with skepticism by a populace that was not oblivious to the highly publicized grave-robbings committed by some of their peers or the autopsies performed on unwilling subjects.[10] In the mid-1850s, for example, the Toronto Asylum was plagued with many charges of abuse and corruption. A number of employees claimed that the steward had impregnated a female patient, while one former attendant, James Magar, charged that he had "known the bodies of the dead to be dissected for the information of Doctors not connected with the Asylum, and their brains kept after the body was interred."[11] Such scandals easily led to the image of the doctor who sacrificed patients in the pursuit of medical knowledge and helped to foster suspicion of all medical establishments.

Moreover, there were other, more flagrant reasons as to why people feared institutionalization in a medical establishment. Because of their unsanitary conditions and the fact that few people left them healed, hospitals were not perceived as therapeutic institutions. Instead, they were seen as places where the most unfortunate went to die and thus were avoided by all except for the very poor.[12] This view of hospitals imbued attitudes towards asylums. Even as late as the 1860s, Wolfred Nelson, inspector of asylums and prisons for the Province of Canada, remarked that "very erroneous views are generally entertained in regard to Asylums" and that they were often viewed with "distrust and alarm."[13] Consequently, institutional officials hoped to dispel negative publicity by advocating that people view their asylums first-hand and see for themselves the progress that had been made in them.

As a means of gaining society's confidence and alleviating skepticism, superintendents and other government officials encouraged visiting in their annual reports, which were reprinted in local papers. The early annual reports of the Provincial Lunatic Asylum at Toronto repeatedly emphasized that the institution was open to visitors from 12 o'clock until 3 and that it was "as open to the public as is compatible with the welfare of the patients and the duties of their attendants."[14] Such promotion was apparently effective since, in 1850, 1,400 visitors reportedly passed through the asylum during that year alone.[15] Even three decades later, in 1880, officials in the province could still be found encouraging the practice in newspapers, including Richard Maurice Bucke, superintendent of the London Asylum, who wrote a letter to the London *Free Press* publicizing that "the Asylum is always open to inspection by the whole public."[16]

As a way of alleviating social stigma, institutional tourism represented an excellent opportunity to educate the broader society on the causes and contemporary treatment of insanity. In their annual reports, officials often referred to the impressions of visitors, thereby highlighting the importance that was granted to public opinion. The chairman for the Provincial Lunatic Asylum in Toronto reported in 1852 that "Large numbers of visitors have ... from time to time, been attended through the building, and these have witnessed the condition of the apartments, the appearance and happiness of the patients, the kindly, but effective discipline, which prevails amongst the afflicted and their attendants. The result has been, so far as is known, a universal satisfaction to visitors, many of whom had been acquainted with similar Institutions in Europe, or the United States."[17] Moreover, many believed that the successful treatment of insanity was dependent upon early committal to an asylum and that the longer loved ones waited, the less likelihood of a cure being achieved. Thus, as Wolfred Nelson pointed out, the "attainment of successful results" was contingent upon the community's "countenance and good opinion."[18]

Mistrust or suspicion was not the only problem with which asylum officials had to contend while negotiating their relationship with the public. As the nineteenth century progressed, asylum expenditure grew, and superintendents were increasingly pressured to justify their efficacy in treating insanity. According to historian S.E.D. Shortt, asylums in Ontario consumed almost 16.5 per cent of the provincial budget in the 1870s, a share that stabilized at more than 19 per cent in the late 1880s. In 1893 this represented twice the combined expenditure on penal institutions, general hospitals, houses of refuge, and orphanages.[19] As James Moran has noted, the "difficulty in raising funds to construct and maintain the province's public asylums" was a persistent problem.[20] As heads of costly institutions, not only were superintendents compelled to highlight their success rates to portray the therapeutic treatments of their institutions as effective, but they also became even more aware of their need for public support.

The dependence of institutions on public funds made many feel particularly vulnerable and pressured to appease taxpayers, thereby placing asylum superintendents in a difficult situation: at what cost did their efforts to win public support through the practice of visiting endanger the mental improvement of patients? While refusing (at least in theory) to open the doors of the Toronto Asylum to the masses, Superintendent Daniel Clark admitted, much to his chagrin, that many people felt they had a right to tour asylums. "It is a public Institution," he lamented, "and it is the privilege of the British subject, if he should happen to be 'a free and independent elector' to look upon an Asylum to the support of which he has contributed his mite of taxes, as a huge menagerie, erected for the purpose of gratifying his morbid curiosity."[21] Although some may have been opposed to the practice, few institutions could afford to, or had the power to, keep the public out entirely. As the superintendent of the Malden Lunatic Asylum explained, "Public opinion is all powerful; and by its help only we can carry into practise the most enlightened principles of management; and by the spread of enlightened principles, only, can we hope for that liberal pecuniary support from the Parliament, which is absolutely essential to the welfare of our asylums."[22]

To understand why those professionally affiliated with asylums would promote public tours, it is helpful to examine the example of Dr Richard Maurice Bucke. Superintendent of the asylum in London from 1877 until his death in 1902, Bucke was Ontario's most outspoken proponent of visiting, and the efforts he made during his career to promote it illuminate why many thought it was such an important practice. As an alienist and superintendent, Bucke believed that part of his role was to rectify public misconceptions of mental hospitals and remove the stigma that was so frequently attached to them. Consequently, in public forums such as newspapers, he endeavoured to redefine popular views of asylums and the tendency to perceive them as little more than dungeons of terror, using for this end the practice of visiting. Hoping to educate the public, Bucke explained in one annual report that was reprinted in a local newspaper:

We have a large number of visitors in the course of the year, both those who come to see friends and relations who are inmates of the Asylum, and those who, having no friends resident in it, come to see the Asylum itself. I always admit these people freely, and I think it is a good thing that they should come and see what sort of a place a Lunatic Asylum is. The people of average education throughout the country have most of them grown up with the idea that a Lunatic Asylum is an immense prison, full of all sorts of horrors. They must consequently, many of them, suffer severely in mind when they have to send a relation to one of these institutions, and I have no doubt that is one cause of the reluctance to send, and the delay in sending patients.[23]

Although he obviously had a professional interest in encouraging favourable views of asylums, Bucke argued that visiting would enlighten the public on the conditions inside insane asylums and ultimately allay fears of committing loved ones. He even went so far as to claim that it was "about the only way that unfortunate prejudice can be removed,"[24] and he would have been pleased with one newspaper account that felt that, because of the "hundreds of visitors to the Asylum each year," "the general public is becoming better acquainted … with the internal management of asylums."[25]

Like Dr Telfer of the temporary Toronto Asylum, who in the 1840s felt that meetings between visitors and those afflicted with mental illness were conducive to the welfare of the latter, Bucke rationalized that institutional tourism also had positive therapeutic implications for the patients themselves.[26] Throughout his years at the London Asylum, Bucke struggled to alleviate the social alienation that institutional life or even mental illness entailed, and whereas many historians have argued that asylum superintendents sought to isolate those labelled insane from outside social interaction, his approach to mental illness, like that of many of his contemporaries, suggests the need to re-evaluate such assumptions. Chastising those who felt the insane should be segregated, he instead argued: "Anyone who would wish to shut out from the wards of an asylum the little healthy mental atmosphere from the outside world that there might be a chance of admitting for fear the contact should wound the diseased susceptibilities of patients, it seems to me would be on a par with the ignorant practitioner of ordinary medicine, who when his patient has a fever, causes all the doors and windows to be shut, and cautions the sick man's friends against giving him a glass of cold water."[27] For Bucke, interaction between patients and the greater populace aided the ill by providing them with "healthy" activities and by distracting them from their confinement. Recognizing that the worst feature of asylum life was its "insufferable sameness and dulness," he stipulated that the "slight change and excitement of the passage of visitors through the halls is, on the whole, both agreeable to, and good for, the patients." Indeed, while emphasizing that his policies would not be dictated by those under his medical supervision, Bucke claimed that patients at the London Asylum did not complain about visitors and that they "never seem to think that they are treated as wild beasts, or made a show of because their fellow creatures ... come to see them."[28]

Not only did Bucke promote public tours of the London Asylum, but like many other superintendents, he also organized a number of social and educational events as a means of fostering relations with the outside world. These activities ranged from cricket matches to theatrical plays and from educational lectures to musical entertainment. Attendants and other members of asylum staff participated in these amusements, which, according to Bucke, kept them "in good heart and in good health, so that [they] may be able to take care" of patients better.[29] These events drew entertainers or educators from the outside; they included minstrel troupes, magicians, and even a hundred local children, who not only performed the operetta *Fairy Grotto* for patients but were treated with a dinner and "went home highly delighted with [their] visit to the Asylum."[30] People from the surrounding community frequently attended these events as well, and advertised through newspapers and posters, they attracted much attention. In 1899, for example, the annual athletic sports for employees and patients drew, as usual, an estimated four to five hundred citizens.[31] As a result, such events helped to make the London Asylum an important locus of social activity and served to strengthen the institution's ties to the world beyond its walls. Clearly, for many superintendents, visiting was not simply perceived as a barbaric tradition that rendered the asylum a human zoo but, instead, was advocated as a means of achieving a variety of both practical and therapeutic goals.

OPPONENTS OF VISITING

In spite of the convictions of those such as Bucke who saw visiting as advantageous, beneficial, and even necessary, there was no consensus surrounding the practice. In annual reports, independent examinations, and government commissions, few failed to address this contentious issue. If some were untroubled by the throngs of people passing through asylums, others perceived visiting as an anachronistic tradition that had no place in contemporary institutions. A number of alienists and other experts affiliated to asylums hoped to see the practice abolished and struggled to prohibit casual visitors from touring their establishments. However, although exclusionary regulations were articulated by such critics, their efforts were usually constrained by the public's insistence on having access to the very institutions they financially supported.

For a society that prized itself on its "enlightened humanity," visiting undermined what many believed to be the very aim of modern asylums: the reformation (or restoration) of character and behaviour. As critics reasoned, if asylums were to cure rather than merely house, then patients should not be treated as spectacles by visitors. For many, the well-being of the institutionalized was paramount, and the presence of strangers in their midst was nothing more than a source of degradation. Superintendents frequently complained of their inability to protect patients and inmates from the hurtful gaze of spectators, and they argued that the people under their care were being taken advantage of by nefarious members of society motivated by the simple desire to gawk at the confined. Perceiving visitors as injurious to patients, Daniel Clark, superintendent of the Toronto Asylum from 1875 to 1905, explained, "It is often pitiful to see the [the patients] hiding in corners, closets, bed-rooms, or any other available place when strangers are approaching, in order to avoid their gaze and questionings. They know their sad condition and naturally desire to flee from the presence of the gaping multitude of curiosity hunters."[32]

Being treated like animals in a zoo, numerous administrators stipulated, resulted in the alienation of those who were already socially marginalized. In the eyes of these critics, there was no therapeutic benefit to the presence of visitors (as Bucke would have insisted); indeed, the progress of curative efforts was actually hindered by them. The public frequently provoked patients, causing distress amongst those suffering from mental illness, and any tranquility or order that transpired in the asylum setting dissolved as soon as visitors traipsed through the wards and across the grounds. According to Superintendent Henry Landor of the Malden Asylum, "Visits of curiosity to the asylum ... are, as all superintendents know, great nuisances, more especially to the patients, who have often told me that they are not wild beasts to be exhibited to every comer, and they invariably try to get out of the way whenever visitors come to the asylum."[33] Superintendents such as Landor argued that those under their care had been institutionalized in part to protect them from the pressures of society, and exposing them to the gaze of onlookers merely contributed to the anguish of insanity. If physicians were to cure mental disease effectively, then they had to have the capacity to shield their patients from stressful situations. To ensure the "recovery and restoration of the insane to society," asylums had to "strictly exclude visitors" as part of the therapy under moral management.[34] Clark explained the importance of this principle, arguing that "a daily influx of strange visitors to the wards causes undue excitement, and thereby retards the recovery of the afflicted under treatment."[35] Moreover, he felt his own position as a medical practitioner was being compromised, explaining, "Very painful to Asylum physicians it truly is, to be called on day by day, to '*show through*' empty-headed visitors, who come to stare, and laugh and wonder at the aberrative manifestations of their fellow beings."[36]

While superintendents could claim that their efforts were thwarted by meddlesome visitors, at the same time they also faced pressure from family members of patients who advocated stringent policies regarding visitors. Indeed, many outside the asylum complained of relatives being gawked at by the public. Not only were these people concerned with the impact visiting had on the institutionalized, but they also feared discrimination if the condition of relatives became public. The brother of one patient in the Toronto Asylum, for example, wrote to the superintendent in 1906 and requested the protection of his sister from sightseers: "I would like you to keep visitors from seeing her or knowing anything about her [. Port Hope] is a small Town and some people are after news to tell."[37] Consequently, even Bucke tried to appease those who might not commit relations to the London Asylum in light of its public openness. Although it is difficult to understand how such a policy could be enforced when the asylum building was open to visitors from 10 a.m. to 4 p.m. six days a week, some could at least choose to believe that "in case of patients whose friends do not desire it, strangers will not be permitted to visit them without a written order."[38]

Albeit less verbose on the topic, Daniel Clark of the Toronto Asylum in many ways represented Bucke's counterpart in the visiting debate. He saw no advantages to the practice and felt that it was nothing more than a voyeuristic pastime engaged in by the general public for non-altruistic purposes. Arguing that "curiosity hunters" inflicted "mentally injury" on patients and caused much distress to their families and friends, Clark stated that he "rigidly excluded" such visitors from his institution. Aware of the unpopularity of his measures amongst many members of the general public, he defended his position by citing the "drain upon the time of the medical staff and attendants."[39] Further challenging the usefulness of the practice, he claimed: "Were the laconic speeches of timid visitors, and the frightened faces of such, productive of power to heal a mind diseased, or even to contribute in a small degree towards recovery, the Asylums whose doors are open to all and sundry should show favourably in striking contrast to the disadvantages of our system of visitation."[40]

While many felt accessibility to public institutions was essential in order to garner the support and trust of the populace, others such as Clark believed visiting in fact accomplished the opposite. Fearful that social prejudice could be bolstered if visitors conversed with unwell patients whose perceptions might distort what conditions were really like inside the asylum, he stated: "[The visitor] pretends to think that there must be 'ways that are dark' and corrupt lurking in an institution within whose walls he is not privileged to air his importance, and carry away his budget of news, gathered from the mad utterances of ones more fortunate, so that their babblings may be the gossip of a whole countryside."[41]

Throughout the nineteenth century superintendents opposed visiting, and generally it has been their voices to which historians have listened. Opponents such as Clark most closely resemble our own sensibilities surrounding the display and spectacle of human beings, and perhaps this affinity encourages the dismissal of visiting as trite and prurient. However, not only do the views of many officials such as Bucke caution us against simplistic interpretations, but the attitudes of visitors themselves further demonstrate that multiple meanings lay behind the practice.

VISITORS TO ASYLUMS

While asylum superintendents such as Bucke and Clark struggled with the issue of visiting, assessing its merits and considering its drawbacks, institutional tourism evolved into an extremely popular activity in Ontario. Consequently, in spite of the condemnation expressed by some, the general populace would not have been easily dissuaded from touring asylums and likely would have protested their closure to the public. Indeed, by the mid-nineteenth century, visiting was far from an uncommon or marginal pastime: thousands of urban and rural dwellers alike flocked to asylums annually. In fact, as the century progressed, the activity became so popular that institutions were frequently overwhelmed on holidays by the "crush and confusion resulting from so many persons being admitted."[42] Thus, while harsh criticism of visiting was voiced and administrators complained of troublesome visitors, few could actually enforce a closed-door policy, and there do not appear to have been any publicly funded asylums in Ontario that could keep the public out entirely. Even if officials were opposed to asylum tourism, they usually had to tolerate the public's presence, and while Clark was officially against sightseers, the practice continued at the Toronto Asylum well into the late nineteenth century, as it did at all other public asylums in Ontario.[43]

Although historians have tended to agree with the attitudes expressed by Clark, the records left by visitors suggest that their motives and experiences were diverse and defy being reduced to voyeurism. Like many other Victorian pursuits, visiting was undeniably rooted in a fascination with those considered deviant and related to the desire to observe or witness the unfamiliar. It was part of the broader "spectacularization" of modern life in the nineteenth century, where "reality seemed to be experienced as a show – an object to be looked at rather than experienced in an unmediated form."[44] However, this phenomenon should not inevitably lead one to conclude that all visitors were merely interested in catching a peep show of the insane. Many visitors certainly treated asylums as human menageries where patients were spectacles to be gawked at and regarded these institutions as entertainment venues that differed little from the circuses and "freak" shows that frequently appeared in their towns and cities. At the same time, although asylum tourism was for many an opportunity to engage in sheer voyeurism, the incentives behind this practice were complex and illuminate the ideological currents and contradictions pervading Victorian culture. Voyeurism was inherent in visiting, yet for a large number of people, institutional tours were a source of self-improvement, "scientific" education, and community pride. Moreover, while its ramifications or effectiveness may be questioned, visiting nevertheless fostered greater exchange and dialogue between the public and the institutionalized and thereby served as an important means through which notions regarding the insane were constructed and defined at the lay level. Thus, by analyzing asylums not as mere physical structures but as tourist sites where popular representations of the "mad" were formed, we can understand these institutions as virtual civic monuments closely connected to the world beyond their walls.

Both Clark and Bucke tended to see all visitors as a homogeneous group, respectively as either voyeurs or responsible citizens. However, those who engaged in asylum tourism were not only guided by an array of incentives but were also from a wide range of social and cultural backgrounds that transcended the lines of gender, class, ethnicity, and age. Local farmers, female leisure travellers, and male bankers visited insane asylums, and children of all ages were exposed to their interiors. As one man remarked on his tour through the Toronto Asylum, "There was a party consisting of a

Lady, Gentleman, and a little Girl going over the establishment, and, as I entered I enjoined them."[45] Visitors lived in the communities connected to these institutions or travelled from other regions and countries, some as far away as Mexico, England, and Germany. In terms of sheer numbers alone, the visitors who recorded their experiences were predominantly of a privileged social stature. Reflecting the cultural and political context of the nineteenth century, the majority of records that exist today were written by white, middle-class males, but, while particular voices dominate the written sources, such individuals did not exercise a complete monopoly over asylum tourism. The fact that many accounts were recorded by a wide range of people who did not fit a particular socio-economic profile is significant, and it thereby provides a more nuanced understanding of community attitudes towards asylums. In addition, while the predominant voice in travel narratives might be middle-class and male, since it was not uncommon for visitors to comment upon members of their tour group, their observations often shed light on the experiences of others.

WHO ENCOURAGED VISITING?

Before exploring motives behind asylum tours, it is important to understand how it is that people were aware that entry could be gained to asylums by the general public and the sources that encouraged them to embark on such avenues of leisurely activity. As literacy increased and both the mass-circulated press and middle-class tourism burgeoned during the nineteenth century, printed material often piqued the interests of potential visitors. For many visitors, guidebooks were a source of inspiration for asylum tours, an increasing number of which were being published; they served, as Jennifer A. Crets has argued, "the same purpose for middle-class travelers as letters of introduction and well-placed family and friends did for wealthier visitors."[46] Canadian guidebooks throughout the nineteenth century frequently advocated the touring of asylums and repeatedly stipulated that certain institutions *had* to be seen by the visitor. Visits to institutions were normalized by the writers of these guides, who portrayed them as a fashionable and essential part of the tourist's itinerary. Museums, government buildings, churches, penitentiaries, historic sites, and universities were commonly presented as areas of interest; invariably, asylums were promoted as "must sees" as well. Such information as physical appearance, location, and visiting hours were generally provided to readers, as were what sights they should expect to see or what architectural features they should be sure to notice. *The Canadian Handbook and Tourist's Guide,* published during the year of Confederation in 1867, was one such source that helped to popularize the practice of visiting. Encouraging travellers to examine the interiors of local institutions, the guide informed its readers that the Provincial Lunatic Asylum in Toronto "is well worthy of a visit by the curious in such matters" and reassured them that there "is no difficulty in obtaining permission to view it."[47] The mass of travel narratives published during the century also promoted sightseeing of asylums, describing these institutions as almost quaint and unthreatening. Indeed, these were far from the oppressive regimes described by Michel Foucault. In addition, attempting to profiteer from society's interest in asylums, transportation companies advertised them as sites of tourism along their routes. With the opening of the Victoria Bridge, the Grand Trunk Railway issued a souvenir note highlighting the Toronto Asylum as one of the "places of interest" along its route to attract potential customers.

A number of other venues rendered institutional tourism desirable. Images of asylums were frequently found in nineteenth-century fiction, and popular authors often made reference to institutional tours. In her novel *Down the River to the Sea* (c. 1894) Agnes Maule Machar wrote of tourists in Toronto who were shown such sights as the Central Prison, the Mercer Reformatory for Women, and the Lunatic Asylum.[48] The works of Charles Dickens, which were pirated with astounding frequency in North America, also likely provoked interest in custodial institutions because of his tendency to focus on the themes of insanity and confinement. Likewise, newspapers ran stories on asylum visits, many of which were presented in a diary-style format that chronicled tourists' trips and frequently reiterated the sentiment that "all news, particularly of a pleasing character, which relates to any of our public institutions (more especially the benevolent ones), ought to form an interesting and acceptable news item in any public journal."[49] Another article stated, "Among the many objects of interest to be seen by the sojourner in London, none will repay him better interest than a visit to the Asylum for the Insane."[50] Newspapers not only encouraged interest in custodial institutions but also provided details about the regulations governing public visits. While the *London Advertiser* informed its readers that the asylum "is always open to visitors between 10 a.m. and 4 p.m., save on Sundays and holidays," it also reassured those hesitant about touring the institution that "not only are [visitors] admitted – they are invited."[51] Moreover, as was discussed above, administrators of institutions frequently promoted visiting in newspapers as well, welcoming tourists, encouraging public inspections of their institutions, and fostering the notion that visitors would be made to feel "at home."[52]

Aside from the printed matter available to the general public, word of mouth and a simple curiosity in one's community institutions likely compelled locals to pursue a tour. Many people had not necessarily read about the phenomenon of visiting but merely assumed that asylums were open to the public for their inspection. Whether encouragement came from a neighbour, a newspaper, or a tourist guide, promoters of asylum tours were quite successful, as even those who had very little time to see all the sights of a particular city generally made time for the custodial institutions. Ishbel Gordon, Countess of Aberdeen and Temair, found herself in Kingston for just two hours, yet under the guidance of a cabman, she still managed to see Rockwood Lunatic Asylum.[53] However the public were informed of the practice, asylums became entrenched as a leisure activity for the inhabitants in their vicinities and also as part of the North American "Grand Tour."

VISITORS' MOTIVES

The public enthusiastically responded to the promotion of asylum tourism and sought to see both the interiors of these institutions and their inhabitants for a variety of reasons that often transcended spectatorship. But this is not to imply that visitors can simply be divided between voyeurs and the well-intentioned, as all who entered into these institutions were voyeurs to a certain degree. Visitors often presented themselves as urban reformers investigating the conditions of institutions, yet, as Judith Walkowitz has argued, "the 'zeal for reform' was often accompanied by 'a prolonged, fascinated gaze' from the bourgeoisie."[54] In order to comment upon the approaches employed in asylums, visitors had to study the institutionalized, but as the power dynamic between these two groups was unequal in that the institutionalized had not made an active "choice" to be viewed by the public, patients were spectacles because of the very nature of such interactions.[55] At the same time, in spite of the fact that there was always a certain power imbalance inherent in these interactions, some visitors were much more inclined than others to view institutional tours as pure amusement and folly. For such individuals, visiting seems to have represented an alluring form of transgression, an opportunity to cross over into the nether world of "abnormal" society and to be risqué by watching, and in many cases ridiculing, the confined.

Visitors mocked patients, taunted them with tobacco, provoked outbursts, and delighted in being able to watch them without necessarily being seen themselves. While some defenders claimed that visiting served an important educational function, others believed these institutions merely offered free, "real-life" amusement. Although the nineteenth century has been characterized as a period in which treatment of the insane was reformed and, in many ways, humanized, a large number of individuals at the lay level continued to perceive asylums as little more than human menageries, in which visiting was an opportunity to gaze at the confined.

The tendency to regard custodial institutions for their entertainment value paralleled many other aspects of nineteenth-century culture. Indeed, the headline for one newspaper article reads like a circus playbill: "The Unsound of Mind. How They are Kept at the London Asylum. A Trip Through the Corridors and Rooms. The Eccentricities of the Patients. Exciting Experiences, Sad Scenes and Amusing Incidents."[56] Until the latter half of the nineteenth century, public executions, "freak" shows, and medical exhibitions encouraged both treatment of the body as an object to be displayed and the perception that the mental and physical suffering of others could constitute a source of amusement. As Vanessa Schwartz has illustrated in her wonderful monograph *Spectacular Realities*, even in death the body was displayed for the purpose of public consumption and popular entertainment. The morgue visiting she documents in Paris was not as common in Ontario, but the popularity of public executions in Canada is a similar phenomenon that certainly attests to the continent's fascination with the human spectacle. For example, when a man sentenced to be hanged committed suicide, city officials in Toronto displayed his body to the public in the morgue in order to appease the thousands who had hoped to witness his execution.[57] Similarly, society's obsession with the physical suffering of others was highlighted in Montreal when tickets to see the last rites being given to a condemned murderer were sold to the public by the sheriff and thousands gathered to watch his hanging.[58] Alongside such popular practices as public executions, visiting can clearly be seen as one element in a rather impressive roster of nineteenth-century voyeuristic, and at times sadistic, pastimes.

Generalizations about the insane were frequently made by voyeuristic visitors, who tended to relay what they perceived as "humorous" anecdotes of female hysterics and childlike men. One journalist, on his tour of the Toronto Asylum under Dr Scott, described the patients he or she saw: the "religious mad ... who will bore you on some knotty point," those "truly pitiable objects" who were suffering from melancholy, with their "down-cast head and look," and others with "much vivacity of manners, loquaciousness of speech, and fondness for narrative." The writer also portrayed one individual who "strutted about attired most ludicrously, fancying herself a Queen."[59] Such visitors saw institutions for the mentally ill primarily as sources of entertainment, and presented the insane as parodies, as characters who could easily have stepped out of a Hogarth print. One popular writer, Susanna Moodie, toured the Toronto Asylum with her daughter and son-in-law, entering areas where "strangers have seldom nerve enough to visit," and proudly relayed her sensationalist impressions and experiences to an undoubtedly dazzled audience.[60]

In spite of the efforts of many asylum superintendents, onlookers motivated by a "perverse" curiosity generally were not prevented from passing through their institutions. As was discussed above, many did struggle with the ways in which such visitors could be kept out. At the same time, though, others were untroubled by the potential presence of visitors who were unsympathetic to the plight of the incarcerated. Dr Sippi, who served as bursar at the London Asylum from 1893 to 1897, complained that the thousands who came through the institution were motivated merely by "idle" and harmful curiosity. However, Bucke refused to stem the flow of tourists, and throughout his career he remained adamant that visitors be allowed into the asylum.[61] Similarly, prior to Daniel Clark's superintendence, the Toronto Asylum was well known amongst many not necessarily for its treatment of the mentally ill but for its receptivity to strangers. After providing a lengthy and rather lurid portrait of the patients in the asylum, one journalist claimed of the superintendent: "Dr. Scott appears to be very attentive to visitors, and gives all information in his power that the most prying could desire." In this institution, the author noted, people could acquire intimate details of patients from asylum personnel, in spite of the fact that some of the lunatics treated visitors "as if they were intruding."[62] Scott may have been oblivious to his visitor's insensitivity, but he clearly was not uncomfortable with members of the "prying" public touring his institution.

As all historians who enjoy peeking into the lives of earlier generations are professional voyeurs in a sense, it is not surprising that the basest of visitors' motives have captured the attention of scholars. However, when visitor narratives are critically examined and situated within their broader cultural context, it becomes apparent that a number of factors stimulated institutional tourism and that focusing on spectatorship obscures the complexities of the practice. In particular, the growing number of people who flocked to asylums in the nineteenth century was related to the socio-economic environment. Urbanization, immigration, and industrialization are traditionally seen as the benchmarks of the nineteenth century, and along with these changes arose an increased anxiety amongst many.[63] Consequently, those who toured asylums often did so in search of a sense of stability and security and as a means of negotiating or mediating the changing urban landscape of the time. In addition, the nineteenth century was an era of reform, a period in which approaches to insanity were being transformed. Moral therapy, as advocated by Philippe Pinel of the Bicêtre in the late eighteenth century and by William Tuke of the Quakers' York Retreat for the insane in the nineteenth, infiltrated the programs of Ontario asylums. As a result, many people wanted to see first-hand the "progress" that had been made in the sphere of health care reform. One journalist in the London *Free Press* highlighted the importance of visiting in this regard and wrote, "Knowing that a great moral and social problem was being worked out at the Asylum, in the success of which humanity's best instincts are interested, to visit it was part of our programme."[64]

In the accounts written by members of the public, there is a strong sense that they believed themselves to be conducting inspections on their tours of asylums. The majority of visitors critiqued the cleanliness and efficiency of institutions, the appearances of patients, and the approaches of superintendents, and also expressed their approval or disappointment with the institution. Consequently, their judgments resonate throughout their writings: "[We] saw nothing to complain of, but on the contrary, plenty to admire" and "beautifully clean and well kept" were typical evaluations of institutions made by visitors.[65] One visitor to the London Asylum noted: "A look through the building is always instructive and while the demented state of the inmates cannot but excite pity, the visitor will be pleased to see the manner in which the unfortunates are cared for."[66] Another visitor to the Toronto Asylum for the annual Christmas feast remarked, "The terrors associated with lunatic asylums made many conceive of them only as abodes of unmitigated wretchedness. The cell, the whip, the strait-jacket, the filth, the food flung to the poor creatures as if they were dogs, are the prevalent notions connected with them; but here we found an Elysium in comparison with those we have read of, and those we have known. The insane were wont to be governed by the law of brutality; now it is the law of kindness, and the influence of it was fully perceived here on Friday last."[67]

Visitors thus frequently claimed that misconceptions were rectified by visits to asylums and that by seeing such institutions and the people inside them, they could understand new approaches to mental illness. Officials of institutions themselves encouraged people to play a role as unofficial visitors, and annual reports frequently referred to the impressions of casual visitors, thereby granting legitimacy to the efforts made by the public.[68]

For example, many superintendents believed the public could gain a better understanding of both insanity and contemporary therapeutic practices merely through custodial tourism and observation. One official in the United States expressed great faith in the people's potential to be astute visitors, and his views were undoubtedly shared by many of his Canadian counterparts. He wrote: "The public, generally, have wrong impressions in relation to the inmates of a Lunatic Asylum. They suppose them to be either idiots, or completely mad, and in both cases incapable of appreciating kindness. If this was true, moral treatment certainly would prove of little avail. But one visit to a well conducted Institution of this kind would be sufficient to correct this error."[69] Moreover, if any lay visitor was an "untrained observer" unsure of how to evaluate custodial institutions, he or she could always consult John S. Billings and Henry M. Hurd's *Suggestions to Hospital and Asylum Visitors* to "learn how to critically inspect [asylums] with a reasonable chance of seeing what is wrong and learning how to value what is praiseworthy," and to learn "*what* to see ... and *how* to see it."[70]

Even if some Canadians feared that insanity was increasing in the nineteenth century, most looked upon the institutions established to deal with this problem not as shameful or demonstrative of social degeneration, but instead, as symbols of progress. As visitor narratives illustrate, asylums were prominent sources of civic pride. Fairs, exhibitions, and holidays – events that are often associated with enhanced expressions of community pride – were particularly popular days for visiting. The London Asylum, for example, drew over 1,700 visitors in just three days during the fall fair in 1877,[71] and it was invariably described as one of the most beautiful spots around London.[72] This sense of civic pride is further evinced by the fact that residents drew the attention of visitors to their asylums, seeing them as important sites of interest and as community landmarks. Hosts and guides often insisted that travellers tour their institutions (occasionally to the chagrin of the tourist), and one newspaper reporter noted that "the average Londoner never fails to ask you with a conscious pride, 'Have you been out to the Asylum yet?' And if you reply in the negative," the author further noted, "you are told, with no little *empressment*, 'You must go!'"[73] Another writer further propounded, "Such institutions, which are amongst the last results of civilization, are an honour to the country which founds and maintains them; they are a credit and ought to be the pride of the PEOPLE to whose wise liberality their existence is due."[74]

In addition to civic boosterism, asylum tourism represented an educational opportunity for many visitors, and in this regard, the incentives behind institutional tourism were inextricably tied to the nineteenth-century impulse towards self-education and self-improvement. John C. Burnham has examined nineteenth-century popular interest in science in relation to the rise of the commercial museum in the United States and has made a number of arguments that are relevant to the phenomenon of institutional tourism.[75] In many ways, asylums constituted living museums that encouraged the diffusion of knowledge through tourism and observation, and even Clark, the staunch opponent of visitors to the Toronto Asylum, supported tours by "professional men having scientific objects in view."[76] Visiting encouraged the public to examine the institutionalized and thus reason with the "experts" about the causes of mental disease, and as one visitor remarked, "a look through the [London Asylum] building is always instructive."[77] Although this particular visitor was touring the Kingston Penitentiary, his belief that information could be obtained "with the evidence of our own eyes"[78] was undoubtedly shared by many asylum visitors as well.

Since education in the nineteenth century was guided by faith in empiricism and the notion that knowledge could be acquired through observation, many people viewed asylums as sites where "scientific" knowledge could be learned. By simply touring the Toronto Asylum and seeing the patients, for example, one writer felt that visitors were given "an idea of the peculiar but lamentable circumstances that conspired to create insanity,"[79] and many felt their tours had enhanced their knowledge of medical practices. After visiting asylums, people often remarked on how the experience contrasted with prevalent assumptions or popular belief, and one writer commented that the most effective way to establish an understanding of asylum management "was to present to their own eyes, to let them see for themselves what had been done, and how it had been done."[80] Embedded as they were in the nineteenth-century culture of looking or visual display, it is clear that when many visitors described different forms of insanity or the impact that institutionalization had on humans, they were expressing a belief in their right to participate alongside other "experts" in current debates, as well as the idea that seeing or observing could foster understanding.

For those interested in contemporary approaches to deviant behaviour, visiting furthermore represented a "safe" opportunity that allowed for the study of the insane in person. One visitor to the Toronto Asylum remarked that the patients were "under such good management ... even a stranger or a child would be unmolested by the worst of them."[81] Visitors often spoke directly to patients, inquiring into the conditions of the respective institution and the causes behind their mental illness, and frequently recorded their conversations with them.[82] Nevertheless, although the desire to better comprehend the mentally ill permeated the writings of asylum visitors, this was not necessarily accompanied by a desire to *freely* mix with them. Through asylum tourism, the public could get close to those deemed mad, yet still maintain a clear boundary between "normal" and "other." Consequently, many who would have felt threatened had they met the institutionalized in the public realm felt comforted by the fact that, in many ways, institutional tours were orchestrated affairs which were not without certain restrictions and parameters. While many sought to understand the plight of the mentally ill, "sane" citizens could feel unthreatened in the controlled context of visiting and could be assured that employees would intervene if the institutionalized became unruly. Asylum attendants stepped in when necessary, barred windows and doors often separated the institutionalized from visitors, and violent cases were frequently restrained or removed from their presence altogether. The lines could become somewhat blurred at asylum social events such as dances, lectures, or athletic games, yet there was always a clear demarcation between the institutionalized and the visitor.

For many visitors, engaging themselves with the work being done for those suffering from mental illness was closely linked to the ideals surrounding philanthropic pursuits and the notion of "Christian duty." Special events at asylums often attracted members of the public, and the writings surrounding such occasions as concerts, fairs, or dances suggest that citizens were expected to attend as part of their civic duty. However, while events such as sports games were open to all, other events such as dances or holiday parties could be more exclusive affairs in which the invited guests were usually of a certain socio-economic profile (generally, prominent members of the middle class), and the moral obligation in attending such social functions was even more prominent. At the Toronto Asylum in 1847, Superintendent Telfer believed that interaction between asylum patients and the outside world was conducive to the welfare of the former, and he accordingly secured by invitation "the attendance of some of the citizens and their families, whom it was reasonable to conceive, would, each and all, be anxious, so far as in them lie, to aid in a work which promised a wide field, not only for 'the good Samaritan,' but for many good Samaritans."[83] While perhaps attending out of a sense of obligation, one newspaper reporter described the London Asylum Ball as a charitable event that was nevertheless enjoyable to all: "One of the most pleasant events in connection with the routine of Asylum life is the annual ball. For years it has been looked forward to with pleasant anticipation by not only the members of the staff and attendants but many in the city, who have either participated in its festivities, and they desired to be present again, or, having heard of its usually pleasant character, were anxious to be among the fortunate invited."[84] Moreover, a number of visitors speculated that such social events had salutary effects on all participants by revealing the efficacy of kind, gentle treatment, and that they could even transform those who had been drawn to asylums out of "morbid curiosity" and generate compassion and empathy for those afflicted with mental illness.[85] Indeed, whereas many initially thought the lunatic ball to be held in Toronto in 1847 was a "strange and cruel hoax," they found that not only was the evening enjoyed by patients and visitors alike, but that they themselves had broadened their knowledge of insanity and its treatment by interacting with the people in the asylum.[86]

The motives behind institutional tourism reveal that not every "free" member of society would experience his or her visit to an asylum in the same way. For some, spending their leisure time visiting was an opportunity to ridicule the suffering of the confined; for others, it was a means to improve oneself, the confined, or society at large. Nevertheless, whether it was for amusement, education, or reform, the practice reveals a society that privileged the visual and upheld the value of the spectacle in a variety of different contexts and for a variety of different purposes. More importantly, the phenomenon of visiting demonstrates that a substantial number of people in nineteenth-century Ontario sought a closer relationship to the asylums around them and actively endeavoured to better understand the people housed within them, thereby rendering these institutions important and familiar sights in the urban landscape.

Many people in the nineteenth century were fascinated by the growing number of asylums found in Ontario and felt compelled to spend their leisure time inspecting them. Individuals embarked on tours that took them through the corridors, rooms, and grounds of asylums, allowing them not only to view the conditions the incarcerated experienced but to observe the patients themselves. The public not only read about asylums in contemporary newspapers, periodicals, and fiction, but they also toured and inspected these institutions themselves. Their interiors, therapeutic practices, and inmates were described, analyzed, and recorded in letters, diaries, and articles by people who were not members of the medical elite but who simply believed that asylums represented something remarkable in society. Asylums were important sites that were visited by thousands of people and, in contrast to traditional interpretations, were deeply embedded within the broader culture of the nineteenth century.

The popularity of visiting was maintained throughout the century, and even those superintendents who strongly opposed the practice found it very difficult to entirely exclude casual visitors and to disregard the advantages that institutional tourism offered. Some superintendents wanted to keep casual visitors out of their establishments and sought to bar their entry, yet sightseers continued to be a presence in asylums in spite of these employees' wishes. Visiting did not entirely dissolve boundaries, but its pervasiveness reveals that the asylum walls were frequently penetrated by those on the outside, and that the desire of some superintendents to remove the mentally ill from all contact with the "free" world did not automatically materialize into practice. Officials of institutions could voice their opposition to the practice, but the efforts to abolish visiting usually did not amount to more than being able to set certain parameters, such as restricting the hours in which the institution could be seen by the public. The thousands of people who toured Ontario's asylums reveal that these institutions were not as isolated from society as many have thought, and it is these moments of interchange that allow us to better understand popular perceptions of the insane and the asylum, as well as the impact the general public had upon the development of these institutions. While attitudes of both the public and asylum officials varied, the practice of visiting nevertheless illustrates that the relationship between asylums and the larger community beyond their walls was at times characterized by interaction and fluidity, rather than unilateral segregation and alienation.

NOTES

This chapter is drawn from my PhD dissertation, "'As in a Menagerie': The Custodial Institution as Spectacle in the Nineteenth Century" (York University, 2004). I would like to thank the Associated Medical Services, Inc., for the funding I received in the form of a Hannah General Scholarship. As well, I would like to thank the editors, anonymous reviewers, and Marlene Shore for their comments and suggestions.

1 E. Katharine Bates, *A Year in the Great Republic* (London: Ward and Downey, 1887).

2 Archives of Ontario, MU 840 1-D-4, Diary of Thomas Dick (1867–1905).

3 The terms "insane" and "lunatic asylum" are used in this article as part of the lexicon surrounding mental illness in the nineteenth century. Their usage is not meant to be disrespectful of those suffering from mental illness in any way.

4 This article stems from a broader study. See my *"'As in a Menagerie.'"*
5 Jennifer A. Crets, "'Well Worth the Visitor's While': Sightseeing in St. Louis, 1865–1910," *Gateway Heritage* 20, no. 3 (Winter 1999–2000): 18; Patricia Allderidge, "Bedlam: Fact or Fantasy?" in W.F. Bynum, Roy Porter, and Michael Shepherd, eds., *The Anatomy of Madness: Essays in the History of Psychiatry*, vol. 2, (London and New York: Tavistock Publications, 1985), 24. Similarly, many historians have provided only cursory references to visitors. See, for example, Pamela Michael, *Care and Treatment of the Mentally Ill in North Wales, 1800–2000* (Cardiff: University of Wales Press, 2003), 88.
6 Erving Goffman, *Asylums: Essays on the Social Situation of Mental Patients and other Inmates* (Garden City, NY: Doubleday Anchor Books, 1961), 14; David J. Rothman, *The Discovery of the Asylum: Social and Disorder in the New Republic*, rev. 2nd ed. (Boston: Little, Brown, and Co., 1971), xxv. Also see Michel Foucault, *Madness and Civilization: A History of Insanity in the Age of Reason*, trans. Richard Howard (New York: Pantheon Books 1965) and Andrew Scull, *Museums of Madness: The Social Organization of Insanity in Nineteenth-Century England* (London: Allen Lane, 1977).
7 S.E.D. Shortt, *Victorian Lunacy: Richard M. Bucke and the Practice of Late Nineteenth-Century Psychiatry* (Cambridge: Cambridge University Press 1986); Ellen Dwyer, *Homes for the Mad: Life Inside Two Nineteenth-Century Asylums* (New Brunswick, NJ, and London: Rutgers University Press, 1982); Peter McCandless, *Moonlight, Magnolias, and Madness: Insanity in South Caroline from the Colonial Period to the Progressives Era* (Chapel Hill and London: University of North Carolina Press, 1996); James E. Moran, *Committed to the State Asylum: Insanity and Society in Nineteenth-Century Quebec and Ontario* (Montreal and Kingston: McGill-Queen's University Press, 2002); and Geoffrey Reaume, *Remembrance of Patients Past: Patient Life at the Toronto Hospital for the Insane, 1870–1940* (Oxford: Oxford University Press 2000).
8 Peter Bartlett and David Wright, eds., *Outside the Walls of the Asylum: The History of Care in the Community, 1750–2000* (London and New Brunswick, NJ: Athlone Press, 1999), viii.
9 "Report of the Medical Superintendent for the Toronto Asylum," *Journals of the Legislative Assembly of the Province of Canada* (1852), appendix J.
10 See, for example, R.D. Gidney and W.P.J. Millar, "'Beyond the Measure of the Golden Rule': The Contribution of the Poor to Medical Science in Ontario," *Ontario History* 86 (1994): 219–35.
11 "Report of the Medical Superintendent of the Provincial Lunatic Asylum at Toronto," *Journals of the Legislative Assembly* (1856), appendix OO.
12 On public views of North American hospitals, see: Judith Walzer Leavitt, "Politics and Public Health: Smallpox in Milwaukee, 1894–1895," in Judith Walzer

Leavitt and Ronald L. Numbers, eds., *Sickness and Health in America: Readings in the History of Medicine and Public Health*, 2nd ed. (Madison: University of Wisconsin Press, 1985), 374. Only in the early twentieth century, with technological and therapeutic changes, would hospitals be transformed into "respectable" and curative institutions used by the middle class. See, for example, Charles Rosenberg, "Community and Communities: The Evolution of the American Hospital," in Diana Elizabeth Long and Janet Golden, eds., *The American General Hospital: Communities and Social Contexts* (Ithaca: Cornell University Press, 1989), 3–17; and Joel Howell, *Technology in the Hospital: Transforming Patient Care in the Early Twentieth Century* (Baltimore: Johns Hopkins University Press, 1995).

13 "Separate Report of Wolfred Nelson for 1861," in *Second Annual Report of the Board of Inspectors of Asylums, Prisons, &c. 1861,* Canada (Province), *Sessional Papers*, no. 19 (1862).

14 "Report of the Medical Superintendent of the Provincial Lunatic Asylum at Toronto," *Journals of the Legislative Assembly of the Province of Canada* (1852), appendix J.

15 "Report of C. Widmer, Chairman," *Journals of the Legislative Assembly for the Province of Canada* (1852), appendix J; ibid. (1850), appendix C.

16 London *Free Press*, 8 June 1880.

17 "Report of C. Widmer, Chairman," *Journals of the Legislative Assembly for the Province of Canada* (1852), appendix J.

18 "Report of the Inspector of Asylums and Prisons for the Province of Canada," *Sessional Papers*, no. 19 (1862).

19 Shortt, *Victorian Lunacy,* 26.

20 Moran, *Committed to the State Asylum,* 49.

21 "Report of the Medical Superintendent of the Asylum for the Insane, Toronto, for the Year Ending 30th September, 1876," Appendix to "Report of Inspector of Asylums, Prisons, and Public Charities for the Year Ending 30th September, 1876," in Ontario, *Sessional Papers*, 1877, ix, part 1, no. 2 (Toronto: Hunter, Rose, & Co., 1877): 208.

22 "Report of the Medical Superintendent of the Malden Lunatic Asylum," appendix to "Report of Inspector of Asylums, Prisons, and Public Charities for the Twelve Months Ending 30th September, 1869," Ontario, *Sessional Papers*, 1869, ii, no. 4 (Toronto: Hunter, Rose & Co., 1869): 60.

23 "London Asylum: Report of the Medical Superintendent and Statistical Information 1876-7," appendix to "Tenth Annual Report of the Inspector of Asylums, Prisons and Public Charities for the Province of Ontario, for the Year Ending 30th September, 1877, Ontario, *Sessional Papers*, 1878, x, part ii, no. 4 (Toronto: Hunter, Rose and Co., 1878): 281.

24 University of Western Ontario Archives, "Asylum Scrapbook," undated and unnamed newspaper article.

25 Ibid.

26 *British Colonist*, 8 January 1847.

27 "Annual Report of the Medical Superintendent for the London Asylum," reproduced in *Sarnia Canadian*, 24 July 1878.

28 "Asylum for the Insane, London. Report of the Medical Superintendent for the Year Ending 30th September, 1879," appendix to the "Twelfth Annual Report of the Inspector of Asylums, Prisons and Public Charities for the Province of Ontario, for the Year Ending 30th September, 1879," Ontario, *Sessional Papers*, 1880, xii, part ii, no. 8 (Toronto: C. Blackett Robinson, 1880): 316.

29 *Sarnia Canadian*, 19 March 1877.

30 London *Free Press*, 12 January 1878.

31 London *Free Press* 29 September 1899.

32 "Report of the Medical Superintendent of the Asylum for the Insane, Toronto, for the Year Ending 30th September, 1876," 208–9.

33 "Report of the Medical Superintendent of the Malden Lunatic Asylum," 60.

34 New York Public Library, Cp v 1711. Theodric Romeyn Beck, *An Inaugural Dissertation on Insanity* (New York 1811): 27–34.

35 According to Clark, "The desiderata in the choice of a site for an asylum are, quietness and seclusion; to avoid exposure and publicity. Apart from the unpleasant character which a city Asylum must always possess, as one of the 'sights' to be seen by visitors whom curiosity alone impels to examine it, is the consideration that diseases of the brain require absolute quietude and place as curative agents." See "Ninth Annual Report of the Inspector of Asylums, Prisons, and Public Charities for the Province of Ontario, for the Year Ending 30th September, 1876," Ontario, *Sessional Papers*, 1877, ix, part I, no. 2 (Toronto: Hunter Rose and Co., 1877): 27.

36 "Report of the Medical Superintendent of the Asylum for the Insane, Toronto," appendix to "Report of Inspector of Asylums, Prisons, &c., for the Year Ending 30th September 1873," Ontario, *Sessional Papers*, 1873, no. 2 (Toronto: Hunter, Rose and Co., 1874): 160.

37 Reaume, *Remembrance of Patients* Past, 195.

38 *London Advertiser*, 1 July 1880.

39 "Report of the Medical Superintendent of the Asylum for the Insane, Toronto, for the Year Ending 30th September, 1877," appendix to the "Tenth Report of the Inspector of Asylums, Prison, and Public Charities for the Province of Ontario, for the Year Ending 30th September, 1877," Ontario, *Sessional Papers*, 1878, x, part ii, no. 4 (Toronto: Hunter, Rose and Co., 1878): 258.

40 "Report of the Medical Superintendent of the Asylum for the Insane, Toronto, for

the Year Ending 30th September, 1878," appendix to the "Eleventh Annual Report of the Inspector of Asylums, Prison, and Public Charities for the Province of Ontario, for the Year Ending 30th September, 1878," Ontario, *Sessional Papers*, 1879, xi, part iii, no. 8 (Toronto: Hunter, Rose and Co., 1878): 292.

41 "Annual Report of the Medical Superintendent of the Asylum for the Insane, Toronto, for the Year Ending October 1st, 1885, appendix to "Lunatic and Idiotic Asylums. Eighteenth Annual Report of the Inspector of Prisons and Public Charities for the Province of Ontario, for the Year Ending September 30th, 1885, Ontario, *Sessional Papers*, 1886, xvii, part 1, no 2 (Toronto: Warwick and Sons, 1886): 44.

42 Archives of Ontario, MS 717, Journal of the Superintendent for the Kingston Asylum, 21 September 1882, 157–8.

43 For example, E. Katharine Bates claimed to have toured the Toronto Asylum with Clark, whom she described as "most kind and good-natured" and relying chiefly on "moral control." See Bates, *A Year in the Great Republic*, 26–7

44 Vanessa Schwartz, *Spectacular Realities: Early Mass Culture in Fin-de-Siècle Paris* (Berkeley: University of California Press 1998), 11.

45 Archives of Ontario, John Symons Family Papers, F 786–2–0–1, box 2, Manuscript book of travels through the United States and Canada West (1852).

46 Crets, "'Well Worth the Visitor's While,'" 5.

47 *The Canadian Handbook and Tourist's Guide* (1867), 111 and 133.

48 Agnes Maule Machar, *Down the River to the Sea* (New York: Home Book Company, c.1894), 73–4.

49 *Sarnia Canadian*, 19 March 1877.

50 *Sarnia Canadian*, 24 July 1878.

51 *London Advertiser* 1 July 1880.

52 London *Free Press*, 11 March 1877.

53 Ishbel Gordon, Marchioness of Aberdeen and Temair, *Through Canada with a Kodak* (Edinburgh: W.H. White, 1893), 39.

54 Judith Walkowitz, *City of Dreadful Delight: Narratives of Sexual Danger in Late-Victorian London* (Chicago: University of Chicago Press 1992), 16.

55 However, this is not to say that the institutionalized passively allowed themselves to be gawked at. Rather, as my dissertation argues, the insane often actively resisted being treated as compliant exhibits and used the presence of strangers to their own benefit.

56 London *Free Press*, 22 November 1880.

57 Toronto Reference Library, Mickle Family Diary, S 27, William Mickle to father, February 1864.

58 Montreal *Pilot*, 1 May 1845.

59 *Bathurst Courier*, 16 August 1850.

60 Susanna Moodie, *Life in the Clearings Versus the Bush* (1853), reprint (Toronto: McClelland and Stewart, 1989), 272.

61 University of Western Ontario Archives, Diary of Dr Charles Sippi, bursar of the London Insane Asylum, 20 September 1893, 20 September 1894.

62 *Bathurst Courier*, 16 August 1850.

63 Pioneering works that correlate the rise of the asylum with social anxiety are Rothman, *The Discovery of the Asylum*, and Michael Katz, Michael J. Doucet, and Mark J. Stern, *The Social Organization of Early Industrial Capitalism* (Cambridge and London: Harvard University Press, 1982).

64 London *Free Press*, c. end of June 1878.

65 *British Whig*, 12 April 1848; Bates, *A Year in the Great Republic*, 26.

66 *London Advertiser*, 1 July 1880.

67 *British Colonist*, 29 December 1846.

68 For example, one annual report for the Toronto Asylum stated, "It has been the desire of the Directors to have the Asylum as open to the public as is compatible with the welfare of the patients and the duties of their attendants. Large numbers of visitors have therefore, from time to time, been attended through the building, and these have witnessed the condition of the apartments, the appearance and happiness of the patients, the tender, but effective discipline, which prevails amongst the afflicted and their attendants. The result has been, so far as is known, a universal satisfaction to visitors." See "Report of C. Widmer, Chairman," *Journals of the Legislative Assembly for the Province of Canada* (1852), appendix J.

69 *Annual Report of the Alms House Commissioners, Comprising Reports from the Several Departments Embraced in the Institution* (New York, 1848), 62.

70 John. S. Billings and Henry M. Hurd, *Suggestions to Hospital and Asylum Visitors*, intro. S. Weir Mitchell (Philadelphia, 1895), 5–6.

71 University of Western Ontario Archives, E 16, Black Box 3; R.M. Bucke, Medical Superintendent's Journal.

72 See, for example, *London Advertiser*, 1 July 1880.

73 London *Free Press*, c. end of June 1878.

74 *Sarnia Canadian*, 24 July 1878.

75 John C. Burnham, *How Superstition Won and Science Lost* (New Brunswick, NJ: Rutgers University Press, 1987).

76 "Report of the Medical Superintendent of the Asylum for the Insane, Toronto, for the Year Ending 30th September, 1876," 208.

77 *London Advertiser*, 1 July 1880.

78 *British Whig*, 12 April 1848.

79 *Bathurst Courier*, 16 August 1850.

80 *London Free Press*, 9 June 1898.

81 *Bathurst Courier*, 16 August 1850.

82 For example, see John MacGregor, *Our Brothers and Cousins: A Summer Tour in Canada and the States* (London: Seeley, Jackson and Halliday 1859); and George Moore, *Journal of a Voyage across the Atlantic* (London: Printed for Private Circulation, 1845).

83 *British Colonist*, 8 January 1847.

84 *London Free Press*, 21 January 1881. This particular ball was deemed "the greatest assemblage in the history of the institution" and attracted 125 people from the city.

85 *British Colonist*, 8 January 1847; see also Toronto *Globe*, 9 January 1847.

86 *Toronto Examiner*, 13 January 1847; see also *British Colonist*, 29 December 1846.

2

"For Years We Have Never Had a Happy Home"

Madness and Families in Nineteenth-Century Montreal

THIERRY NOOTENS

MADNESS, FAMILIES, AND DISTURBED RELATIONSHIPS

During the transition to industrial capitalism in the nineteenth century, many families were forced to make important decisions at one point or another in their history. To emigrate, to take advantage of professional opportunities, to find satisfactory residential accommodation, to adapt to changing demographic behaviour – these were only some of the areas where a family's capacity to choose, and hence to influence its future, was put to the test. Families that lived in Montreal had to come to terms with a difficult environment, one that included insufficient income for many of them, economic crises that affected commercial and industrial activity, seasonal unemployment, a poor property market, inadequate sanitary conditions, and a high rate of sickness and mortality. Of course, the ability of families to respond to these problems depended in good part on their socio-economic status. But on the whole, life in the nineteenth-century urban milieu was marked by risk and a widespread structural uncertainty.[1] Given this context, it is particularly interesting to pose questions regarding the relationship of families to disorder and misfortune.

Some Montreal families were faced with the mental disorder of a family member or with behaviour that was considered insane. Most of the time, the embarrassing situations and conflicts experienced by such families preceded a request for help from the justice system and from formal institutions. At this essential stage in the "careers" of mental deviance, the actions of individuals judged "abnormal" thwarted the expectations, demands, and plans of families. Moreover, much of this challenging behaviour had an impact, sometimes quite severe, on the functioning, reciprocal exchanges, affective relationships, and distribution of power among Montreal families.

Several studies in the history of mental health have examined the familial circumstances leading to the decision to institutionalize family members. Richard Fox was perhaps one of the first researchers to emphasize that mental illness represented a considerable burden to families and their neighbours.[2] Other research on the process of institutional confinement has demonstrated that institutionalization followed the exhaustion of kin and the punishing situations sometimes experienced by families.[3] The asylum constituted the last resort of a family at the end of its tether.[4]

If, in this article, we are going to examine the concrete problems posed by mental illness and the solutions put in place by families, it must be achieved outside the traditional perspective of institutionalization, as discussed in the recent edited volume entitled *Outside the Walls of the Asylum*,[5] the first work to specifically address the question of the management of madness in the community. The forces at play in the community phase of the care of lunatics must be better understood. In order to address the problem of the relationship between madness and families, we must consider both the process of the social reproduction of families and a relational model of the sociology of deviance. Briefly put, social reproduction can be defined as the aggregate of concrete efforts and attempts by families to achieve the necessarily unpredictable but desirable goals of self-perpetuation, the maintenance of social status, and (if possible) the experience of social promotion (notably by the advances of their children). In the nineteenth century the dynamic generated by property and income was central to this general process. Within the working classes this dynamic was marked by a daily resourcefulness and by the contribution of all the members of the family to household income,[6] while within middling and wealthier families the preservation and transmission of inheritance played a fundamental role. As will be shown, instances of mental deviance challenged the abilities of families to engage in their social reproduction process.

According to the sociological theory of "labelling," deviance and its "treatment" depends above all upon social reactions to specific behaviour, and the subsequent labelling of such behaviour by elite groups within society, during specific encounters.[7] These reactions provide essential evidence of the social experience of madness upon which the researcher must base his or her conclusions. However, the different theoretical perspectives on the labelling of behaviour have a tendency to neglect an important element: that problematic behaviour may have existed from the outset.[8] The potential burden of deviance can not be ignored.[9] Consequently, labelling theory needs to be understood within a more functionalist framework tied to the dynamic of familial social reproduction. The relational consequences of certain states and situations need to be considered. As Sheldon Ekland-Olson explains, we can define deviance as "a particular kind of relational disturbance – a breach in normative ties ... [and] assume that normative disruptions are frequently accompanied by changes in the strength of affective ties and patterns of exchange resulting in strained or weakened relationships ... [and] define the severity of any normative breach as the total amount of relational disturbance created."[10] The family is made up of a web of connections and ties of immediate interaction, of reciprocal (although not always equal) exchanges that aim at affective as well as economic benefits, which ultimately constitutes and permits its existence. Its everyday existence is made up of power relations and continual negotiations. In the nineteenth century what were the repercussions of certain behaviours on the functioning of the family vis-à-vis daily survival, the care of children, the management of inheritance, and the transmission of property?

The petitions and testimonies produced by judicial procedures of "interdiction" have much to tell us about the situation of Montreal families facing insanity in their midst. Through this civil law recourse, the kin of individuals considered insane could ask for the removal of the individual's capacity to manage his or her own affairs and for the assignment of a person judged more competent to take responsibility for the lunatic's property (this person being named curator or curatrix).[11] All interdiction files concerning Montreal dwellers created between 1820 and 1895 (330 case files) were examined for the purposes of this study.[12] Certain individual and familial trajectories affected by mental illness have been subjected to detailed scrutiny.[13] This chapter will first consider the connections between the impact of madness and the role of individuals judged to be insane within the context of their families. The familial and community reactions to madness will be examined afterwards.

MADNESS AND FAMILIAL ROLES: THE SITUATION OF MONTREAL WIVES

Mental deviance highlighted the specific conjunctures and the disturbances of social and familial roles.[14] It precipitated an imbalance in the relationships closest to the individual affected. The situation of women whose spouses were unable to fulfill the requirements of their role illustrates this phenomenon well. It was certainly one of the most punishing domestic situations within nineteenth-century Montreal society. Many wives had to struggle to compensate for their husbands' disorder by assuming specific economic functions within the patriarchal household structure.

These dramatic situations were notably distinguished by a lack of consistent earnings: spouses were also burdened with the task of generating household income, a situation that in the nineteenth century had in many ways not been "anticipated." Bettina Bradbury has already provided evidence of the major difficulties encountered by working-class women following the death of a husband and the "survival strategies" that they adopted.[15] A similar situation arose for women whose husbands survived but were burdened with considerable incapacity. Such dependence represented a heavy burden on the ability of Montreal families to reproduce economically, whether they were poor or rich, although it goes without saying that the latter were not directly menaced by hunger.

David M. was a jeweller who had suffered from madness for a long time, according to his spouse, Philomène, who demanded his interdiction. With the help of her husband's parents, she placed him in the Brattleboro Lunatic Asylum in Vermont. After a stay of several months, he was diagnosed as "incurable." Not having the means to pay for a long stay in the institution, Philomène returned him home to Montreal. The couple had five children, whose ages ranged from fifteen months to fourteen years. The applicant said that she did not have the necessary resources to get by "unless put in the position to carry on the business of her husband either personally or through another as conseil or curator." Philomène was named curatrix, from that moment she acquired the prerogative to manage the affairs of the household.[16] Adeline L., the spouse of another institutionalized man, Athanase M., was likewise in difficulty at the beginning of the 1870s: "since the sickness of her husband she had often had to take the recourse of the goodwill of her parents in order to get the necessary means for the subsistence of her family, as she had not yet had the authorization to touch any of the monies belonging to her husband." The couple had four young children. She was also named curatrix.[17]

These are two examples of the problems brought upon a young family by the advent of mental illness: the eventual absence as a result of an institutional stay, the lack of resources occasioned by the halting of formal economic activities, young children who became difficult to feed, a spouse forced to carry on in the face of her own legal incapacity. This incapacity was in part counterbalanced by the assignment of the spouse as curatrix. But this new legal status did not provide supplementary resources for the support of the family. By examining other legal acts relative to an interdicted individual, we can follow the progressive financial collapse that very often accompanied the incapacity of a husband. In this way it is also possible to illuminate the phenomenon of role compensation by the spouse.

In March 1836 Michel D., a master cooper, was interdicted because of attacks of madness. The nominated curator, Francois T., was not a member of the family. A little time after the court proceedings, this guardian presented a request to be authorized to take out a loan with the purpose of making repairs to houses owned by the household and in order to repay certain debts. Michel's madness had probably not favoured the good financial health of his family. The curator also desired to be authorized to use the rental income from the same houses to support the affected man and his relatives. But in February 1837 Julie M., Michel's wife, asked for the dismissal of the curator before the Court of King's Bench. She said that, at the moment of her husband's interdiction, he had real estate whose rents "were sufficient to support Michel, your supplicant, and her children (who number nine) in a decent lifestyle." However, two houses possessed by Michel had burned down in October 1836 and "were not insured by any fire insurance through the negligence and grave fault of Francois T. curator." From all available evidence, these houses represented the principal resources of the interdicted man; after this fire, his revenues had declined dramatically. Michel was at this time residing in the Quebec Madhouse;[18] thus Julie was not able to ask for his assistance in any way.

One of the members of the family council, reunited on the occasion of this request to remove the curator from his duties, maintained that Julie could be trusted with the guardianship because she was very thrifty. She was named guardian. A little later, she submitted a request to be authorized to sell some real estate; she also desired to take out a loan to rebuild one of the burnt houses, because it represented the principal source of revenue for the household. This request was also granted. However, several months later (in August 1837), she requested a new authorization to sell. Of three out of four properties that she was authorized to sell by the preceding act, she only succeeded in selling one for £156, of which £75 were directed "to paying a few small debts and to providing household objects necessary for putting her in a position of keeping a boarding house, the only means now left to her for supporting her family." To madness and fires one must add a lack of success in selling the properties. Julie thus turned to one of the few practical options for women in the nineteenth century to acquire income –

taking in boarders.[19] The couple had by then become indebted to the amount of £270 "by the small debts which your supplicant had to contract in order to support her family, because of a lack of success of her boarding house."

On 16 April 1839 Michel D. was relieved of his interdiction at the request of his wife. Unfortunately, he died soon after on 22 October of the same year. Thus Julie was left alone with seven young children under her care, children whose ages ranged from five to eighteen years (three older children of the couple had left the province). Faced with such a situation, she was authorized to sell their only remaining property in order to pay off persistent debts. Thus the rough financial situation that this household faced persisted, despite all the efforts of the spouse, who had fought the management of the first guardian, whom she judged to be too costly, assumed the management of the property of the couple, and tried to create new sources of revenue in the form of a boarding house.[20] The sexual division of tasks and the patriarchal structure of the family had ultimately defeated her.

The spouse who was forced to find a solution to the financial problems created or amplified by mental illness sometimes had to face behaviour that hindered her efforts. The deviant, it is important to remember, most of the time remained within the household. Joseph P., a merchant, had six children. According to his spouse, Éloïse, his madness and "the bad business decisions that he made had ruined his livelihood … his mania consisted of buying horses at any price." For this reason, he was interdicted a first time in the district of Joliette. Éloïse then came to Montreal "to establish a boarding house in order to ensure the means of supporting her said husband and her family of six children." Joseph, having appeared to improve, was relieved during this time of his legal incapacity. The family subsequently returned for a while to L'Assomption hoping for better success. But in a request for a new judicial intervention presented in 1867, Éloïse affirmed "that today they are all back in this city [Montreal] in order that your applicant could maintain a private boarding house, to meet the needs, some basic and some urgent, of her family." At this point, it should be remembered, her husband was in complete possession of his civil rights. But then, "unfortunately, her husband had begun again to make bad deals, exposing your applicant and her family to all sorts of problems and the little of the household that remains to your applicant might be seized from one moment to another." Éloïse was nominated curatrix, which gave her, from a legal perspective at least, the direction of the household affairs.[21]

Curatorship made some pitfalls disappear and added a certain legal capacity to maternal resourcefulness. That a spouse would be nominated curatrix and given control over the affairs of her husband created an unusual situation within the context of nineteenth-century society. It had the impact of overturning social-legal structures that underpinned the institution of marriage. In civil law, the married woman figured amongst those who were legally incapable, a group that also included minors and the interdicted. It is probable that the judicial system and the family circle, which played an important role in the choice of curator or curatrix through the mechanism of the family council, recognized the difficult situation of women and their competence to assume, in exceptional circumstances, the management of the household. On the other hand, this recognition did not necessarily rectify the situation: a legal emancipation was not the equivalent of an emancipation from need! In fact, judging from the preceding cases, the difficult and "declining" economic condition of women appeared to be constant in the interdiction files of married men. The family occasionally suffered tensions that could bring it to the point of disintegration.

This analysis of the overturning of social roles and the disruption of relationships could be perhaps be applied to other "figures" of madness and to the specific tensions that accompanied them. For example, cases of mental retardation created a stress related to the management over the long term of such vulnerable individuals, who were incapable of taking care of themselves; "idiots" were not able to meet the expectations of their parents (in the context of a professional situation, legal capacity, or the social expectations of adulthood).[22] Honore G. was not able to "provide for his subsistence and had never taken his first communion and had lived at the expense of his brothers and his parents, spending several weeks and several months alternatively at the home of one or the other."[23] For their part, aged and senile persons challenged the very delicate familial transition that was inheritance transmission. Old age was sometimes accompanied by a decline in intellectual faculties that might have necessitated the appointment of a curator. However, certain familial disputes look like inheritance conflicts preceding the death of a testator. These incidents testify to an often overlooked and far from brilliant aspect of the role of the aged in nineteenth-century Montreal society: that of the provider of a long-awaited inheritance.[24]

THE FAMILY CIRCLE AND COPING

The means by which the family circle dealt with madness outside the formal recourse to institutionalization clarifies the dynamics within the family that were precipitated by different types of mental alienation. Above all, these reactions were very significant with respect to the responsibility and the power of the family circle in the management and control of mental illness.

This chapter will not utilize the concept of family "strategies." To a certain extent, the idea of strategies implies that the individuals involved acted in a comprehensively rational way, that they understood their predicament well, and that they were capable of predicting the future consequences of their actions. The term also tends to imply that families always did what they had to do (despite their poverty, their apparent difficulties, etc.) or, rather, that they did something that was inherently "natural" to them. As a result, the family strategy concept tends to interpret human actions of the past as evident and spontaneous objects. In the present case, arrangements put in place by the families of the mentally ill were, most of the time, incomplete, improvised, and mixed in their results.

The term "coping" better conveys the complex dynamics that comprised the behaviours and attitudes of familial actors responding to situations of mental alienation. The kin of the mad had to contend with the disorder and to face the consequences of the situation. Confronted by madness and the disturbances that it elicited, parents and friends faced the problem and searched for an arrangement, a solution that was satisfactory and the least damaging for the continued social reproduction of the family. These actions further complicated the existing burden and anxieties already inflicted on the family and contributed to the reformulation of intra-familial relations. What is more, coping did not operate in a vacuum. Its operationalization depended on certain factors. [25] Evidently, the severity and the duration of unsettling behaviour gave some indication of the challenge at hand and of what had to be accomplished. The status of the deviant person was also significant: for example, to confront a middle-aged father who knew how to make himself feared was not the equivalent of having to find a pension for an orphaned niece who had been an idiot from childhood. Moreover, all families did not have the same financial and human resources upon which to draw. The problems and the conflicts could also arise unexpectedly at almost any stage of the family life cycle. That fact, in turn, influenced the human resources available (older children could play a variety of roles) and the more or less dramatic nature of the situation.

The familial reactions to mental illness in nineteenth-century Montreal assumed many diverse forms. There were not only the life histories of those affected by mental troubles: the family also had a life history of its own, a history of management of an embarrassing person for whom it had to care for. The familial responses also evolved over time. [26] Therefore familial reactions will be distinguished here principally by their relationship to time, but this is not to suggest that the different actions and attitudes followed one another. They can be divided into four subgroups: advice; informal negotiations and sanctions; compromise and cohabitation; ad hoc reactions; and palliative and long-term measures.

The painful situations indicated in the case files did not develop overnight. These troubles were certainly preceded by a considerable history of worry, meetings, advice, negotiations, and threats, of which the archival documents can only yield rare examples. In certain cases, these essentially verbal interactions probably represented a very important part of the non-institutional experience of deviance. A half-sister of Édouard G., who was declared incapable in 1893, said to him, "You are often drunk; and it is not wise to carry as much money"; to which the man responded, "I am not mad; I am capable of taking care of it."[27] Advice was probably often mixed with, or followed by, injunctions. Charles S. "has entirely lost his mental control and would not pay regard to the wishes or desires of those who were with him and his relations, and they could in no way control him or make him act reasonably."[28] Evidently, since the relatives finally asked for a legal interdiction – the withdrawal of the individual's civil capacity – it is not surprising that family members mentioned that their advice had not brought about the desired result.

In the face of ineffective familial advice and reprimands, kin could accommodate themselves to the problem over a period of time, if this accommodation was not too destructive to daily life, if the familial position occupied by the deviant was important, or if the alternatives were impractical. One of the most usual aspects of coping consisted of cohabitation with the deviant. But this co-residence covered many sundry situations that were, in many respects, ambiguous.

Would an aged mother have been accommodated by her daughter, regardless of the presence or absence of mental disorder? Probably. Joseph G., a former employee of the Grand Trunk Railway Company certified as mentally unsound in 1865, had become "for several months following fatigue and sickness ... feeble-minded and imbecilic." He stayed at home.[29]This circumstance is not surprising at first glance; but one fact remains: in a considerable number of cases, the person judged incapable was living with other members of his family circle or had become accommodated somewhere. An elderly man, interdicted in 1825, lived with his daughter who took care of him.[30] At the other end of the century, an elderly widow of eighty-three years also lived with her daughter.[31]

In other cases, it is clear that cohabitation or lodging was directly tied to the problematic condition of the person. A son of a first marriage, an adult (but imbecilic) man, lived with his remarried mother.[32] This taking charge of the incapacitated is even more evident when the documents mention the care given to the individual. Alfred M., clerk who was declared mentally incapable in 1891 and who "had completely lost use of his reason," was "for a long time under the care of one of his brothers."[33] The family remained the first line of defence with respect to sickness and poverty in Montreal throughout the nineteenth century. The residential accommodation that could be arranged played an important role in ameliorating particular problems or crises.[34]

With the emergence of the asylum system, such cohabitation no longer seemed obligatory. The Saint-Jean-de-Dieu Asylum was officially founded in 1873.[35] Situated at the eastern end of the island of Montreal, it subsequently witnessed a dramatic growth. Yet, as the preceding examples show, this strengthened institutional presence did not signify the end to housing those deemed mentally incapacitated in households. Although the asylum solution became more and more popular, it never fully replaced the family as the principal locus for the care and control of the mad.[36] In this sense, the asylum merely added to the variety of options available to Montrealers, in certain circumstances, for the regulation of deviance.[37]

While sometimes cohabitation with a person considered mad could last for years or an entire lifetime, necessitating an adjustment in daily life, other situations were marked by a need to act more immediately and often in an ad hoc manner. In certain cases, a more active surveillance had to be put in place around the individual concerned. This surveillance could be an onerous task; its possibility depended on the financial and human resources that could be dedicated by the family for an indeterminate period of time. Joseph L., a grocer, interdicted in 1857, was also considered dangerous. He was overseen by two men, his brothers-in-law. He was finally locked up in the district prison.[38] Elsewhere, an "attendant" was assigned to an aged man. The latter managed to escape his guardian and get lost in the middle of the day.[39]

Family members clearly found themselves physically threatened on certain occasions. The dangerousness of uncontrollable men constituted a real problem. Luc Q., a mason, "comported himself with great excess by striking his wife, Julie [L.], and even threatened to kill her … she lately discovered that he had a knife hidden on him with which he tried to achieve that end." A day labourer who lived in the same house had to remove a hatchet from Luc's hands as the latter threatened his wife.[40] However, ad hoc gestures did not exclusively involve the dangerousness of lunatics. A man who knew Émerante R. for a long time, a woman who was considered insane, thought "that without the help of neighbours she would have died of hunger or frost in her house."[41] Did Montrealers show a greater degree of patience during manifestations of madness that were not very threatening? Julien P. stole an object from the store of an auctioneer who knew him well. The proprietor "allowed this matter to remain [unsettled] from a conviction that said [P.] was not sane."[42]

Sometimes the violent crises of several lunatics were followed by one of the most spectacular familial reactions: confinement in the home itself. Evidently, it was not a very practical solution, but certain Montreal families had to urgently sort things out, at least until the institutional resources of the region were more abundant (that is, after the third quarter of the nineteenth century). The interdiction files, in fact, give the impression that this form of control later disappeared.

We have already spoken of the financial problems encountered by the spouse of Michel D., the individual who was interdicted in 1836. In addition to the economic setbacks of the couple, his wife revealed that he had had his "freedom restricted" for her safety and that of their children. A neighbour who lived in the lower half of the house had assisted in locking up Michel in "a small apartment prepared for his reception," a place where he was tied. This quasi-internment did not make cohabitation with the lunatic any easier, as is evidenced by the same neighbour, who said that he screamed "[like] a mad man" and made noise almost every day. Moreover, the curator named in the first instance (before Michel's spouse replaced him) had been chosen principally for his physical size. Shortly after his interdiction, Michel stayed in the Hôpital général in Quebec City.[43] Why so far away? The Soeurs Grises of the Hôpital général of Montreal had refused in 1830 to receive new lunatics into their cells (*loges*), which left an institutional void for the reception of the mentally ill in the Montreal area in the 1830s (until the opening of the Montreal Lunatic Asylum in 1839).[44] During this interval, the only institutional option in the district was the prison.[45]

In other circumstances, kin could try to find a convenient long-term arrangement, in order to ensure the management of the deviant and the satisfactory functioning of the family. These actions comprised certain measures employed to protect patrimony (outside the interdiction procedure itself), some juridical acts (legacies, transfers of goods, and other financial arrangements), and the pensioning off of the lunatic.

The financial situation of many interdicted Montrealers and their families depended strongly on their interest in real estate, inheritances, and

income from rents. All these sources of revenue had a real importance for
city dwellers who, even in modest circumstances, did not depend solely on
salaries and expedients to survive. In the case of the mentally ill and their
families, if the trouble was severe, these resources were even more essential.[46]

Montrealers certainly sought to protect their inheritance and income.
Interestingly, some measures that were similar to a curatorship of goods
(though lacking a legal sanction) were often applied over a significant span
of time. But changing circumstances ultimately led to resorting to a curatorship proper. David M., a jeweller whom we have already discussed, had
a flourishing business, "which with the kind assistance of his friends has
been partially kept up and continued during his illness."[47] Evidently, this
kind of informal administration was less safe than a real curatorship, and
it was clearly impractical if important deeds had to be ratified or if judicial
procedures were necessary and imminent.

Other solutions were more juridical in their orientation. Some testamen-
tary clauses and other financial arrangements indicate a desire to ensure
longer-term maintenance of an individual whose mental incapacity had
been ascertained for quite a while. For example, Francois G. was interdicted in 1832. His brother, Jean-Baptiste, was obliged by their mother's
will to lodge him and furnish him with an annuity. The brother, however,
found this responsibility too onerous. The curator of Francois G. (his first
cousin) believed that "It would be dangerous to remove the said Francois
(G.) to another family; considering that he has all his habits and affections
with this one, where he is moreover treated with particular attention,
where he is also quiet in mind, and if he were forced to live elsewhere, he
would be irritated by this annoyance, which would probably render him
fully insane."

The curator indicated in this way his marked preference for the care
given by kin. Financial adjustments were made so that Francois's boarding
with his brother would continue. The latter agreed to "look after all his
needs, be it in health or in sickness [and to] make the necessary funeral
arrangements after his death."[48] Marie V. was "lodged, fed, and maintained" by her curator and brother-in-law following the death of her
mother. However, the only resource at her disposal was a modest sum of
£93 from her father's estate. Her curator offered by contract "to lodge her
with him and his family and to feed and maintain the said Marie and to
care of her for the rest of her life, be it in sickness or in health," in exchange
for the said sum (including interest). His request was granted.[49]

This type of agreement implies cohabitation with an embarrassing or vulnerable individual. A residential arrangement led occasionally to the removal of the person concerned. On the one hand, some behaviours may have been so disruptive that kin chose to endure them no longer. On the other hand, the human resources of the family were not always able to accommodate the often heavy task of care and domestic surveillance. Moreover, the family finances had to be able to support a remedy of this kind. In one case at the end of the century, sending to the countryside, or boarding out, preceded institutionalization. Olivine T., a widow interdicted in 1895, "had always resided with her husband in Montreal, except when, given her demented state, she was transferred to the countryside in Beauharnois" for two years. She was then admitted as a public patient at the Saint-Jean-de-Dieu Asylum.[50] Sufficient funds gave the opportunity for the family to avoid taking care of the deviant. Several upper-middle-class interdicted persons found themselves placed in boarding houses at the end of their lives, a recourse that appeared to be specific to them.[51] These boarding-house placements demonstrate the diversity of the residential solutions applied to madness, outside institutional avenues of care and control.

As all of these family manoeuvrings testify, mental deviance was not just a specific "career" of an individual. A situation full of difficulty and/or conflict influenced, more or less, the trajectory of the family itself. Furthermore, according to specific circumstances, the kin likely had recourse to a variety of measures. The typology outlined thus far imperfectly conveys the relationship between familial reactions and time. One especially detailed family trajectory will illustrate this dynamic.

John C. was interdicted in 1895. In this case, elements that were likely to influence the family reactions to mental illness are clear: the status and family role of the individual considered insane, the severity of the deviance, the extent of familial resources (human and financial) available. This "gentleman" of sixty-eight years, head of his family and endowed with a considerable fortune (his wealth would approximate $200,000), seemed strongly authoritarian; his behavioural troubles lasted for several years (for eight to ten years, according to his children) and made living with him impossible. All his children were adults; one of the daughters was married and established outside the household. This particular combination of factors (a severe head of household, a very problematic behaviour, and a family circle composed of several adults) had contributed to much conflict over power in this Montreal household. And given the particular era in which this story was played out – the end of the nineteenth century – the use of the asylum was a possibility.

From 1880 John C. seemed to indulge in heavy drinking. Yet it was chiefly his violence, his paranoia (he believed that someone wanted to kill him), and his coarseness (he called his daughters prostitutes) that made things untenable. Because of his behaviour, one of his daughters affirmed, "For years we have never had a happy home." His brother concurred by stating, "I always liked him when he was reasonable ... but since he has been so bad to his wife and children I have not spoken to him; I have not spoken to him for years on account of that." A neighbour had similarly stopped visiting the family as a result of the stress it was going through. The impact of a certain type of madness, the disruption of exchanges of which families and their sociability were made, are rendered clear in this case.

The family's nights were constantly troubled by the mayhem and the fear that the man would provoke. He entered the children's bedrooms and lit matches above their heads. These nocturnal events precipitated practically a domestic guerrilla warfare. His son, Sarsfield, testified, " I used to keep a pillow on the floor at the foot of the door ... You know that if you open a door with a pillow against it that way it will get under the door and jam it, and whenever I heard him coming I would wake right up." The same son, who was said to be the protector of the family, had to contribute with his physical strength to control John C. The son had even once come to blows with his father, when the latter sought to strike his mother and one of his sisters.

John C. was also the subject of negotiations and threats. With his spouse, "he would begin scolding and then after a long time Mrs [C.] would say to him for God's sake to give her ease or she would have to leave the house to him." What is more, we find an attempt to confine madness to the private sphere, notably by keeping the doors of the residence closed. The sense of shame and embarrassment may have constituted one of the important motivations of family reactions to madness. Families made an effort to refrain from having the madness of one of their members become public knowledge.[52] In fact, for his brother James, John was a disgrace "to the name of the family, and he is considered by everybody to be a fool." Reputation and honour were crucial components of the relations between family members; the actions and gestures of an individual implicated and bound the rest of the family.[53] Montreal families tried at all cost to avoid material, as well as symbolic, falls from grace. And in the city, public space was more immediate, thus hastening interventions against deviance.[54]

Because John C.'s family was not able to address the problem of his behaviour at its foundation, the failure of informal negotiations and reproaches and of ad hoc measures that only prevented certain troublesome consequences of the head of family's conduct rendered the continuation of ordinary daily living impossible. The deviant behaviours overturned the resources and the cohesion of this family group. When things no longer worked, one could try to banish the madness or to withdraw oneself. The daughters of the couple passed their evenings outside the home and returned home at a late hour. The son, the defender of the rest of the family, left the house three times before finally never returning. The wife and children found refuge at the home of the married daughter, reconstituting themselves outside the original family household. The husband of the latter declared, "I might say that my house was a kind of house of refuge for the members of the family one after another owing to the treatment they were getting from their father."

On 11 September 1895 John C. was confined as a dangerous lunatic at the Saint-Jean-de-Dieu Asylum. In fact, the confinement of the troublemaker had already been anticipated many years previously, which merely illustrates the perseverance of his family. Once confined, he was placed under the prerogative of his wife, who was named curatrix the same day. However, he did not stay without a fight. After an appeal, he obtained a reversal of his interdiction on 23 December 1895, and an order was granted for his release from the asylum seven days later.[55]

CONCLUSION: MADNESS AND THE FRAGILITY OF LIFE IN THE NINETEENTH CENTURY

The experience of madness is first and foremost a familial experience in the nineteenth century. On kin devolved direct responsibility to compensate for the breach that the presence of insanity represented to the exchanges, contributions, and norms which made up families of this period. Mental alienation unsettled the routine of daily life. It undermined financial situations that were sometimes already precarious, plans made for children, and efforts to move upward through Montreal's social and symbolic hierarchy. Two dynamics of time and action thus collided: that of the lunatic's behaviour, contingent and irregular as it was, and that of the ordinary and immediate workings of the family and its long-term plans. The intensity of this upheaval varied according to the incapacity of the deviant to assume his social role, from the viewpoint of the expectations and needs of his family circle and with regard to the socio-legal framework of this era. The dramatic situation of women who were faced with the prolonged incapacity of their spouses bears eloquent testimony to this disruption.

Yet the family circle faced the situation. As the interdiction case files have revealed, this involvement of family members proceeded from the worry of maintaining patrimony and income and avoiding misery or the decline of the household, but also from the desire to ensure a certain form of care for the mental deviant, as different legal acts have shown. The implementation of coping measures, whether immediate and urgent or longer-term in nature, depended on several identifiable variables – the severity of the troubles, the position occupied by the deviant in the household, and the human and financial resources available. These different tactics demonstrated simultaneously the great burden that responsibility for certain individuals entailed, the immense role of the family in the management of mental deviance, and the limited effectiveness of the solutions upon which Montrealers could draw.

These lunatic-family encounters speak of an era. Over the course of the nineteenth century, the interdiction files generally denote few changes with regard to the management of madness outside institutions. This phenomenon needs to be explained. The fundamental importance of property and income for Montreal families persisted throughout the nineteenth century despite the transition to capitalism or, rather, in accordance with it. In spite of the spread of waged work and the increased division of labour, there remained very few protections for Montreal families. Nineteenth-century Montreal remained a locus of precarious living. Death and sickness struck hard, as did commercial bankruptcies. Although the economy was becoming greatly transformed, family ties interwoven with wealth and income remained necessary and strong, as these ties were essential to familial survival and also to the maintenance of status and honour. This interweaving of the familial and the material is a central fact of the experience of deviance in the nineteenth century. If historians characterize this era as one of change par excellence, one also finds continuity, tied, of course, to the new global logic of regulation that transformed it.

Even at the end of the nineteenth century, the impact of deviance continued to be equally devastating, perhaps even accentuated on account of the transition to capitalism, with more and more pronounced familial dependence on the income of the male breadwinner, a dependence that grew with urbanization as well as with industrialization. This dependence rendered families more vulnerable, among other things, to their income being diverted towards the purchase of alcohol.[56] The history of madness, then, like that of other deviances, forms part of the history of the hazards experienced by social formations in the past.

NOTES

This chapter is drawn from my doctoral thesis: "Fous, prodigues et ivrognes: internormativité et déviance à Montréal au 19e siècle" (PhD thesis, Université du Québec à Montréal, 2003). This research has benefited from generous grants from the Social Sciences and Humanities Research Council of Canada and from Associated Medical Services. This chapter has been translated from the French by David Wright and James Moran, with assistance from the author.

1 John Modell, "Changing Risks, Changing Adaptations: American Families in the Nineteenth and Twentieth Centuries," in Allan J. Lichtman and Joan R. Challinor, eds., *Kin and Communities: Families in America* (Washington: Smithsonian Institution Press, 1979), 119.

2 Richard W. Fox, *So Far Disordered in Mind: Insanity in California, 1870–1930* (Berkeley: University of California Press, 1978), 10, 11, and 163.

3 See, for example, Cheryl Krasnick Warsh, "The First Mrs Rochester: Wrongful Confinement, Social Redundancy and Commitment to the Private Asylum, 1883–1923," *Canadian Historical Association/Société historique du Canada, Historical Papers/Communications historiques*, 1988, 148; Nancy Tomes, *A Generous Confidence: Thomas Story Kirkbride and the Art of Asylum-Keeping, 1840–1883* (Cambridge: Cambridge University Press, 1984), 13.

4 This fact has been revealed by many studies. The article that pays special attention to the question of the family-asylum interface is David Wright, "Getting Out of the Asylum: Understanding the Confinement of the Insane in the Nineteenth Century," *Social History of Medicine* 10, 1 (1997): 137–55.

5 Peter Bartlett and David Wright, eds., *Outside the Walls of the Asylum: The History of Care in the Community, 1750–2000* (London: The Athlone Press, 1999).

6 Bettina Bradbury, *Familles ouvrières à Montréal: Âge, genre et survie quotidienne pendant la phase d'industrialisation* (Montréal: Boréal, 1995).

7 Howard S. Becker, *Outsiders: Études de sociologie de la déviance* (Paris: A.-M. Métailié, 1985), 32–3.

8 Michael S. Goldstein, "The Sociology of Mental Health and Illness," *Annual Review of Sociology* 5 (1979): 387–8.

9 Contemporary studies have clearly demonstrated the negative impact for the family of bouts of mental illness; see, for example, Kenneth G. Terkelsen, "The Meaning of Mental Illness to the Family," in Agnes B. Hatfield and Harriet P. Lefley, eds., *Families of the Mentally Ill: Coping and Adaptation* (New York: Guilford Press, 1987), 128–50.

10 Sheldon Ekland-Olson, "Deviance, Social Control and Social Networks," *Research on Law, Deviance and Social Control* 4 (1982): 282.

11 The procedure of interdiction is described in detail in Nootens, "Fous, prodigues et ivrognes," chap. 1.

12 Tutorship and curatorship collection of the Superior Court of the judicial district of Montreal (collection CC 601 of the Archives nationales du Québec à Montréal, hereafter ANQM). This series is almost complete with the exception of a very few dossiers.

13 These reconstructions are based on other judicial files concerning interdicted persons, files from the tutorship and curatorship collection, or files from other civil lawsuits.

14 David Mechanic, "Some Factors in Identifying and Defining Mental Illness," in Thomas J. Scheff, ed., *Mental Illness and Social Processes* (New York: Harper and Row, 1967), 28.

15 Bradbury, *Familles ouvrières à Montréal*, chap. 6.

16 ANQM, CC 601, 11 December 1868 (date of the act), no. 496 (no. of file). For similar situations see ANQM, CC 601, 29 August 1866, no. 318, or 14 November 1888, no. 623.

17 ANQM, CC 601, 23 May 1872, no. 279.

18 This was very likely the *loges* at the Quebec General Hospital.

19 Bradbury, *Familles ouvrières à Montréal*, 263–4, 275, and 277.

20 For the story of Michel D. and Julie, see ANQM, CC 601, 29 March 1836, no. 281; 10 June 1836, no. 454; ANQM, collection of the Court of King's/Queen's Bench of the judicial district of Montreal (henceforth cited as TL 19), February 1837 term, no. 443, *ex parte* [M.]; ANQM, CC 601, 22 February 1837, no. 102; 31 March 1837, no. 210; 18 August 1837, no. 498; 16 April 1839, no. 290; 5 November 1839, no. 727; 16 November 1839, no. 758.

21 ANQM, CC 601, 16 May 1867, no. 209. For other examples of this combination of insane husband and obligated wife resorting to the operation of a boarding house or a business, see ANQM, CC 601, 28 February 1873, no. 86; 21 November 1878, no. 467. See also the trajectory contained in the following documents: ANQM, CC 601, 16 December 1895, no. 695; 8 July 1898, no. 380; 5 December 1899, no. 720.

22 See David Wright, "Childlike in his Innocence: Lay Attitudes towards Idiots and Imbeciles in Victorian England," in David Wright and Anne Digby, eds., *From Idiocy to Mental Deficiency: Historical Perspectives on People with Learning Disabilities* (New York: Routledge, 1996), 131.

23 ANQM, CC 601, 9 September 1890, no. 500.

24 Nootens, "Fous, prodigues et ivrognes," 177 and following.

25 These factors are examined in Diane T. Marsh, *Families and Mental Retardation:*

New Directions in Professional Practice (New York: Praeger 1992), especially 81–2.

26 Kenneth G. Terkelsen, "The Evolution of Family Responses to Mental Illness through Time," in Hatfield and Lefley, eds., *Families of the Mentally Ill*, 151–2.

27 ANQM, Files of the Superior Court, Montreal Record Office (henceforth cited as TP 11), 1893, no. 2131, Brady vs. Dubois.

28 ANQM, CC 601, 12 January 1891, no. 18.

29 ANQM, CC 601, 17 March 1865, no. 93, and 17 March 1865, no. 94.

30 ANQM, CC 601, 11 January 1825, no. 7.

31 ANQM, CC 601, 16 August 1895, no. 448. In the following cases there was co-residence without this corresponding clearly to the close management of a troubled individual: ANQM, CC 601, 12 April 1850, no. 225; 4 February 1862, no. 34; 31 July 1869, no. 275; 14 December 1894, no. 697; 14 January 1895, no. 14.

32 ANQM, CC 601, 9 November 1850, no. 625.

33 ANQM, CC 601, 31 August 1891, no. 442. For other cases in which lodging is linked to the mental trouble or incapacity of an individual, see ANQM, CC 601, 22 February 1850, no. 53; 17 February 1865, no. 58; 14 July 1891, no. 351.

34 Bradbury, *Familles ouvrières à Montréal*, 85 and 87. In England in the nineteenth century, the nuclear family was the first line of defence in the management of idiots. See David Wright, "Familial Care of Idiot Children in Victorian England," in Peregrine Horden and Richard Smith, eds., *The Locus of Care: Families, Communities, Institutions, and the Provision of Welfare since Antiquity* (London: Routledge, 1998), 178.

35 Denis Goulet and André Paradis, *Trois siècles d'histoire médicale au Québec* (Montréal: VLB éditeur, 1992), 99–100.

36 Peter Bartlett and David Wright, "Community Care and Its Antecedents," in Bartlett and Wright, eds., *Outside the Walls of the Asylum*, 4 and 5.

37 James E. Moran, *Committed to the State Asylum: Insanity and Society in Nineteenth-Century Quebec and Ontario* (Montreal and Kingston: McGill-Queen's University Press, 2000), 79, 80, 99 and 170.

38 ANQM, CC 601, 21 January 1857, no. 28.

39 ANQM, CC 601, 21 May 1885, no. 259.

40 ANQM, CC 601, 13 May 1823, no. 190.

41 ANQM, CC 601, 12 April 1850, no. 225.

42 ANQM, CC 601, 5 July 1845, no. 461.

43 For this story, see note 20 above.

44 Peter Keating, *La science du mal: L'institution de la psychiatrie au Québec, 1800–1914* (Montréal: Boréal, 1993), 47–8.

45 Moran, *Committed to the State Asylum*, 17.

46 See especially ANQM, CC 601, 9 November 1850, no. 625; 12 October 1894, no. 561; 14 January 1895, no. 14.

47 ANQM, CC 601, 11 December 1868, no. 496; see also 18 May 1886, no. 257.

48 ANQM, CC 601, 3 February 1832, no. 61, and 21 June 1839, no. 422.

49 ANQM, CC 601, 1 October 1833, no. 1094; 1 October 1833, no. 1098; 8 October 1833, no. 1128; 11 October 1839, no. 675.

50 ANQM, CC 601, 4 September 1895, no. 486.

51 See the history constituted by ANQM, CC 601, 22 May 1832, no. 328; 15 February 1833, no. 187, and 30 April 1833, no. 610 B, or the case constituted by ANQM, CC 601, 24 July 1893, no. 347; TP 11, 1894, no. 265, Breton vs. Warren *es qual.*; ANQM, CC 601, 27 September 1898, no. 517.

52 Akihito Suzuki, "Enclosing and Disclosing Lunatics within the Family Walls: Domestic Psychiatric Regime and the Public Sphere in Early Nineteenth-Century England," in Bartlett and Wright, eds., *Outside the Walls of the Asylum*, 119 and following.

53 On the ties between honour and group belonging, see Maurice Daumas, *L'affaire d'Esclans: les conflits familiaux au XVIIIe siècle* (Paris: Seuil, 1988), especially 81–2.

54 Mary Ann Poutanen, "The Geography of Prostitution in an Early Nineteenth-Century Urban Centre: Montreal 1810–1842," in Tamara Myers *et al.*, *Power, Place and Identity: Historical Studies of Social and Legal Regulation in Quebec* (Montreal: Montreal History Group/Groupe sur l'histoire de Montréal, 1998), 102 and 127.

55 ANQM, CC 601, 11 September 1895, no. 502; TP 11, sub series *ex parte*, 1895, no. 93, *ex parte* John C.; TP 11, *ex parte* register, 1895–97; TP 11, judgements of 1895, vol. 6, p. 60, C. vs S.; TP 11, sub series *ex parte*, 1895, no. 90 A, *ex parte* John C. vs Dame J.S.

56 Jack S. Blocker, *American Temperance Movements: Cycles of Reform* (Boston: Twayne Publishers, 1989), 20.

3

Patients at Work

Insane Asylum Inmates' Labour in Ontario, 1841–1900

GEOFFREY REAUME

In 1879 the provincial inspector of insane asylums for the province of Ontario, John W. Langmuir, wrote that to "implant and cultivate in that class of patients a taste for work ... is of infinitely greater importance, than any other portion of Asylum work and supervision."[1] When he made this statement, Langmuir was laying the groundwork for the intensification of patient labour, which would see an increase in the rate of patient labour at Ontario's mental institutions from one-third in the late 1870s to 75 percent of the entire inmate population by 1900.[2] The motives that influenced this policy were rooted in both Anglo-American ideas of work as therapy and the need to pay for the maintenance of more mental institutions in the province in the second half of the nineteenth century.[3] With increasing costs, administrators advocated the increased participation of unpaid patient labourers, a policy that literally paid off by saving untabulated thousands of dollars for the province. This article will focus on what patient labourers actually did and how many were engaged in what was called "employment," even though they were not paid. While at the beginning of the period, the level of work in Ontario's insane asylums was barely perceivable (insofar as the sources are able to tell us), it rose in a steadily growing crescendo of activity during the next six decades.

Before I discuss the actual nature of the toil done by patient labourers, it is necessary to address the rationale for work therapy as part of moral treatment from the perspectives of asylum operators. As James Moran and Steven Cherry have shown in reference to nineteenth-century proponents of moral treatment in Ontario, Quebec, and England, doctors provided a physiological basis for their claim that putting patients to work helped them to recover their sanity. Physical exercise brought about by certain types of work, such as agricultural labour or working in a laundry, was viewed as an essential way of redirecting a person's "alienated mind" from their troubles onto the task at hand. As well, doing regular, steady work would supposedly lead towards regular, steady, and above all, rational habits and away from mad thoughts. A good diet was essential to this work regimen, all of which, it was argued, would help to improve a person's physiological functions through invigorated brain activity and a healthier flow of bodily fluids which physical labour could help to regulate.[4] As Yannick Ripa has written in regard to women inmates in nineteenth-century France, from the asylum officials' point of view, the rationale for work was that it "focused attention on the concrete tasks of everyday life and dispelled their fantasies."[5] Physical and mental health were therefore linked with the positive reinforcement of each leading to a sane mind. That was the theory. Of course, there were other ideas that motivated this work, as the writings of provincial asylum superintendents reveal. As will be seen below, the reality of patient labour and the impetus for pushing it forward on a wide scale in Ontario as the nineteenth century wore on was quite different from the theory that justified it.

THE EARLY YEARS: 1841–1860

For most of the initial decade of this study patient labour is not well documented. Between 1841 and 1850 the first Provincial Temporary Lunatic Asylum operated in Canada West, or Ontario, as the province was named after 1867. It was located in various facilities in Toronto. The first superintendent, William Rees, wrote in 1842 that it was his desire to implement "medical and moral treatment" in the treatment of insane asylum patients, who at that time averaged thirty-six men and women. Though he refers to their being engaged in "labours of various kinds," nothing is specified beyond fishing along the shore of Lake Ontario in the company of an attendant.[6] While evidence for patients' labour during these early years is scant, what evidence does exist reveals a practice that would reoccur in years to come: using asylum inmates to help get a new institution ready for later arrivals. In October 1849 male patients from the Temporary Asylum worked on making the grounds level at the new permanent provincial asylum in Toronto, several months before the first patients arrived in January 1850.[7]

From this time on, a more detailed picture begins to emerge of patients' labour in Ontario. Superintendent John Scott's words would be repeated time and again by asylum administrators over the next fifty years when he wrote in the annual report for 1850, "As a general rule, all who are capable are kept employed." He also defended the use of patients' work in words that would be echoed down the years by his successors. When he claimed that it was beneficial, not exploitative, the intent was to consider this practice a benign form of moral therapy: "In no case is labour made compulsory or painful, the patient who at first may be averse to work, becomes persuaded by his attendant, or stimulated by the example of others to make a beginning and in a very short time realizes the advantages and pleasures resulting. It is to be understood that the labour of patients is not reckoned on as a source of gain or profit, but simply as a means likely to promote their well-being of body and mind."[8] The prevention of "idleness," as Andrew Scull has noted, was a "leading principle" of moral treatment.[9] Individuals who went against this basic premise were duly criticized in annual reports and, one assumes, in person.

Those who did not work were described as "indolent and moping." Whether they objected to not being paid is impossible to know. However, the moralizing judgment towards patients who were capable of work but did not do it, is clear from the earliest report and permeates much of this history. Patients' labour in 1850 included "cutting and preparing firewood"; kitchen, laundry, and ward work; male patients mending their clothes; and among women, needlework. Indeed, one report boasted that "among the females many are excellent needle-women and are so industrious as to perform all the work required in this Institution." When conditions allowed, forty to fifty men – about a third of all male patients – "engaged in digging, levelling, draining and in cultivating a large crop of vegetables." As an added incentive, coffee and bread were provided to patient field labourers around three in the afternoon.[10] Use of incentives, or bribes, to get people to work was not unusual. Ellen Dwyer had recorded the use of similar tactics in New York State's Willard Asylum during the nineteenth century.[11]

It is hard to imagine what incentive might have been used to get patients to do one particularly odious job a few years after the permanent asylum opened in Toronto. During the year 1853, diarrhea and dysentery frequently affected the patient population. The source of this recurring health problem was discovered to be a huge cesspool that had accumulated for several years underneath the basement floor as a result of a faulty drainage system. From November 1853 to January 1854, Joseph Workman, the recently appointed superintendent, had male patients clean it up. It was in an underground area measuring six hundred feet long by thirty to sixty feet wide with the sludge measuring three to five feet in depth. The work was done under the direction of attendants and included the removal of "several hundred cartloads" of what Workman later wrote of as "reeking filth." According to the superintendent, the "tedious, tiresome and sickening work" was done by "hard-worked lunatics." New gravel and drains were laid so that waste from the laundry, kitchen, and elsewhere would no longer collect beneath the asylum basement. This episode reveals how patients' working conditions could, at times, have been anything but "therapeutic." Though the superintendent reported that he had delayed this work until the cold weather to lessen the chance of the spread of disease, Workman reported that "the health of the inmates … [and staff] … was much affected" during the cleanup operation.[12]

In contrast to the cesspool cleanup, the benefits of outdoor labour were repeatedly emphasized. Most of this work would have been reserved for males. While statistics are absent for most of the 1850s about who did what, a reference to "the want of employment" for men patients during the winter indicates that alternative indoor jobs were not yet available for most of them. Nevertheless, by the mid-1850s some twenty to thirty patients of both sexes worked daily in the sewing room, where their work was overseen by a seamstress and a tailor. This work saved the asylum money by having all the "needle-work" and men's coats made on the premises.[13]

While gender-specific tasks are mentioned in these early reports, one such example was quite unusual for an insane asylum: caring for a newborn baby. A baby boy was born under dreadful conditions to asylum inmate Catherine L. on 11 June 1856. This baby was taken from the mother and was looked after with "great tenderness" by the matron and nurse, who were "aided by a female patient."[14] How long this arrangement lasted is not stated; nor is there information about what eventually happened to mother and baby. The fact that a woman patient helped to care for this baby is evidence of how some asylum inmates took on nursing duties.

The use of patients as unpaid supplemental staff was practised elsewhere during the nineteenth century. Yannick Ripa has noted that in French asylums staff would occasionally use the "healthiest patients" to assist them in supervising other inmates at work. At the Pennsylvania Hospital for the Insane, Nancy Tomes records how some patients watched over fellow patients to ensure that they followed regulations on the ward.[15] In short, some patients were put to work as unofficial attendants, responsibilities that would have given them a degree of power over their peers, creating a "hierarchy" among inmates, as Ripa observes. However, the absence of any reference to this happening with any frequency in the Ontario records from the same period suggests that this was not a typical job for most patients. Instead, more common forms of physical work were emphasized.

Unquestionably, it was male farm labour that was repeatedly stressed by asylum officials during the 1850s as being most valuable from both a therapeutic and a financial perspective. This was so even though it was also claimed that more land was needed to realize the full potential of patients' agricultural labour.[16] The first clear statistics of how many patients worked overall during this period were offered by Joseph Workman for 1858. Noting that more patients could have been put to work if the means were available – that is, a larger farm – he observed that there were 196 "industrious" asylum inmates in Toronto, 41 per cent of the total. Workman boasted: "I do not believe there is any Asylum on this Continent in which so large an amount of work is done by the patients; indeed I have seen few that will compare advantageously with it."[17] The following year, the composition of this workforce changed in a way that reveals much about the value of patient labour to the provincial asylum system.

In 1859, to alleviate overcrowding at Toronto, a branch asylum was opened in Amherstburg, in the southwestern part of the province near Windsor. It was situated in the unused British military barracks at Fort Malden, along the bank of the Detroit River, and thus was called Malden Asylum. In order to get it ready for later occupants, "twenty of our most industrious" male patients were sent on 14 July 1859 to Malden with Dr Andrew Fisher, the superintendent. Workman wrote that the "change produced by the removal" of these patients from Toronto "has been very palpable ... but I trust that our new stock will, under careful and kind treatment, soon present sufficient material to recruit our working forces."[18] As will become evident in later reports, Workman was one of many in the asylum bureaucracy who used the rhetoric of moral treatment as a recruiting mechanism for their own internal economy needs. Indeed, Dr Fisher clearly regarded these patient labourers very highly when he wrote: "Each of these patients would perform as much work as an ordinary labouring man, and their loss must have been seriously felt at the [Toronto] institution."[19]

The work of these men patients was so "energetically" pursued that within three months a larger group of both men and women patients was sent from Toronto to live at the Malden Asylum. In what would become a frequent refrain over the next forty years, the use of unpaid patient labour was lauded by officials for saving the public money.[20] Using work therapy as cheap labour was also mentioned in published reports during the late 1850s at the Norfolk Lunatic Asylum in England.[21] Thus asylum proprietors on both sides of the Atlantic were not shy about stressing how supposedly therapeutic benefits of work for patients could also benefit the finances of mental institutions.

Work completed by patient labourers at Malden during the early months of its operation included preserving and repairing the main buildings; developing a drainage and water-supply system; installing new "water-closets," window guards, baths, furnaces, boilers, roofing, and eaves; fencing in fifty-eight acres of asylum farm land; grading surfaces; planting trees; and driving wooden piles into the Detroit River behind which stones were placed to create a stronger breakwater defence against soil erosion. Agricultural work also quickly became a prime feature of this facility. This is hardly surprising given the emphasis on this type of outdoor work under the tenets of moral treatment and the fact that this part of Ontario has some of the most fertile soil in the province. As men worked outside, women worked inside, making over 1,400 items in 1860 ranging from quilts to chemises to window blinds.[22]

While patients toiled to get the Malden property into shape for their peers, building a new asylum from the ground up was part of the work of another group of inmates. In Kingston, efforts were underway to construct a permanent asylum for people found to be criminally insane. Ordinary convict labour was used for much of this work, though there are also references to criminal "lunatic labour" being used for "bricklaying, painting, glazing" as well as farm and garden work.[23] Still other patient labourers elsewhere worked to build brick walls around the grounds upon which they lived. In 1860, ten years after it opened, permission was granted by the Provincial Board of Inspectors for "the work of building the wall to enclose the Asylum at Toronto, a work in which the patients themselves have been employed."[24] What more poignant example of patient labour can there be than that of insane asylum inmates building the very walls behind which they were confined?

MALDEN AND ORILLIA INSANE ASYLUM
PATIENT LABOURERS DURING THE 1860s

The most consistently detailed reports on patient labour in Ontario during the 1860s concern the Malden and Orillia insane asylums.[25] Both these facilities closed in 1870 after eleven and nine years of operation respectively. A brief survey of patient labour at these two smaller institutions provides a good idea of the amount of work done by a relatively small labour force prior to any central directive being extensively pursued across the province on this issue. Keeping statistics on patients' overall labour was left to the whim of the superintendent during the 1860s, with the result that detailed data on the entire working population is sporadic, though there is some useful information. In 1861 it was reported that out of 196 patients at the Malden Asylum, 89 people, or 45 per cent, were "industrious," while the rest were listed as "idle."[26] By the end of the decade, the number of patient labourers at this facility oscillated between a low of 25 per cent of 208 patients in 1868 to 84 per cent of 159 people the following year. It is hard to know how reliable these figures are. In the very same report that clearly tabulates two-thirds of all males at Malden as employed, Superintendent Henry Landor wrote that an average of half were "daily doing something." He further subdivides this group into two-thirds "working in the proper sense of the word," while the remaining third of male working patients do "slight things."[27] However, as will be evident below, there is no doubt as to how valuable this labour was.

The Orillia Branch Asylum, housed in an old hotel, was located on far less property than any other facility – six to eight acres along Lake Couchiching. Thus there were a smaller number of patients to work a smaller property. But work they did. The only patients' labour statistics for Orillia during the 1860s were for 1862, when 30 per cent of 128 patients were listed as working – 40 per cent of the males, 32 per cent of the females.[28] At both facilities, women patients did sewing and knitting, mending all the clothes and creating thousands of new articles. Perhaps the most unusual items that female inmates at both Malden and Orillia made were straitjackets – 6 of these out of 1,639 articles made at Malden in 1861. During the first five months of Orillia's operation that same year, when 25 women were housed there, they, along with female staff, made: 112 quilts, 128 sheets, 98 bed ticks, 86 pillow ticks, 219 pillow slips, 49 dresses, 65 cotton and flannel shirts, 92 cotton and flannel chemises, 76 cotton and flannel petticoats, 11 tablecloths, 25 pairs of socks, 6 stocking pairs, 46 women's caps, 7 towels and rollers, 12 night gowns, 5 straitjackets, and 400 gallons of soft soap.[29]

In 1863, women at Orillia made more than 3,000 gallons of soft soap, 800 pounds of hard soap, and 50 pounds of candles.[30] These lists grew longer as the decade wore on; so much so that the Orillia superintendent was not exaggerating when he wrote in 1869, "Independent of the list of articles as given above, the mending and repairing allow little idle time for either nurses or patients."[31]

The list of jobs done by male patients at both Orillia and Malden during the 1860s is similarly extensive, and in the latter instance it included building the medical superintendent's residence. Patient labourers also built a laundry and bakery in 1861 at Malden; it still stands today, over 140 years later, as the interpretative centre and museum for Fort Malden National Historic Site, though the history of the people who built it is nowhere acknowledged within its walls.[32] The following list is a typical example of patients' labour recorded at these largely forgotten insane asylums from the 1860s. In addition to plastering, painting, carpentry, and laying floors, making benches, tables, cupboards, ladders, picture frames, a pantry, and a water-stand, creating new openings for doors and fireplaces, glazing lights, and shingling, twenty "industrious" men patients and their "keeper" at Orillia in 1862 also worked on the farm, built fences and a piggery, laid drains, paved 787 yards of farmyard, and made a 76-yard-long road, among other things.[33] Farm and garden produce at Malden was especially plentiful and profitable, with twenty-two items listed for 1862 valued at $1,645.45. The value of this yield rose to $3,000 by 1865. So successful was the Malden farm that residents had more grapes than they could consume; so the grapes were ground down and made into wine, "which will be fit for use in a year or so."[34] The same year, patients contributed to saving the Malden Asylum from being burnt down when they helped to operate the asylum fire engine, in which they had been trained in case of emergency.[35] As will become increasingly evident, beside saving buildings, patients also saved the asylum a good deal of money, even though officials offered contradictory views on how much they valued patient workers.

THE VALUE PLACED ON INSANE ASYLUM INMATE LABOUR
DURING THE 1860S AND 1870S

The abilities of patient labourers were acknowledged by provincial authorities. However, this acknowledgment also proved patients were better workers than could sometimes be claimed, thus leaving asylum proprietors open to charges of exploitation for not paying them. James Moran has noted that at Quebec's Beauport asylum in 1849, the family of patient Jean Dupont charged that this man was "kept in the asylum in a state of 'slavery' because he was a good worker whose labour was of great value to the institution." He was subsequently released though asylum officials defended themselves by claiming that asylum inmate labour "does not pay."[36] In France exploitation charges included reference to the tiring nature of inmate labour and the primacy given to saving money as being more important than therapeutic benefits for patient workers.[37] One way around this charge of exploitation was praising individual workers while making general statements about the whole group. Yet evidence of patients' unpaid labour that contributed significantly to keeping provincial asylums operating clearly undermines broad statements about their supposed unreliability. After listing the immense amount of work they did in 1862, Orillia superintendent John Ardagh claimed these same workers were "fickle and whimsical," though his own reports and those of his contemporaries offer a different picture. In 1863 the floor of the Orillia laundry was in need of serious repair: "One of our patients, a mason, undertook the task of remedying it," with the result that it became "an excellent floor, hard and durable."[38] A year later Ardagh wrote of a male patient who was in charge of the men's dining room as being "more exacting with rules than if he were a paid attendant, and his assistants obey his rule and order."[39]

Rockwood Asylum superintendent Litchfield paid tribute to the labour of four patients judged criminally insane, about whom he wrote that "the value of their services to the Institution cannot be questioned." One of these men, a sixty-year-old cook who reliably served all meals to fellow patients, assisted by "insane attendants," was described thus: "I do not know where it would be possible to get paid labour to execute the work so well."[40] The savings to the public by getting patients to do so much of this work within the asylum is repeatedly stressed in annual reports during the 1860s, a clear indication that officials recognized how they could use "therapy" to their own financial benefit. Indeed, hiring outside help was seen as a waste of money when so many free patient labourers were around to do the job. For part of 1862 a tailor was employed at Malden, but this post was "abolished" when Superintendent Fisher realized it "did not pay"; thereafter all clothes for male patients were made by women patients "and the saving thus effected has been considerable."[41] By the end of the decade the Malden Asylum steward calculated the worth of two asylum patient farm workers as the same as one paid employee. With the value of farm produce more than meeting their expenses, they were able to realize "a very handsome profit." Patients laboured two thousand days on the farm the preceding year, six hours per day; at the unpaid rate of 50 cents for "ordinary day labour," the overall annual value of their work was estimated at $1,000.[42]

Although they were unpaid, an occasional "privilege" to asylum patient workers was recorded. Malden Asylum working patients, presumably men, were given beer to supplement their diet.[43] When it was time for some of these same inmates to move to a new asylum, fifteen to twenty of those who were considered among the most trusted inmates were sent to the

London, Ontario, asylum farm to plant spring crops in 1870. Half a year later this facility opened, after which the Malden Asylum was closed and the remaining patients were transferred to this new institution.[44]

Within two years, just over half of the 496 patients were toiling away in the farm, garden, shops, and wards of the London Asylum, a steady figure into the mid-1870s.[45] Yet these numbers "give no adequate idea of the amount of work done," according to Superintendent Henry Landor, who was out to prove wrong a claim that patients under his charge were too "idle."[46] To assist with accomplishing this goal, a London Asylum bylaw had earlier stipulated, "Patients must be employed as much as possible," and attendants who "heartily" carried out this task would be looked upon more favourably by their employers.[47] Evidently, the results were very satisfactory for more than just the presumed goals of moral therapy. For the year 1874 Landor reported "Everything is charged for and against, except labour of patients, which, of course, is abundant every year and tells strongly in favour of our balance sheet."[48] Inspector J.W. Langmuir also had an eye on the balance sheet, though he expressed his suspicions about patient labour as well when he wrote during the early 1870s that "all who are not mentally incapable of labour, are sufficiently sane not to care about working without wages."[49] As will be seen, these suspicions did not get in the way of a massive patient labour program that he advocated a few years later.

By the late 1870s there were four independent provincial insane asylums operating in the province – Toronto (1841), London (1870), Kingston (known as Rockwood from 1856 until it was transferred from federal to provincial control in 1876), and Hamilton (1876) – as well as one asylum for the "feeble-minded" in Orillia (1876).[50] With the establishment of a larger network of asylums than had ever before existed in Ontario, provincial authorities, in particular Inspector Langmuir, became noticeably more insistent about promoting the "Employment of Patients," a category that came to be systematically reported for each facility in every annual report beginning in 1879 and which continued to be reported until 1907. Thus the most detailed information for this study comes from this later period. Langmuir's emphasis on economy and efficiency was first felt in asylum laundry departments, which by 1878 had switched from hand to mechanized labour at all facilities.[51] Reduced laundry costs were realized by speeding up and increasing the volume of cleaning clothes as well as the fact that this mechanization resulted in two laundry maids losing their jobs to machines that unpaid patient labourers could operate at the Toronto Asylum.[52] Not only was it important to economize with unpaid patients' labour inside the asylum, but it was essential to economize in outside work as well. In 1879,

Langmuir noted that provincial patient farm and garden labour "very materially reduced the cost of maintaining Asylums" in this particular year to the tune of $32,490.62.[53] So that his point would not be lost on medical officials, he continued: "It is clear therefore from the standpoint of pubic economy, and leaving out of the question the beneficial and healthful results accruing to the insane from land cultivation, that as large an area of land should be attached to asylums as can be profitably worked."[54]

A few years earlier, Superintendent Landor of the new London Asylum had also put a price on the value of this type of patient labour. Though he claimed that three working patients were the equivalent to one paid labourer, he nevertheless wrote in 1871 that the farm and garden work which patients had done that year "yielded more than double the cost of cultivation."[55] Several years later the bursar of the London Asylum estimated that five agricultural patient labourers were worth one paid worker, which he estimated saved the asylum $3,425.26 in the farm and garden category.[56] In 1878 the newly appointed London Asylum superintendent Richard M. Bucke said asylum patients only did half the work of "a sane person," though "still the aggregate amount of work done by the patients in a year at this Asylum is enormous."[57] Thus during the 1870s, patient labourers' worth, compared to ordinary paid work, was rated by provincial asylum officials as being in the range of two-to-one, three-to-one and five-to-one. All of this number crunching, however variable, indicates that patients' labour was clearly recognized as being of prime economic benefit in keeping costs down, even while the operators of the asylum undervalued their unpaid workforce in relation to hired workers. It is notable that the practical effect of getting paid for one's work is not mentioned in these calculations as having had any influence on the level of output by patient labourers in contrast to regularly paid employees.

This devaluing of patients' labour compared to that of non-patients reached perhaps its most extreme form when the prospect of inmate help in one area was noted as being almost tantamount to a public health threat. In 1875 London Asylum superintendent Landor wrote that while patients were all right to clean up after the cooks and baker, they should not entertain any culinary ambitions, for "I decidedly object to eating or making others eat food prepared by patients."[58] No other asylum superintendent expressed similar 'gastronomical terror' of patient food preparation during the period examined here.

In spite of this sort of occasional reluctance to employ patients in certain jobs, there is no doubt that Langmuir's entreaties to economize with an increase in patient labourers reached receptive ears among asylum superintendents by the late 1870s. In 1877 J.W. Wallace of Hamilton Asylum reported that an average of twenty male patients worked daily in a quarry "breaking stones for the roads," as well as on other outside jobs. A year later he wrote that "all the tailoring, dressmaking, mending and darning for the Asylum" were done by women patients who also worked in the laundry and kitchen, while men patients farmed, shovelled coal, did landscaping, and continued to work in a nearby quarry.[59] However, this was not enough, for he wrote, "I hope in a short time to have a stronger force of working patients."[60] As the next two decades would reveal, this creation of a "stronger force of working patients" was pursued as never before throughout all provincial asylums in Ontario as pressure was exerted on asylum superintendents to cut costs for an ever-expanding asylum inmate population.

THE INTENSIFICATION OF PATIENT LABOUR
IN ONTARIO, 1880–1900

Statistics taken from five sample years between 1880 and 1900 reveal a wide variation in how many patients were employed at each facility (see table 3.1). However, by the mid-1880s there was one figure that stayed consistent: never less than 70 per cent of patients were working at all provincial insane asylums combined (these figures do not include the Orillia Asylum for the Feeble-Minded). Thus in the six years since Inspector Langmuir's call for the widespread use of patient labour in 1879, the provincial rate had climbed over 100 per cent from one-third to over two-thirds by 1885, or 74 per cent. These figures are reflected in the operation of individual asylums. The London Asylum was consistently in either first or second place in overall patient employment during this period, with the largest proportion of patient workers – 95 per cent – recorded in 1885, an increase of almost twice the ratio of only five years before. Superintendent Bucke noted in his report that patients worked "most of them nearly every day, during the year, exclusive, of course, of Sundays."[61] Eventually, the overall patient labour rate at London stabilized in the upper 70 to low 80 per cent range during the 1890s. London also had the largest farm operation of all the institutions then in existence – two hundred acres, plus a twenty-acre garden.[62] Thus Langmuir's call to use patients as agricultural labourers was able to be efficiently implemented at this facility, which was situated on prime farm land.

Yet even at an asylum such as Kingston, which had poor agricultural land and so was less successful in implementing farm labour, statistics show that there was more than enough work to be found for inmates. This

Table 3.1   Asylum inmate labour in Ontario, 1880–1900

		Toronto	London	Kingston	Hamilton	Mimico	Brockville	Average
1880								
Days worked	M	52.5	50	62	29.5	–	–	48.5
by gender	F	47.5	50	38	70.5	–	–	51.5
as percentage								
No. of patients								
who worked		225	445	268	115	–	–	1053
% of total		30	49	54.5	20	–	–	39.5
1885								
Days worked	M	47	48	49	50	–	–	48.5
by gender	F	53	52	51	50	–	–	51.5
as percentage								
No. of patients								
who worked		469	983	488	371	–	–	2311
% of total		57	95	87	51	–	–	74
1890								
Days worked	M	62	51	48.5	57	–	–	54
by gender	F	38	49	51.5	43	–	–	45
as percentage								
No. of patients								
who worked		504	802	669	790	–	–	2765
% of total		52.5	76	84.5	75.5	–	–	72
1895								
Days worked	M	32	47	51	52	59.5	49.5	48.5
by gender	F	68	53	49	48	40.5	50.5	51.5
as percentage								
No. of patients								
who worked		772	966	549	861	398	136	3682
% of total		89	82	76	77	54.5	65	76
1900								
Days worked	M	41	51	52.5	51	45.5	51	49
by gender	F	59	49	47.5	49	54.5	49	51
No. of patients								
who worked		580	924	537	899	546	392	3878
% of total		68	80	82.5	78	77.5	61	75

SOURCES: All figures are from the annual report for each year and have been rounded off to the nearest decimal point. The numbers of patients who worked are not broken down by gender in the annual reports. All averages are based on the category "Total number of Asylum registers and actually under treatment in each Asylum" and not the lower "Number of patients remaining in Asylums on 30th September," as this latter figure does not include all patients resident for a given year, while the earlier one does.

included having male patients clear rocks from their "rough" farm land.[63] Except for 1895, Kingston competed with London for either first or second place between 1880 and 1900 in the proportion of patients employed among Ontario's provincial asylums. Not having a good farm was no impediment to the employment of patient labourers. The increase in patient labourers at Hamilton was in some ways even more notable. The proportion of employed patients rose two and a half times between 1880 and 1885 and almost four times in ten years, from 20 per cent in 1880 to 75.5 per cent in 1890. Superintendent Wallace's goal of creating a stronger workforce was realized during his tenure and under his successor, James Russell, when Hamilton went from the smallest workforce among Ontario's insane asylums to a consistently strong third place by 1890. This pattern continued in 1895 and 1900, when there were six insane asylums operating in Ontario.

Overall work among patients at the Toronto Asylum was much less stable, rising from 30 per cent in 1880 to just over half in 1890, when it was last among four provincial insane asylums, to a peak of 89 per cent by 1895, the highest rate in the province. However, this rate declined by 1900, when there were just over two-thirds of patients working, making Toronto fifth out of six insane asylums. This generally lower rate was due to the objections of relatives of paying patients who did not want their family member working, since it was viewed "as derogatory to the social status of the patients."[64] But some of them did work. Since 89 per cent of the patients were employed at Toronto in 1895, some had to be from among the paying patients, who made up 37 per cent of the asylum population, the highest ratio in Ontario, with London's paying population next in line at 20 per cent.[65] Unlike at other facilities, this high rate of private patients in Toronto had been identified since 1883 as an obstacle to raising the number of working patients there.[66]

Thus it is not difficult to surmise that it was the poorest class of patients who contributed most to the internal economy of provincial asylums. Yannick Ripa reached a similar conclusion in her study of madwomen in nineteenth-century French asylums, where the poorest class of patients was recorded at that time as comprising "the majority of productive workers."[67] Studies of the Toronto and London asylums reveal these class biases in another way. Greater value was placed on lower-class patients who worked than on inmates who did not work regularly or who did no work at all.[68] Favouritism was also practised towards working patients at the asylum in London where "privileges are given to patients who work, and withheld from those who do not," and at the Toronto Asylum, where there was "bribing with something of a trifling nature," such as tea, coffee, and tobacco.[69] Between 1880 and 1900 the figures remained fairly stable for the number of public charges in Ontario's insane asylums – 87 per cent in 1880 and 85 per cent in 1900.[70] Thus the vast majority of people who worked as patient labourers in Ontario were "free patients." This term became something of a misnomer, since it became increasingly clear that officials expected most of them to pay for their room and board as well as to reduce costs to the province through their own toil. Thus the poorer the patient, the more work he or she was expected to do. Nineteenth-century middle-class views, which judged a person's worth by whether she or he was a good, reliable worker, was very much part of moral therapy during this period and influenced how the abilities of asylum patients were characterized.[71]

Without any doubt, the cheap labour and high-quality working abilities of insane asylum inmates saved provincial asylums a bundle of money. The per capita cost to the province of maintaining patients in Ontario's asylums was repeatedly referred to by administrators as being quite low; in fact, they boasted about how low maintenance rates were, clearly indicating how much was saved through patient labour. The average weekly maintenance rate for patients during the last decades of the nineteenth century was reported at Kingston as ranging from $2.32 in 1878 to $2.61 in 1895, when Superintendent C.K. Clarke wrote that "the maintenance rate is exceedingly low" and, he cautioned, should not be reduced further.[72] At the London Asylum, R.M. Bucke reported in 1885 that "the large amount of labor done by the patients is now beginning to tell upon our maintenance rate ... [T]he labor of the patients has been made to effect more or less saving." After listing various savings produced by patient labour, Bucke wrote that the "large decrease in the maintenance rate" was not all due to patient labour but was also because of various cost-cutting measures, such as lower consumption of meat and flour as a result of the large amount of vegetables on hand – which, he neglected to add, were produced by patients.[73]

Perhaps the best evidence of the bargain that free patient labour provided to provincial asylums was offered by figures from the Hamilton Asylum. Superintendent Wallace wrote in 1885 that this included "food, clothing, furniture, repairs and ordinary alterations of buildings, and all salaries and wages." Over a twenty year period between 1880 and 1900, the average weekly maintenance rate for patients at Hamilton rose from $2.16 to $2.26. Like Bucke at London, Superintendent Russell at Hamilton connected these low maintenance rates to patient labour when he wrote about the 1891–95 period: "[D]uring the five years we had been doing a heavy amount of work ... our average yearly per capita cost was $120.31, or a weekly rate of $2.31. With such results as these I had no hesitation in deciding that we were certainly discharging our proper function and doing it by the most economic methods." Five years later he wrote that the average per capita cost per patient from 1896 to 1900 was $2.24 per week, and he concluded: "The expenditure is far below that of asylums in Britain, Europe and America."[74] Free insane asylum inmate labour, then, was very profitable for the province.

For the patients who toiled away for no compensation, their place of work within the asylum was greatly influenced by gender. For the most part, as in earlier decades, men and women continued working in sex-segregated jobs. This pattern was also typical of asylums outside Ontario during this period. In the United States, Britain, and France as well as elsewhere in Canada, the gendered division of labour in asylums was a standard feature of patients' labour.[75] The gendered nature of asylum inmate labour in Ontario during the period examined here is therefore not surprising. Nevertheless, the extent and significance of their labour deserves far greater attention than has been given in most asylum studies. Women were concentrated in doing indoor domestic work, such as sewing, knitting, and kitchen and laundry work, as well as cleaning the ward. Men were also recorded as doing kitchen work and cleaning on the ward, which is not surprising given that they lived in sex-segregated institutions. Indeed, keeping men and women separate within the institution was extended to the workplace as a matter of policy, and in one instance where this was not done, it was cause for concern. In 1900 Superintendent N.H. Beemer of Mimico Asylum wrote in regard to the laundry that "the incidental intermingling of so many male and female working patients is not entirely free from an element of danger even under the strictest possible supervision." So he recommended structural changes to the workplace that would keep the two sexes apart.[76] Interestingly enough, the laundry appears to be the only area in asylums where the sexes worked together, at least for a time. At the Norfolk Lunatic Asylum in England the laundry became a women-only workplace in 1888 after a female inmate became pregnant on the job site.[77] While some men were employed in laundry jobs, most of this work was done by women: 79 per cent at Hamilton in 1885, 69 per cent at London in 1890, 88 per cent at Kingston in 1895 and 76.5 per cent at Mimico in 1900, where it was reported that eighteen patients processed 270,392 laundry articles during that year alone.[78]

This predominantly female patient labour also cut down costs by allowing administrators to get rid of hired staff to do jobs that patients did for no wage, as in the London Asylum. Superintendent Bucke reported in 1885: "Some saving has been effected by dispensing with hired labor in the sewing-room, the patients now doing nearly the entire sewing of the institution, and the entire knitting."[79] At the time that this report was made, all of the sewing-room work and mending was done by women patients, and women inmates were also reported to have done 98 per cent of the knitting at London that year.[80] The sewing work included making 9,100 new items and repairing 50,289 other items, from blankets to blouses. In addition, 2,102 stockings, socks, mitts, and cuffs were knitted at the London Asylum in 1885.[81] Similarly, women patients were reported as having done nearly all the knitting of stockings at the North Wales Asylum in Britain during this period.[82] Thus Ontario was hardly alone in using moral treatment as a form of cheap labour. Women were also employed as domestic servants for asylum officials, as occurred at the Brockville Asylum in 1900 where two women patients worked an average of 230 days each in the "officers' quarters."[83]

As before, men continued working outdoors. Landscaping, ditch digging, and large-scale construction work were a part of this routine. In Hamilton it was reported in 1880 that "A drain has been constructed for the cellar of the Farmer's house, necessitating an excavation from four to six feet deep, and upwards of eight hundred feet long. This work has been done entirely by the labour of patients."[84] This heavy work was not at all unusual. A report from the same asylum fifteen years later states: "A new kitchen has been built at the farmer's house, also a kitchen at the gardener's house. The work on the last two buildings, including a cellar to the farmer's kitchen, was done entirely by asylum labor. The excavation for the foundation of the infirmary and kitchen at East House was done by patients' labor. The patients quarried all the stone, and the sand and stone were all hauled by asylum teams. The mason and carpenter work done by our own labor has been especially effective in building and repairing and has effected a large saving in work, which would otherwise have been done under contract."[85]

Male patient construction labour also quite literally built and rebuilt the institutions in which asylum inmates lived, a practice carried on from the beginning to the end of the period examined here. A sixteen-hundred-foot boundary wall, averaging sixteen feet in height on the east and west sides of the property, was rebuilt with patients' labour at Toronto Asylum in the years 1888–89.[86] To help relieve Toronto's chronic overcrowding, Mimico Branch Asylum was opened on the shore of Lake Ontario in 1890 and became independent two years later. It was five miles from the older facility. Before it was opened, male patients were sent back and forth the same day in 1888 to work on the farm. However, this was not a practical way of getting the work done. So, beginning in 1889, the first occupants of the soon-to-be-opened institution were ten male patient labourers and two attendants who were sent out from Toronto Asylum in 1889 to begin to get it ready for the later influx of inmates.[87] During the next few years, male patient labourers helped to build and maintain many of the buildings they and others would live and work in at Mimico, including the large "cottages" that housed up to sixty patients, the superintendent's residence, an Assembly Hall (which doubled as a chapel), storage facilities, sidewalks, and pavilions along the lakeshore. Patients also levelled rough ground for a 150-yard-long cricket oval.[88] Superintendent Beemer boasted in 1897 that the carpenter who directed patients in building the Assembly Hall "proposes to finish the whole structure without any hired help."[89] The skills of these patient labourers who built the boundary walls for the Toronto Asylum and who constructed the buildings and levelled the grounds at Mimico Asylum are still very much in evidence today, more than a century after they completed their work.[90]

One particularly unusual aspect of Mimico was the creation of "subways" underground to connect buildings. In 1892 three male patients worked 517 days in this subterranean world, either moving items from place to place or repairing leaks; by 1899 seven male inmates had accumulated 2,509 days as "subway" workers.[91] Upstairs, patients helped to bake a daily average of 180 loaves of fresh bread at Mimico, the quality of which was reputed to be "everything that could be desired" – a far cry from the "gastronomical terror" of patients' food preparation noted earlier at the London Asylum.[92] Indoor work by men included skilled jobs such as shoemaking, tinsmithing, and tailoring as well as painting both inside and outside the asylum.[93] Skilled artisans could also be put to work in an attempt to improve the appearance of the institution. At the Kingston Asylum the work of patient Peter M. was on display for all to see: in 1895 he cut "a beautiful stone basin," 46 feet long by 20 feet wide, as a fountain in front of the hospital.[94] This fountain too still exists, though without running water. Similarly, other male patients were put to work creating "ornamental gardens" at the London and Hamilton asylums.[95]

In the midst of all this toil by asylum inmates, Toronto Asylum superintendent Daniel Clark expressed reservations in 1885 that too much emphasis was being placed on patient labour.[96] Yet this concern was not taken up elsewhere, even at Toronto, where Clark remained in charge until 1905, as reports from the following years clearly indicate. Instead, enthusiasts such as London superintendent Bucke wanted to go even further. He suggested that a "work colony" be established in the wilds of Ontario, the purpose of which would be to employ the increasing number of patients whom he felt were sure to arrive on the doorsteps of asylums in the years to come. It would "earn its own living" through full-scale patient labour of never less than 80 per cent inmate workers at any time.[97] This scheme did not go anywhere, but it indicates how much medical officials were looking for ways to exploit patients' labour to the maximum benefit of saving the province money. So pervasive and open was this attitude that Superintendent Russell of the Hamilton Asylum proposed formalizing the reality of what asylums had become by a name change from "Asylum for the Insane" to "The School of Mental and Manual Training."[98] This name change did not happen, but the extent of the valuable unpaid work patients did is not in doubt.

In 1900 three-quarters of provincial insane asylum patients in Ontario were employed at their place of residence, and during the previous ten years 75 per cent had been so occupied.[99] These figures clearly indicate that inmate labour had become a central part of institutional life throughout the province and was essential to the internal economy of the mental hospital system. Ontario officials were not any different from their counterparts elsewhere when it came to using patient labour for economic self-interest, while claiming it was "therapy."[100] While asylum inmates in some places, such as nineteenth-century France, were unevenly paid for their labour, this did not happen in Ontario during the same period.[101] At the same time as the province's asylum patients did not get paid for their work, convicts in the prison system were being compensated. Ordinary convict labourers in Kingston were paid 30 cents a day, while convict tradesmen received 40 cents daily. In Kingston in 1859, three hundred convicts were paid at the higher rate for their labour.[102]

One patient, David M., who "does all the blacksmithing" for the Kingston Asylum, did have his $10 travel expenses paid in the late 1890s to go home for an occasional visit to see his family. This reimbursement was agreed to on the basis of his "general and mechanical usefulness" about the asylum.[103] After 1900 there are no further letters about it until 1904, when the inspector wrote the asylum in response to its latest request for travel money for this man: "I am instructed to say that the payment of any sum to patients for services rendered cannot be considered by the Department."[104] Having provided a brief precedent for some kind of compensation in lieu of services, the inspector put a stop to it. It would be the late twentieth century before compensating psychiatric patients for their work became a much more controversial issue in the wider community.[105]

CONCLUSION

There is no escaping the fact that having patients work to economize within the expanding provincial asylum system was the central purpose behind the escalation of patient labour in late nineteenth-century Ontario. The constant emphasis of this point in published reports makes the rationale explicit, even while some officials continued to claim that washing literally hundreds of thousands of pieces of laundry, knitting and sewing thousands of pairs of items, doing domestic work for asylum officers, digging ditches that were hundreds of feet long, planting crops, hauling rocks, and constructing brick walls, all by unpaid, insane asylum-inmate labourers, was, in fact, therapy. Langmuir's successor, Inspector Robert Christie, wrote in 1896 that "the present condition of the institutions ... indicate[s] their advanced and improved state ... These have been done largely by institution labor, and the employment of patients ... The benefit patients derive from this cannot be overestimated, and if outside labor were employed, it is obvious that the expenditure would be largely increased."[106] In essence, this is no different from what R.M. Bucke had stated so simply eighteen years before in 1878: "Every patient who is fit to work is asked to do something, both for the sake of the patient and for the sake of the Asylum."[107]

The twin goals of saving money for the province and "benefiting" patients through unpaid work "therapy" allowed asylum officials to exploit people who were in no position to contest their unpaid status. There is a hint of patient agency in references to trusted workers almost always as male employees during this period, as with the farm labourers sent from Malden to the London Asylum in 1870 or the men who went to prepare the Mimico Asylum for habitation in 1889. Their trusted status was directly related to their work performance, and it indicates how this group of male patients was able to secure a greater variety of work, especially outside jobs, than was ever available to many of their peers, particularly women patients. Yet even here this privilege should not be exaggerated: digging ditches and hauling rocks would not have been fun. For all patients, both men and women, the work they did depended on the needs of the asylum and what type of work they could do.

In 1868–69, Henry Landor wrote that it was a good policy to employ patients in the same job that they had had before entering the asylum.[108] This approach allowed for the most efficient use of asylum labour. It also reflected the theory of early proponents of moral treatment at the York Retreat in Britain, who believed that it was important to provide work to patients based on their past abilities and existing preferences. According to Anne Digby, "This would not only revive the technical skills of earlier employment but also strengthen the moral faculties."[109] The reality of putting this theory into practice, however, has to be held up against the constant refrain of saving money, which was cited over and over as the main reason for the employment of patient labourers, even before the intensification of labour began in the last two decades of the nineteenth century. As the reports indicate, this policy was put into practice quite effectively – for the asylum operators.

It can be argued that destitute public patients who paid no fees were getting a good deal by working for what would otherwise be free room and board in an insane asylum. However, when their situation is compared to that of unskilled day labourers who toiled outside the asylum during this same period, there is a very significant difference in patients' ability to find work and "negotiate," such as it was, with an employer. Day labourers had far greater freedom of movement than did insane asylum inmates to choose where to look for work. They also had far greater opportunity to organize opposition to their exploitation by striking for better wages from their overseers, though of course they did not always succeed.[110] It is also important to note that skilled workers such as Peter M., who cut the ornamental stone basin at the Kingston Asylum, and many others who toiled in asylum workshops would have received a wage for their skilled labour out in the community. They would also have had far greater bargaining power than day labourers with an employer who was not paying them any wages at all. Indeed, in 1900 a copper company inquired at the Toronto Asylum whether one of its recently confined employees, forty-three-year-old coppersmith James W., could be released as the company was in desperate need of his skilled work. Superintendent Clark informed the company that Jim was not well enough to be discharged. As it turned out, Jim was never released. Instead, he worked with the asylum tinsmith until his death in 1928.[111] Had he been working out in the community, this coppersmith would have earned far more than the equivalent of room and board in an insane asylum. Yet neither skilled nor unskilled workers received a wage of any kind in Ontario's asylums. In short, there was an "equality" of wage discrimination, if nothing else, for all classes of inmate labourers.

In her study of the Willard and Utica asylums in New York State, Ellen Dwyer noted that some patients and friends protested that, far from getting a good deal with free room and board, they felt that people who had been involuntarily committed to an insane asylum did not owe the state anything.[112] This is an essential point to consider when examining this topic.

Poor patients, who made up the vast majority of labourers in Ontario's asylums, were not given a choice of where they were to be "employed," unlike day labourers who were not confined behind brick walls. Yet, as has been noted elsewhere in this article, the same state that chose to confine mad people in nineteenth-century Ontario did provide compensation to penitentiary convict labourers. In addition to the many other restrictions a diagnosis of insanity brought, it prevented workers from getting the most basic entitlement they would have received out in the community, a wage for their work.

Ellen Dwyer has concluded that at the Willard Asylum "economic considerations tended to override therapeutic ones ... Clearly employing the largest number of patients for maximum profits was Willard's primary objective."[113] Indeed, this same point can not be emphasized too much as it relates to Ontario's public insane asylums during the nineteenth century. Moral "therapy," when stripped of its therapeutic veneer, was in reality a public works program run on the "free" labour of people confined in insane asylums. As the nineteenth century wore on, it becomes clear from reports of asylum officials that the use of unpaid patient labour in Ontario between 1841 and 1900 was ultimately influenced more by economic factors than by the therapeutic claims of medical officials.

NOTES

I would like to thank the editors of this volume, James Moran and David Wright, as well as two anonymous reviewers, for their very helpful comments on an earlier draft of this chapter. Portions of this chapter have been presented during various psychiatric survivor events in Ontario in recent years. I would like to thank all of the participants for their comments, especially Graeme Bacque, Janet Bruch, Jennifer Chambers, Lucy Costa, Lilith Finkler, Wayne Lax, Ali Lennox, Lynne Moss-Sharman, Randy Pritchard, Mel Starkman, Marianne Ueberschar, and Don Weitz for discussing this topic with me at various times.

1 Archives of Ontario, "Annual Report of the Inspector of Asylums, Prisons and Public Charities," 1879, 20. Note: All annual reports (AR) cited below are in the Archives of Ontario (hereafter AO). They were usually published the year following the period reported. All AR dates below reflect the year being reported, not the year of publication, unless otherwise indicated for pre-1859 reports. From 1859, when reports were published in separate volumes, only AR and year will be cited, except when no pages numbers were printed, in which case the specific asylum issuing the report will be indicated.

2 Langmuir noted that though one-third of patients worked, some did less work than others: AR, 1879, 19. In 1900 Inspector Christie wrote that 76 per cent of patients worked in Ontario's insane asylums and that 75 per cent had done so during the previous ten years: AR, 1900, xiv. However, statistics for the year 1900 show that he made an error in calculation of less than 1 per cent, as 3,879 working patients out of 5,149 insane asylum inmates equals 75.31 per cent. These figures do not include the Orillia Asylum for the Feeble-Minded. For data, see AR, 1900, xvi–xvii, xxxvi–xxxvii.

3 The history of moral therapy is a well-trodden field, though few historians have delved in detail into exactly what it was that asylum inmates did over an extended period of time in the jobs assigned to them. Most of the focus has been on the ideas behind moral therapy, as opposed trying to grapple with patients' labour as a worthwhile subject in itself. In addition to sources cited elsewhere in this article, one of the standard studies on this topic is Anne Digby, *Madness, Morality and Medicine: A Study of the York Retreat, 1796–1914* (Cambridge: Cambridge University Press, 1985). Canadian studies that address aspects of this topic include Cheryl Krasnick Warsh, *Moments of Unreason: The Practice of Canadian Psychiatry and the Homewood Retreat, 1883–1923* (Montreal and Kingston: McGill-Queen's University Press, 1989); Geoffrey Reaume, *Remembrance of Patients Past: Patient Life at the Toronto Hospital for the Insane, 1870–1940* (Toronto: Oxford University Press, 2000); and James E. Moran, *Committed to the State Asylum: Insanity and Society in Nineteenth-Century Quebec and Ontario* (Montreal and Kingston: McGill-Queen's University Press, 2000).

4 Moran, *Committed to the State Asylum*, 92; Steven Cherry, *Mental Health Care in Modern England: The Norfolk Lunatic Asylum/St. Andrew's Hospital c. 1810–1998* (Suffolk: Boydell Press, 2003), 66.

5 Yannick Ripa, *Women and Madness: The Incarceration of Women in Nineteenth-Century France*, trans. C. Menage (Cambridge: Polity Press, 1990), 125.

6 AO, AR, 1842, *Journals of the Legislative Assembly of Upper Canada* (hereafter *JLAUC*), vol. 2, appendix U. Reports for 1845–48 make no reference to patients' labour: AO, 1849, *JLAUC*, vol. 8, appendix 3, QQQQ.

7 AO, RG 10, MS 640, 20-B-5, vol. 2, [Commissioners'] Minute Book, 13 October 1849. Cited in Pleasance Kaufman Crawford, "Subject to Change: Asylum Landscape," in E. Hudson, ed., *The Provincial Asylum in Toronto* (Toronto: Toronto Regional Architectural Conservancy, 2000), 72–3.

8 AO, First Annual AR [1850], *JLAUC*, vol. 10, appendix C, 1851.

9 Andrew Scull, *The Most Solitary of Afflictions: Madness and Society in Britain, 1700–1900* (New Haven: Yale University Press, 1993), 150.

10 AO, First Annual AR [1850], *JLAUC*, vol. 10, appendix C, 1851.

11 Ellen Dwyer, *Homes for the Mad: Life inside Two Nineteenth Century Asylums* (New Brunswick, NJ: Rutgers University Press, 1987), 133.

12 AO, *JLAUC*, 1854–55, vol. 13, appendix H [AR, 1853–54]; Joseph Workman, "A Description of the Pestilent Condition of the Toronto Lunatic Asylum in 1853, and the Means Adopted to Remove It," *The Sanitary Journal* 2, 1 (January 1876): 1–6. Certain details regarding physical dimensions vary between these two sources. Thanks to John Court, archivist, Centre for Addiction and Mental Health, Toronto, for providing me with a copy of the 1876 article.

13 AO, *JLAUC*, 1856, vol. 14, appendix 2 [AR, 1855].

14 AO, *JLAUC*, 1857, vol. 15, appendix 12 [AR, 1856]. This reference is in an 8 July 1856 report of Workman, who is responding to charges of abuse of this woman patient, Catherine L., who was three months pregnant upon admission. The Commissioners supported the superintendent's views.

15 Ripa, *Women and Madness*, 109–10; Nancy Tomes, *The Art of Asylum-Keeping: Thomas Story Kirkbride and the Origins of American Psychiatry* (Philadelphia: University of Pennsylvania Press, 1994), 207.

16 AO, *JLAUC*, 1857, vol. 15, appendix 12 [AR, 1856]. See also AO, *JLAUC*, 1857, vol. 15, appendix 12 [AR, 1856]; *JLAUC*, 1858, vol. 16, appendix 9 [AR, 1857].

17 AO, *JLAUC*, 1859, vol. 17, appendix 11 [AR, 1858].

18 AR, 1859, 46. An earlier branch asylum was opened in Toronto in 1856, known as the University Branch, which operated until 1869. The Malden Insane Asylum was a branch of Toronto Asylum from 1859–1861 and an independent facility from 1861–1870.

19 AR, 1860, 97.

20 AR, 1859, 46; AR, 1860, 84. See also Fisher's comments in this regard in his Malden Asylum report for 1860, 100. Besides saving money, he also valued patient labour as inducing discipline, a reference to moral treatment concepts.

21 Cherry, *Mental Health Care in Modern England*, 66–7.

22 AR, 1860, 96–100.

23 AR, 1859, 79; AR, 1861, 163.

24 AR, 1860, 10. Portions of this 1860 boundary wall still exist and are therefore the oldest surviving evidence of asylum patient labour in Ontario. Efforts were under-way when this chapter was written to preserve this wall and remember the people who built it on the grounds of the present-day Centre for Addiction and Mental Health, Toronto.

25 Including branches, Ontario asylums in the 1860s were the following: Toronto, University Branch, Malden, Rockwood (federal ownership), and Orillia. Workman reports little about patient labour at Toronto for the 1860s.

26 AR, 1861, 112. Males comprised 48 per cent and females 41 per cent of Malden patient labourers.

27 AR, 1868–69, 60, 73. The huge difference between the 1868 and 1869 force of patient labourers is likely due to the change in superintendent in July 1868. Fisher

left and Landor took over, having found the Malden Asylum, except the farm, in a state of neglect and collapse. Patients did an enormous amount of work getting the place back into shape. For reference to the problems of statistical interpretation regarding patient labour, see Dwyer, *Homes for the Mad*, 133.

28 AR, 1862, Orillia Branch Asylum [no paging].

29 AR, 1861: Malden, 115; Orillia, 123. How many women patients worked out of 25 at Orillia is not specified.

30 AR, 1863, 62.

31 AR, 1868–69, 80.

32 AR, 1861, 117; Malden AR, 1862 [no paging]. The author last visited this national historic site in August 2003. The only acknowledgment that this former British fort was for eleven years an insane asylum is a brief reference in a tourist pamphlet. The building housing the site's museum has wide-ranging displays about the fort's history during the nineteenth century, but in a telling omission, nothing is included about the people who built and laboured inside the very structure that is now a museum; nor is there any public interpretation about the history of the insane asylum period – yet another example of the hidden history of psychiatric patients that needs to be publicly acknowledged.

33 Orillia AR, 1862 [no paging].

34 Malden AR, 1862 [no paging]; AR, 1865, 59. Malden had sixty acres of cultivated land.

35 AR, 1865, Inspector E.A. Meredith's report, 10.

36 Moran, *Committed to the State Asylum*, 93.

37 Ripa, *Women and Madness*, 126.

38 Orillia AR, 1862 [no pages]; 1863, 60. The laundry floor measured 29 by 19 feet.

39 AR, 1864, 133.

40 AR, 1866, 130–1.

41 AR, 1863, 71.

42 AR, 1868–69, 71, 76.

43 AR, 1868–69, 74.

44 AR, 1869–70, 44; 1870–71, 73.

45 AR, 1870–71, 168; 1872–73, 177–78; 1874, 176.

46 AR, 1874, 168

47 AR, 1872–73, 22.

48 AR, 1874, 169.

49 Inspector Langmuir's Report, AR, 1872–73, 25.

50 These dates can be found in AR, 1896, xi–xii.

51 Langmuir's emphasis on economy and efficiency can be found in AR, 1875, 18. Reference to the mechanization of provincial asylum laundry facilities can be found in AR, 1878, 26.

52 AR, 1877, 239.

53 AR, 1879, 21.

54 Ibid.

55 AR, 1870–71, 161.

56 AR, 1875, 237.

57 AR, 1878, 317.

58 AR, 1875, 226. Interestingly enough, at the Norfolk Lunatic Asylum in England during this same period, baking bread and brewing beer were not deemed appropriate jobs for patient labourers. See Cherry, *Mental Health Care in Modern England*, 67.

59 AR, 1877, 309; 1878, 348. No labour statistics are mentioned for 1878.

60 AR, 1878, 348.

61 AR, 1885, 66.

62 AR, 1880, 314.

63 AR, 1880, 335.

64 AR, 1894, 6.

65 AR, 1895, 35.

66 AR, 1883, 13–14, 66.

67 Ripa, *Women and Madness*, 107.

68 Cheryl L. Krasnick, "'In Charge of the Loons': A Portrait of the London, Ontario Asylum for the Insane in the Nineteenth Century," *Ontario History* 74, 3 (September 1982): 168–9; Reaume, *Remembrance of Patients Past*, 143–4.

69 AR, 1883, 86; AR, 1885, 45.

70 These figures do not include the Orillia Asylum for the Feeble-Minded, only the provincial insane asylums. When Orillia is added, there is no change of any note: the figures stay the same in 1880. In 1900 this figure increases by 1 per cent to 86 per cent of all inmates who were public charges. These figures were arrived at by adding the total paying patients in each year and then subtracting this number from the overall asylum population: AR, 1880, 18, 28; 1900, xvi–xvii, xlvii.

71 Andrew Scull, "Moral Treatment Reconsidered," in Andrew Scull, ed., *Social Order/Mental Disorder: Anglo-American Psychiatry in Historical Perspective* (Berkeley: University of California Press, 1989), 89–94.

72 AR, 1878, 330; 1895, 73. The maintenance rates for 1890 and 1895 are recorded in yearly figures, unlike for other years cited here. The weekly rate is thus calculated by dividing the yearly figure by 52 weeks to come up with the amount indicated.

73 AR, 1885, 66.

74 AR, 1880, 349; 1885, 114; 1895, 117; 1900, 87. The theme of low maintenance costs was also mentioned in the 1890 Hamilton Asylum report, where it was noted that "our expenditure is still low, and well within the appropriation in

every department" (AR, 1890, 124). Though not part of this overall study, it is worth noting that at the Orillia Asylum for the Feeble-Minded (which opened in 1876, six years after the insane asylum there closed) Superintendent A.H. Beaton was especially pleased about how low the patient maintenance figures were for this institution. In 1895 he reported the amount was at a "low water mark" as it had dropped from a yearly per capita rate of $118.58 a year earlier to $105.18 that year, "a figure, I venture to say, that has never been equaled by any similar institution in the world" (AR, 1895, 213).

75 Gerald Grob, *The Mad among Us: A History of the Care of America's Mentally Ill* (New York: Free Press, 1994), 67; Dwyer, *Homes for the Mad*, 134–5; Anne Digby, "Moral Treatment at the Retreat, 1796–1846," in W. Bynum, R. Porter, and M. Shepherd, eds., *The Anatomy of Madness, Volume II, Institutions and Society* (London: Tavistock, 1985), 63; Cherry, *Mental Health Care in Modern England*, 67, 135; Ripa, *Women and Madness*, 109–10; Reaume, *Remembrance of Patients Past*, 139–42; Moran, *Committed to the State Asylum*, 83, 92–3.

76 AR, 1900, 114.

77 Cherry, *Mental Health Care in Modern England*, 135.

78 AR, 1885, 131; 1890, 91; 1895, 106; 1900, 126, 130.

79 AR, 1885, 66.

80 AR, 1885, 83.

81 AR, 1885, 90–1.

82 Pamela Michael, *Care and Treatment of the Mentally Ill in North Wales, 1800–2000* (Cardiff: University of Wales Press, 2003), 71.

83 AR, 1900, 149.

84 AR, 1880, 350.

85 AR, 1895, 122.

86 AR, 1888, 4; 1889, 5; 1890, 42–3.

87 AR, 1888, 4–5; AR, 1889, 6.

88 AR, 1891, 5; 1892, 10–11; 1893, 132, 156; 1894, 142; 1895, 159–60; 1896, 193–5, 224; 1897, 178, 207; 1898, 193, 222; 1899, 153, 173.

89 AR, 1897, 178.

90 Plans are underway to preserve and publicly memorialize the Toronto Asylum patients' labour and social history along the east and west boundary walls, which they re-built in 1888–89 (along with remaining portions of the 1860 patient-built south boundary wall) at the present-day Centre for Addiction and Mental Health, Toronto. The Mimico Asylum closed in 1979, when it was known as the Lakeshore Psychiatric Hospital. It is now part of Humber College, Toronto. A massive refurbishing campaign has made the old wards into class-rooms and the Assembly Hall into a public arts and community centre. The cricket oval that was levelled by patients and one of the patient-built pavilions

continue to be well used, while the superintendent's former residence housed people until recently.

91 AR, 1892, 134; 1899, 168.
92 AR, 1897, 179.
93 The statistical tables that list the "Employment of Patients," 1879–1900, identify these various jobs. For example, for Hamilton, see AR, 1890, 141.
94 AR, 1895, 74.
95 AR, 1880, 314; 1890, 124.
96 AR, 1885, 45.
97 AR, 1895, 39–42.
98 AR, 1895, 125.
99 For figures from 1900, see note 2 above.
100 Nancy Tomes, *A Generous Confidence: Thomas Story Kirkbride and the Art of Asylum-Keeping, 1840–1883* (Cambridge: Cambridge University Press, 1984), 285.
101 Ripa, *Women and Madness*, 110.
102 AR, 1859, 98, Report by D. McIntosh, clark, Provincial Penitentiary, 31 December 1859; AR, 1860, 137, E. Horsey, Architect, Provincial Penitentiary, 21 January 1861.
103 AO, RG 63, A-1, vol. 135, file 4820, Kingston Asylum – Compensation to Patients, 1894–1904: Dr Clarke to Inspector Christie, 15 June 1897; Inspector Christie to D. Miller, 16 June 1897.
104 Ibid. Inspector Christie to Dr Clarke, 27 July 1904.
105 Geoffrey Reaume, "No Profits, Just a Pittance: Work, Compensation and People Defined as Mentally Disabled in Ontario, 1964–1990," in S. Noll and J.Trent, eds., *Mental Retardation in America: A Historical Reader* (New York: New York University Press, 2004), 466–93. See also a recent report related to this issue: Arthur O'Reilly, *The Right to Decent Work of Persons with Disabilities* (Geneva: International Labour Organization, 2003).
106 AR, 1896, xxiv–xxv.
107 AR, 1878, 317.
108 AR, 1868–69, 61.
109 Digby, *Madness, Morality and Medicine*, 62.
110 Bryan D. Palmer, *Working Class Experience: The Rise and Reconstitution of Canadian Labour, 1800–1980* (Toronto: Butterworth, 1983), 72–3.
111 Reaume, *Remembrance of Patients Past*, 154.
112 Dwyer, *Homes for the Mad*, 133.
113 Ibid., 135. Dwyer also notes that this goal of putting patients to work on a large scale "enjoyed wide popular support" outside the asylum.

4

The Uses of Asylums

Resistance, Asylum Propaganda, and Institutionalization Strategies in Turn-of-the-Century Quebec

ANDRÉ CELLARD

AND MARIE-CLAUDE THIFAULT

In 1824 the report of a special committee commissioned by the government of Lower Canada to investigate (among other things) institutions responsible for caring for people with a deranged mind very clearly set out the new role the government planned to adopt with regard to the mentally ill. The report stressed: "It is almost impossible in private families with a mentally deranged member to provide the supervision his condition requires, for his own sake and for the well-being of the family and society in general. It therefore is necessary in almost every case to remove him from the home."[1] This new philosophy clearly differentiated itself from that which had guided the previous system, and it marked a revolution in the maintenance and care of the mentally ill in Lower Canada (later Quebec). This revolution witnessed the replacement of the family with the state institution as the central locus of care for the mentally ill. Barely seventy-five years after this report, the number of mentally ill people in the care of the state in Quebec had grown by a factor of forty. This change can be partly attributed to the social-regulation measures that accompanied the transition to capitalism early in the nineteenth century, as well as to the enthusiastic promotion by physicians of institutional treatment.[2]

There is no denying the role played in this fundamental change by government officials and by the most fortunate members of society, both of whom were concerned about potential urban disorder.[3] However, the reform movement's involvement in asylum promotion and construction cannot fully explain this development. This institutional revolution was made possible by the support of another important segment of society: the family. Since families had traditionally cared for members who were coping with mental problems, they were primarily responsible for transferring custody of their mentally ill members to the state.

Over the past fifteen years, a new historiography of madness has emerged that is less concerned with the socio-economic determinants of the asylum and other institutions of social regulation and more focused upon the mentally troubled – their identities, origins, and social and familial ties. This focus has demonstrated that complex social interactions operating beyond the asylum's sphere of influence altered the course of confinement of the insane.[4] This chapter adds to this perspective by examining the relationship between the family dynamics of nineteenth-century Quebec and the integration of the asylum as a means of managing those suffering from mental disorder.

This chapter will show that families did not passively accept institutionalization of a mentally ill relative, but displayed resistance and a form of reappropriation of asylums that had a strong influence on the phenomenon of institutionalization in the nineteenth century. We will see that although use of asylums increased spectacularly, this growth occurred in several waves throughout the century. In the first half of the nineteenth century, the population in the earliest asylums consisted primarily of poor and indigent mentally ill persons whose families could not care for them. Later in the century we find that the history of internment of the mentally ill was met with resistance by other families, who were better able to cope with the burden of a mentally ill member. Finally, we will see that this resistance dissolved as families gradually reappropriated asylums.

RESISTANCE AND ASYLUM PROPAGANDA

Urban Pauperism and Institutionalization

The steady growth of cities, fluctuations in the economy, and the urban suffering that emerged in the transition to capitalism in the nineteenth century not only concerned the ruling classes but also placed increasing pressure on families, especially those with dependent indigent members. Caring for a mentally disturbed relative was enough of a challenge in the country, but this role encountered special obstacles in an urban setting. For example, while a person with mild mental illness in a rural area might participate in the family economy, he quickly became a burden in the city. Similarly, family members could go about their work in the country while supervising a mentally ill relative, but this became virtually impossible in the city, where they often had to leave the home to earn a living. Having close neighbours also posed another obstacle in the city because of increased perceptions of danger and the possibility of disturbing others or even shaming the family, at a time when mental illness was increasingly viewed as a moral danger to the surrounding community.[5]

The archives of the provincial curator and provincial secretary of Quebec are filled with passages describing the disruption faced by some families coping with a mentally ill member and seeking assistance from the authorities.[6] They often had no choice but to leave their relative in prison or, worse, in the street when, for example, the head of the family fell ill or when the loss of a job forced the family into poverty. The statistical data available on the earliest cases of institutionalization provide extensive details on the origin of the mentally ill who became wards of the state. In the early decades, most came from urban areas.

Banning and curatorship constituted a civil procedure at the time for family members and friends of an insane person to protect his estate by removing his or her authority to manage that estate and entrusting it to a relative. A study of almost five hundred cases of guardianship (*curatelle*) for the districts of Montreal and Quebec City from 1801 to 1845 reveals that 25.5 per cent of urban residents who resorted to the banning procedure[7] in the first half of the nineteenth century used institutional confinement of a mentally ill relative, compared with 1.4 per cent of those living in the country. The 1851 census confirms this fact since 87 per cent of the 153 patients then in Beauport came from Quebec City and Montreal, at a time when these cities accounted for about 10 per cent of the province's population, which was 85 per cent rural at the time.[8]

Banning records for 1801–45 also reveal that 37.2 per cent of this demand for institutionalization originated from anglophones, compared with 19.1 percent from Francophones. Anglophones also accounted for the majority of internees at the Quebec City General Hospital from 1800 to 1845.[9] Admissions data for the Montreal Lunatic Asylum,[10] where francophones represented just 23.4 per cent of patients compared with 75.6 per cent for anglophones, also confirm this clear trend. During this period, anglophones were concentrated in Montreal, Quebec City, and the Eastern Townships and represented less than 25 per cent of the total population of Quebec.

This striking contrast in the habits of anglophones and francophones caring for the mentally ill appears to be the result of several factors. It is caused in part by the concentration of anglophones in the province's largest

Fig. 4.1   Ethnic origin of the Montreal population and of inmates at the Montreal Lunatic Asylum, 1839–1844

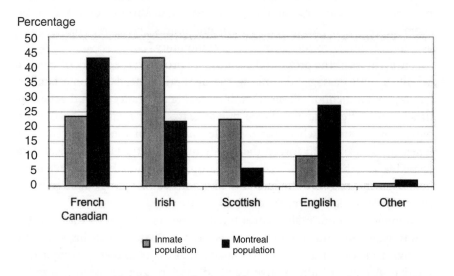

cities, but we attribute this statistical disparity primarily to the shortage or lack of family support networks for newly arrived residents and the grinding poverty faced by the large wave of English-speaking immigrants, mainly from Ireland and Scotland, from the 1820s to the 1840s. While caring for a mentally ill relative could be demanding for a family in the city, we can only imagine what it would be like for a new arrival whose family links were tenuous or simply non-existent and who lacked the means to maintain this person in the home. For two centuries, French Canadians had developed solid networks to lighten the burden of a family in need, and thus fared better. The breakdown of admissions data for the Montreal Lunatic Asylum also shows under-representation of mentally ill patients from England (see fig. 4.1). Since the Conquest in 1760, these emigrants to Canada, who often belonged to the upper class in Quebec society, were better able than their Scottish and Irish "cousins" to cope with the burden of an indigent relative.

It should also be noted that most admissions to the Montreal Lunatic Asylum were from prison. This was also the case for the Beauport asylum in the 1840s, 1850s, and 1860s, since a high proportion of patients came from prisons in Quebec City and Montreal. Once again, this pattern clearly illustrates the extent to which in the early decades of its appearance in Quebec an asylum was primarily an institution of last resort.[11] Finally, the data available show that the first patients institutionalized usually had no stated occupation and were unmarried. In 1851, two-thirds of mentally ill internees were unmarried, which once again confirms the importance of family support in the public custody of a mentally ill person.[12] Thus in the mid-nineteenth century the typical profile of an institutionalized mentally ill person was an urban indigent, usually an English-speaking immigrant, who was unmarried and who became a ward of the state in an asylum because of limited family support or the poverty of his home community, often following imprisonment of some duration.

Resistance to Institutionalization

In their early years, asylums clearly were used primarily to institutionalize the poorest members of society, from the most vulnerable segments of the population, while those with even minimal family support and care remained in the home or the community, despite pressure from asylum advocates from the 1850s to the 1880s. The reports of these advocates, echoing those of government inspectors, constantly voiced serious concerns about the reluctance of relatives to place family members in the care of strangers:

How is it that the relatives of these unfortunates fail to clearly understand the pressing need for prompt intervention in mental illness and the urgent need to provide appropriate treatment as quickly as possible?
It is difficult to become accustomed to the thought of removing a family member from the home, and when false sensitivity takes precedence over reason, these unfortunate relatives lack the courage to entrust the mentally ill person to those dedicated to treating these unfortunate souls ...
In the interim, asylums are filling up with poor miserable creatures whose spark of reason has probably been extinguished forever.[13]

Asylum advocates were concerned because they had quickly realized that asylums and moral treatment were not meeting the initial objective of providing a cure. They concluded that this was because the mentally ill people sent to them, whether from prison or from families, had suffered mental disorders for too long and were now incurable, and nothing more could be done for them. Wrote one director, "It is unfortunate to find that families keep their ill members in the home so long before sending them to a hospice; ... often only when pushed to the limit do these families relinquish care of their mentally ill members, so these unfortunate people quite often come to the asylum in a totally incurable condition."[14]

To overcome this reticence, advocates published the content of the annual reports they were required to produce for the government. A few were published as monographs, while others were reprinted in whole or in part in several of the province's daily newspapers. The comments about families occasionally were also quite strident: "This is the place to lament once again the deliberate negligence of families in obtaining treatment for unfortunate people affected by mental illness. Usually, the mentally ill are not interned until they have become a burden on the family and a danger to society, months and years after the start of the illness and after any chance of a cure has disappeared."[15] This resistance, if not repugnance, by families to relinquish a relative for whom they had always been responsible was directly rooted, according to asylum advocates, in the system of family and community support. In 1856 Dr James Douglas, director of the Beauport asylum, explained it in these terms: "This reluctance to place insane persons and idiots in an asylum is also attributed to the strong parental feelings, and the close ties of the Habitants." The asylum advocates focused in particular on rural families, which continued to resist the urban setting of an asylum: "Even in the country, where the presence of the abnormal might appear to escape all the difficulties and vexations that everything seems to generate in large cities ... While the unfortunate insane in the city more quickly become the target of public ridicule and torment, in the country they more quickly become a vagabond without hearth or home."[16]

Not only were relatives or friends much more reticent to institutionalize their relations and neighbours, they also did not always use the asylum as advocates would have hoped. It appears that many only turned to an asylum in an emergency and constantly clamoured for the release of those they had placed in the care of an asylum. The Beauport asylum directors put it this way:

We do not blame the honourable sentiments these families may experience around bringing home, as soon as possible, a member taken away by a regrettable disease; but we wish to point out that most accidents caused by an insane person who has been released are almost always attributable to the stubborn urgings of relatives to release these people from asylums even before they are cured. They believe they are acting honourably in the interest of these unfortunates, and take upon themselves a responsibility that may cause them harm... A mistake! A futile pretext that just further demonstrates the incompetence of families in such matters.[17]

These arguments about the perils of early release were further emphasized by the occasional horror story in which, to take one example, a family

Fig. 4.2   Ethnic origin of the general population and of inmates at the
Beauport asylum, 1857

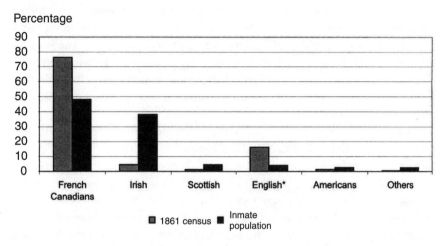

member resting quietly was decapitated by a relative prematurely released
from the asylum.[18] In the late 1850s, twenty years after the appearance of
asylum institutions in Quebec, the population profile for the provincial
asylum in Beauport clearly illustrates the extent to which francophones,
who still accounted for only 48.2 per cent of internees compared with 49.3
per cent for anglophones, were still reticent to send a family member to
these institutions (see fig 4.2).

Changes in Family Resistance and Reappropriation of Asylums

Not until the last quarter of the nineteenth century, when the Saint-Jean-
de-Dieu and Verdun asylums in particular opened, do we find an increase
in institutionalization leading to a notable change in the typical profile of
institutionalized patients. The growing urbanization of Quebec society
contributed to this process, as family strategies clearly changed to reap-
propriate asylums. Families gradually developed a certain culture of relying
on the institution and learned to use it to meet their needs. Admittedly,
advocates would argue for a few more years that families remained reticent, but it also becomes clear that after this time, internment gradually
ceased to be viewed as a solution of last resort for the destitute with no
family support. In the 1870s this change led Drs Landry and Roy, asylum
advocates at Beauport, to say: "When our facility [the Beauport asylum]
began, only as a last resort, when forced by poverty or imminent danger,

were we given custody of a furious patient, and only then did families decide to ask the authorities to take in the patient. Since then, however, the organization of asylums has improved and the earlier prejudice in families has changed to well deserved trust, as patients have arrived from all parts of the country, regardless of family, means, or occupation."[19] The statistical data available, especially the 6,110 or so admissions to Saint-Jean-de-Dieu between 1873 and 1900 (as well as a total of 4,631 cases from Verdun and Saint-Jean-de-Dieu for 1900–21, used on an ad hoc basis here),[20] support their claim.

First, at Saint-Jean-de-Dieu we find an increase in the proportion of children admitted under thirteen years of age in relation to the interned population as a whole. The child clientele, mainly orphans and abandoned children, rose from 3.5 per cent of the total in 1874–78 to 4.9 per cent ten years later, between 1884 and 1888. Not only did this trend become clear at Saint-Jean-de-Dieu, but at this time we also see the opening of institutions specifically intended for insane children or "idiots or imbeciles from birth," such as Saint-Julien (1872) and Sainte-Anne de Baie-Saint-Paul (1889).

Admission records for Saint-Jean-de-Dieu also show a decline in unmarried patients – from two-thirds to half of patients admitted – and a corresponding rise in admissions of married patients. While single patients accounted for 65.1 per cent of admissions between 1874 and 1878, their proportion declined steadily to 52 per cent of admissions in the five years between 1894 and 1898. The proportion of married people admitted to the same institution rose from 27 per cent between 1874 and 1878 to 41.3 per cent from 1894 to 1898 (a study of our sample reveals that this trend continued into the early twentieth century: in 1921, unmarried patients represented 48 per cent of admissions, compared with 38.2 per cent for married people, at Saint-Jean-de-Dieu, while in Verdun, the proportions for single and married people were 42.7 and 47.7 per cent respectively). We therefore find that in the last quarter of the century, a strong family bond such as a parent-child or husband-wife relationship was no longer sufficient in and of itself to prevent confinement. The next statistical data show that patients gradually ceased to come solely from the poorest segments of society. This change is reflected in the proportion of skilled workers admitted to Saint-Jean-de-Dieu, which doubled in twenty-five years, from 10.2 per cent in 1874–78 to 19.3 per cent of new admissions between 1894 and 1898. In 1912 the proportion of skilled workers admitted to Saint-Jean-de-Dieu was 25.3 per cent, compared with 21.6 per cent in 1921. It was 28 per cent in Verdun for the same year (which also had more than 10 per cent admissions from the lower middle class). The proportion of unskilled workers in turn declined from 49.9 per cent between 1874 and 1878 to 29.3 per cent of admissions in 1889–93.[21] Asylums therefore were no longer seen as the solution of last resort and ceased to be the catch basin for prisons. For Beauport between 1867 and 1883 and for all asylums in Quebec in 1890, the proportion of mentally ill patients transferred from prisons fell from 48.1 per cent in 1867–69 to 10.5 per cent in 1890.[22]

Institutionalization extended to all elements of society as rural residents[23] and francophones[24] came to use asylums in proportions similar to their representation in the general population. Rural residents, seriously under-represented in the Beauport asylum between 1845 and 1872, when they accounted for 30.8 per cent of internees although they represented some 85 per cent of the population of Quebec, increased their proportion in the Beauport and Saint-Jean-de-Dieu asylums to 44.1 per cent between 1894 and 1903, although, overall, they then represented only 60 per cent of Quebec's total population. In turn, francophones' proportion in Quebec asylums rose from 56 per cent between 1845 and 1873 to 76.4 per cent between 1894 and 1898 (for the Saint-Jean-de-Dieu, Verdun, and Beauport asylums).

INSTITUTIONALIZATION STRATEGIES

These statistics indicate that when the life of members of a family unable to cope with the difficult reality of caring for a mentally ill person was seriously affected, internment in an asylum was gradually seen as a necessity. The worry and shame resulting from lascivious acts, immoral remarks, and threatening, violent gestures by an insane person moved many families to bring their ill relatives to Quebec's mental institutions.

By reading the many letters from parents, children, or spouses of women and men interned at Saint-Jean-de-Dieu, as well as the replies from successive medical superintendents between 1873 and 1921, we can learn about the world of applicants as it related to the ill relative they placed in the care of asylum staff. This evidence indicates that the internment of a wife or husband in an asylum was considered the best treatment to cure insanity at the end of the nineteenth century, whether the person was hysterical, catatonic, depressed, or affected by acute mania.

We examined the medical records from Saint-Jean-de-Dieu hospital (stored in the medical archives of Louis-H. Lafontaine hospital) from 1873 to 1921 to gain perspective on the pre-internment lives of patients and of members of their families. The discovery of correspondence full of emotion toward the women and men interned at Saint-Jean-de-Dieu provides a glimpse into the private life of many families separated from their ill members, and thus a better understanding of a family member's expectations about the treatment administered to his or her child, spouse, or parent. The motives for excluding, isolating, or interning a woman or man showing signs of insanity through agitation, violence, mania, persecution, or attempted suicide, are also explained in these documents.

Exhaustion of Family Resources

Hundreds of women and men diagnosed with mental illness were interned at Saint-Jean-de-Dieu. Many were taken there by their families, by municipal authorities, or by order of the recorder. Despite fatigue, fear, and discouragement, the family sought to control the unwanted and often unpredictable actions arising from the imagination, delirium, dementia, or violence present in the disruptive, exasperating person. The family (as well as those around it) survived the patient's crises until the day when exhaustion, despair, and distress forced it to face the inevitable – internment in an asylum. In many cases, this option was delayed until the illness became extreme and when internment became an unavoidable solution to control these men and women who had become very embarrassing in an urban setting, but who were primarily uncontrollable in either city or countryside.

Applications for admission, usually submitted by a family member or by the parish priest or village doctor if the family lacked the ability to fill out the form, reflect the main problems faced by these families. As the following examples demonstrate, these letters, addressed to the medical superintendent of the asylum, reveal the fear, worry, discouragement, and exhaustion of long-term care and management of the mentally troubled. In the first example, a daughter explains the domestic and social difficulties resulting from her mother's unusual behaviour:

She is worse then ever ... Her insanity has her believing that everyone is stealing her clothes, myself as well as others, and for this she causes a scene with me every day, to the point that I am no longer mistress of my own home. Everything belongs to her, she rummages through everything and I am forced to keep the furniture locked. If I don't do that she may empty the drawer 15 times a day, she insults everyone, so I can no longer have any visitors, woman or child, much less a man. She tells people I mistreat her, that I hit her, she plays the martyr and no longer wants to stay with me, I am forced to watch her night and day. This situation cannot go on, my health is changing and if I fall ill, I really do not know what will happen. Also, I have to earn a living, and as long as my mother is in this condition, this is impossible. I am truly discouraged.[25]

In another plea for institutional confinement, the view of the asylum as a safe and secure alternative to family and community care is clearly made: "You have no doubt read in the newspaper that a mentally ill person in Saint-Constant attempted suicide a few days ago by slashing his throat with a razor. He is now in full recovery, and the family would like to have him interned in an asylum since he is a constant danger to himself and his family, and they cannot maintain continual surveillance of him as you can do in your institution."[26]

As the following example demonstrates, the physical violence attending mental illness was not exclusive to men: "On Sunday the 18th, she suddenly suffered a nervous breakdown, pulling out her hair, crying, saying she was damned, etc. Each day since this time brings great excitement, and despite the sedatives she is given, it can take as many as four men to subdue her."[27] Finally, the following example shows the potential dangers of managing certain mentally unsound individuals while at the same time documenting the fact that women were most often confronted with the burden of caring for them:

I am Charles's wife. I live with him on the second floor in my brother Julien's home and I am forced to care for him. I have to watch him constantly. He always wants to break things. I cannot rest, he often rummages about for part of the night and I cannot let him out of my sight, I cannot say a word to him without making him angry and incurring threats that he will hit me. He has punched me twice and if I had not fled, I would have been hit many times. He often tells me, "If I had my axe, I'd cut you up into pieces." He charged me with a knife. I am forced to hide the table knives.[28]

Clearly, the lives of these families were disrupted. To live with Maria was to live in fear of the threats of death she uttered night and day;[29] with Marie-Rose it meant following her every step, to prevent her from seriously injuring herself with self-inflicted wounds;[30] with Louis it entailed preventing him from hitting, tearing, at and assaulting everyone he met;[31] with Magloire it meant enduring constant social embarrassment.[32] The relatives and friends of these patients were constantly alert to signs of danger and disruption. Their lives were never-ending battles against the potential fallout from socially unacceptable behaviour. But no one could devote an entire life to monitoring an insane person. Other family members had to be cared for, the home needed to be maintained, meals prepared, clothing mended. In the city, family members had to leave the home to earn a living.

Therapeutic Isolation and Family Support

The medical records of Saint-Jean-de-Dieu patients between 1873 and 1921 often contained correspondence between the medical superintendent and a family member of the insane person discussing the health of the patient. There are enough of these letters to show that families did in fact maintain contact with their sick relative during internment. These letters also reveal the main concerns of the husband, mother, sister or son about the patient interned behind the asylum's stone walls.

With confidence or apprehension, men and women from all walks of life and every generation engaged in the art of writing to maintain family ties. Letters by the hundreds were delivered to Saint-Jean-de-Dieu from saddened, anxious, disappointed, discouraged, or angry relatives. Simple postcards, onionskin, foolscap, or business letterheads conveyed a range of messages, some difficult to understand and some written with style and clarity. In either case, the medical superintendent was careful to answer these missives with dispatch.

Some patients had barely left the family home before relatives were demanding updates from the superintendent. Others wanted to bring their loved ones home, even though they were still disturbed. These were very startling turns of events considering the problems, frustrations and hazards caused by these patients before internment. These family members usually found that their interned relative's health was very slow to show signs of improvement. Disappointment, discouragement, and loss of hope plagued husbands, fathers, daughters, and sons, who became increasingly skeptical about the effectiveness of treatment based on isolation in an asylum that separated them from their wife, child, or father. Typical of this skepticism, and of the disparity between the prognosis of the insane person's relative and the medical superintendent, is the correspondence between a husband and the medical superintendent of Saint-Jean-de-Dieu. On 7 March 1915 the husband wrote: "I am hereby asking you as a favour to release my wife from the Saint-Jean-de-Dieu asylum, so I can see whether she might live with her family in the future." Two days later the medical superintendent responded by warning him: "I must tell you that Marie-Anne's condition ... has shown no improvement. She is very moody, tries to lash out and rebels at the least contradiction. It would be impossible to keep her in the room. She is in fairly good physical health. It would not be wise to grant her leave at this time."[33] In another case, the letter of Arthémise to Dr Chagnon of 3 June 1898 clearly articulates the worries that many held about asylum treatment of the insane:

Dear Doctor,
You gave me great hope last Friday when I saw you regarding my brother Ernest. There was no doubt in my mind that he is in his right mind. The two times I have seen him since he entered the asylum, in March and on the 27th last, I found both times that he had a good memory, recalling all facts correctly. He chats and jokes as usual. I found nothing about him that is out of the ordinary. So I find it odd that my family decided to leave him there in the asylum in these conditions. Since I know that nothing pleases you more than helping your patients and those interested in them, I am asking whether you would be kind enough to talk to him a little every day. I plan to return to Montreal next week to see him again, and you can tell me what you think. My greatest desire is to get him out right away.
Please excuse me if I am taking advantage of your kindness
Your very humble Arthémise[34]

With tension, uncertainty, and disappointment, over the weeks, months, and sometimes years following internment of their family member, these people often received discouraging results from the medical superintendent regarding their loved one. Disillusionment quickly took over from hope for a cure. This reality of internment inevitably raised many questions about the effectiveness, relevance, and usefulness of the therapy provided in the closed world of an asylum. Internment definitely provided care for the insane, but beyond this control exerted over asylum patients, the therapeutic results were unconvincing. Asylums clearly excelled in caring for patients in crisis who posed a danger or who were "deranged," but once these insane characteristics were controlled, the institution may have had nothing more to offer than the family home in which the patient, in the best cases, was treated with attention, vigilance, and kindness.

Asylums may have had the usefulness of providing a respite or short rest for exhausted families unable to provide adequate supervision of their loved ones. Less than two weeks after the internment of some patients, the superintendent was already receiving requests to release these recently hospitalized patients. Unexpectedly, letters from families carried the same message that they wanted to bring their relative home. Distanced from the storm the patient could cause, they began to miss their loved one or feel guilty about abandoning him or her in an institution, and this was probably enough to persuade a mother, husband, or brother to demand the return of someone taken out of the family's life. In another way, the family's interest in seeking the return of their ill relative (regardless of that person's contribution to the family economy) may be traced to the fact that families probably realized fairly quickly that, in contrast to the words of asylum staff, these institutions had little to offer patients and that, ultimately, the best place to recover their health was in the family home.

If an individual case of asylum confinement was put into question, a petitioner could have a patient released back into the family context, in the form of a "probationary discharge"[35] This procedure permitted a next of kin to keep a daughter, wife, husband, or parent for a period of three months, whether or not the state of the patient had improved or not, so long as the patient did not present a danger to him or herself or to others. The advantage of this process was that if it was unsuccessful, the patient could be readmitted to the asylum without requiring a new round of application procedures.

The use of probationary discharge by a tormented spouse, an anxious mother, or a chagrined daughter who wanted to place the asylum patient back in his or her "natural" setting – the very setting which, according to asylum alienists, was likely responsible for the onset of madness – nevertheless allowed families to gauge the benefits, up to that point, of institutional confinement. Without probationary discharge, there is no doubt that many patients would have experienced longer stays at the asylum – longer stays that would not have necessarily benefited these patients therapeutically. Indeed, the following letter written by Dr Devlin concerning the confinement of a patient named Irma suggests that patients for whom there was no family to take them back on a probationary basis were largely forgotten at the asylum: "Dear Sir, I write you with reference to Irma, who has been in your institution since last May, who I understand is well enough to leave but having no relatives in this country to come to her aid is perhaps the reason for her detention there so long."[36]

In 1890, about 1 per cent of female admissions to Saint-Jean-de-Dieu benefited from a probationary discharge; by 1906 the percentage of patients leaving the asylum on this basis had risen to 30; and by 1928, 53 per cent left the asylum as probationary patients during the course of their confinement. These figures are especially surprising because at the end of the nineteenth century the rising use of this procedure speaks to the power of families who were able to control the timing of patient discharge in order to meet their desires to take their institutionalized relations back into the family setting. Although the reasons put forth for requesting a temporary probation varied according to the sex of the patient, in a general way, there was much overlap in the rationales behind the requests. According to a sample of one year in three from 1903 to 1912, 28 per cent of females and 29 per cent of males left the asylum on probationary discharges. In general, the discharge of asylum patients was requested when it was felt that they could be again cared for within the family. But the return of wives was clearly also connected to a desire for them to re-establish their responsibilities as female heads of households, including their cleaning and cooking functions in the home and their educational duties towards their children. For the unmarried and for widows, their discharge was a more complicated matter, which loosely corresponded to familial desire for them to care for other family members or to take on the myriad tasks specific to individual family contexts. For their part, regardless of their societal status, male patients were requisitioned by their wives, their mothers, and their sisters to help provide for the needs of their families.[37]

Despite the principles of asylum advocates who encouraged the removal of the insane person from their home environments, the home care of a mentally ill relative was a way for families to be actively involved in the therapeutic treatment of their loved ones. In the twentieth century these family initiatives were increasingly authorized by the superintendent, and they show that medical staff who were overwhelmed by the excessive number of patients in fact relied on help from families to relieve them of many patients for whom they had to care. In this way, families took on an important role in asylums. They made strategic use of asylums and were by no means poor victims. Husbands, parents, and children assumed the role of applicant and used asylums to meet the needs of their ill relative, based on the cycle of episodes of mania or depression. Over the course of the twentieth century, families developed their own patterns for using asylums to compensate for resources lacking within the family. They let go of some responsibility for their mentally ill family member without totally disconnecting and ending their relationship with this relative.

CONCLUSION

Asylums began as an instrument of social regulation to manage, supervise, and control marginal and marginalized people. The statistical results presented in the first section of this chapter clearly show that family resistance to these new state-regulated institutions subsided in the last quarter of the nineteenth century. As a result, the profile of asylum internees gradually changed from urban indigents with no family ties to a group representing the general characteristics of Quebec society. Admittedly, mainly francophone families in rural areas initially resisted placing a family member in the care of an asylum. Allowing strangers to care for their ill relative clashed with their family values. Once they overcame this barrier and acknowledged and accepted the need for care by asylum staff, however, families coping with a mentally ill member agreed to entrust this person to the care of specialists.

Yet families developed strategies over the twentieth century for using asylums in their own way. Rather than being victims of a regulatory system that forced them to relinquish an ill relative, they agreed to place this person in the care of asylum staff while maintaining some involvement in the therapeutic process.[38] Finally, patients who enjoyed the attention and support of their family certainly were those best served by their internment. They also had the best hope of release.

NOTES

Quotations from French-language sources have been translated by the authors.

1 "Rapport du Comité spécial," *Journal du Conseil législatif* (Quebec, 1824), appendix 1.
2 See A. Cellard, *Histoire de la folie au Québec, 1600–1850* (Montréal: Les éditions du Boréal, 1991).
3 On this subject in the Anglo-American context see, for example, David Rothman, *The Discovery of the Asylum: Social Order and Disorder in the New Republic* (Boston: Little Brown, 1971); Andrew Scull, *Museums of Madness: The Social Organization of Insanity in Nineteenth-Century England* (London: Allen Lane, 1979).
4 For a study of this recent historiographical trend, see Roy Porter's introductory survey in Roy Porter and David Wright, eds., *The Confinement of the Insane, 1800–1965: International Perspectives* (Cambridge: Cambridge University Press, 2003). In a more geographically proximate study, David Wright, James Moran, and Sean Gouglas have produced an excellent historiographical synthesis of the history of madness and institutionalization in Canada. See "The Confinement of the Insane in Victorian Canada: The Hamilton and Toronto Asylums, 1861–1891," in Porter and David Wright, eds., *The Confinement of the Insane, 1800–1965*, 100–28.
5 A similar argument for the United States has been made by Gerald Grob in *The Mad among Us: A History of the Care of America's Mentally Ill* (New York: Free Press, 1994), 24.

6 A qualitative analysis of curatorship can be found in André Cellard, *Histoire de la folie au Québec,* chapters 2 and 3. James Moran in turn explored the same themes through the archives of the provincial secretary in his book *Committed to the State Asylum: Insanity and Society in Nineteenth-Century Quebec and Ontario* (Montreal and Kingston: McGill-Queen's University Press, 2000).

7 For details, see André Cellard, "La curatelle et l'histoire de la maladie mentale au Québec," *Histoire sociale/Social History* 19 (1986): 443–50.

8 Canada (Province), Board of Registration and Statistics, *Census of the Canadas for 1850–1851* (Quebec, 1853), 585–6.

9 Cellard, *Histoire de la folie au Québec,* 190.

10 The Montreal Lunatic Asylum was the first institution for the insane in Quebec. This temporary facility closed in 1845 when the province's first permanent asylum opened in Beauport. Before 1839, the mentally ill were confined to the Montreal, Quebec City, and Trois-Rivières general hospitals or placed in prison.

11 In the late 1860s, 205 of the 426 patients admitted to the Beauport asylum came from prison, especially the prisons in Quebec City and Montreal (See annual reports of the Bureau des inspecteurs de prisons, asylums, etc., for 1867, 1868, and 1869, *Documents de la session* [Québec, 1869–71]). This high proportion of admissions from prison greatly concerned asylum staff because in most cases (34 of 50 patients admitted from prisons in Quebec City and Montreal in 1868, 39 of 58 patients admitted for Quebec as a whole), nothing was known about them "[We] know nothing about the background of a patient the police have found in the street and arrested as a vagabond incapable of accounting for his conduct or providing the least information about himself" ("Rapport des propriétaires de l'asile de Beauport pour l'année 1868," *Documents de la session* [Québec, 1869], Doc. no. 23, 2).

12 Canada (Province), *Census for 1850–1851,* 585–6.

13 "Rapport annuel des propriétaires de l'asile d'aliénés de Beauport pour l'année 1869," *Documents de la session* (Québec, 1870), Doc. no. 12, 44.

14 "Rapport de l'asile d'aliénés de Québec pour l'année 1883," *Documents de la session* (Québec, 1884), Doc. no. 15, 244.

15 "Rapport sur le service de l'asile d'aliénés de Québec pour l'année 1882–83," *Documents de la session* (Québec, 1884), Doc. no. 9, 8.

16 "Asiles d'aliénés de Québec, 1881," *Documents de la session* (Québec, 1882), no. 35, 14.

17 "Asiles d'aliénés de Québec, 1873," *Documents de la session* (Québec, 1873), Doc. no. 5, 67 and 69.

18 Ibid.

19 "Asile des aliénés de Québec, 1873," *Documents de la session* (Québec, 1873), Doc. no. 5, 28.

20 Saint-Jean-de-Dieu was the only major asylum in the Montreal area in the last quarter of the century, until the Verdun institution, which we discuss later, opened in the early 1890s. These data were gathered as part of a history project on marginalized populations in Montreal in the years 1850–1921, by the Centre d'histoire des régulations sociales. The authors wish to acknowledge the contribution of Éric Chalifoux, Daniel Dicaire, and Bruno Therrien, who entered the data and prepared them in statistical form.

21 We find the calculation of the proportion of unskilled workers somewhat more random, however, than that of skilled workers because it often appears to vary according to the interpretation of those filling out the forms. These people appeared to make no distinction when applying the terms "day labourer," "with no fixed work," "unknown," or "no work" to casual or farm workers. This lack of uniformity generates significant variations from year to year. The proportion of unskilled workers generally ranges from 33 to 40 per cent in our sample for Saint-Jean-de-Dieu for 1900–21.

22 It proved fairly difficult to obtain a continuous statistical series for admissions from prison in the second half of the nineteenth century. We had to choose the years 1867–69, 1872–74 and 1881–83 for the Beauport asylum, since these were the only groups of years available through the *Documents de la session*. For 1890, we counted 52 individuals transferred from prison to the asylum, compared with 526 admissions to Beauport and Saint-Jean-de-Dieu. We did not count admissions at Verdun for this year, since virtually all were for Saint-Jean-de-Dieu and Beauport. For 1893, we counted 43 patients from prison for 385 admissions to the province's three main asylums.

23 These last two charts were obtained from broken series, and while we have confirmation of the start and end data, the data presented between the beginning and end of the periods must be viewed as indicative. For the proportion of rural patients, the first data (1845–72) originate from the annual reports of asylum staff at Beauport and can be considered reliable. It should be noted, however, that in this instance we use the "districts" entry compared with that for "cities," "prisons," and "hospitals" to produce this statistic. This approach suffered the drawback of slightly underestimating the proportion of rural patients since a small number of people admitted from prison were also from rural areas. For 1873–83, we used only the entries for Beauport, because we found that those for Saint-Jean-de-Dieu might skew the totals, given the large number of transfers when that institution opened. For 1884–93 and 1894–1903, we used the data from the registers of patients at Saint-Jean-de-Dieu, since no such data were available for Beauport. For the 1894–1903 period, we did not have the entries for 1899, 1901, and 1902.

24 The data on ethnic origin or language spoken by patients admitted are more reliable and frequent. We used the session documents for data on Beauport and Verdun, starting in 1890, as well as the "Registre des aliénés" for Saint-Jean-de-Dieu from 1874 to 1898. We had to subtract transfers from Saint-Jean-de-Dieu and Beauport from the totals for Verdun.

25 Archive de l'Hôpital Louis-H. Lafontaine. Correspondence, medical record: 13899, 21 March 1933. The spelling in the French text reflects the original document. We did not want to encumber the text by adding the notation "[sic]" wherever the methodology would dictate. The same approach has been used for all quotations from this text.

26 Ibid., medical record: 5589, 9 December 1896.

27 Ibid., medical record: 7243, 27 January 1903.

28 Ibid., medical record: 6013, 22 July 1898.

29 Ibid., medical record: 8358, 1906.

30 Ibid., medical record: 7243, 27 January 1903.

31 Ibid., medical record: 5621, 7 April 1897.

32 Ibid., medical record: 6476, 15 December 1903.

33 Ibid., medical record: 12039.

34 Ibid., medical record: 5856.

35 Formule J: Demande de garder temporairement un aliéné en conge d'essai.

36 Archive de l'Hôpital Louis-H. Lafontaine. Correspondence, medical record: 13726.

37 See Marie-Claude Thifault, "L'enfermement asilaire des femmes au Québec: 1873–1921" (thèse de doctorat, Université d'Ottawa, 2003).

38 As we mentioned at the beginning of this article, several authors have, for a few years, underlined the importance of interventions located outside the walls of the asylum. Many researchers in both Europe and North America have come to similar conclusions as those reached by us here. Studies that most readily come to mind are Akihito Suzuki, "Enclosing and Disclosing Lunatics within the Family Walls: Domestic Psychiatric Regime and the Public Sphere in Early Nineteenth-Century England," in Peter Bartlett and David Wright, eds., *Outside the Walls of the Asylum: The History of Care in the Community, 1750–2000* (London and New Brunswick, NJ, 1999), 115–31; and Bill Forsythe and Joseph Melling, eds., *Insanity, Institutions and Society: New Research in the Social History of Madness, 1800–1914* (London: Routledge, 1999). One can also consult some of the work of Michael MacDonald; see, for example, his "Madness, Suicide and the Computer," in Roy Porter and Andrew Wear, eds., *Problems and Methods in the History of Medicine* (London: Croom Helm, 1987), 207–29. See also Nancy Tomes, "The Anglo-

American Asylum in Historical Perspective," in C.J. Smith and J.A. Giggs, eds., *Location and Stigma: Contemporary Perspectives on Mental Health and Mental Health Care* (Boston: Unwin Hyman, 1988). More recently Patricia Prestwich has published a very interesting article in this regard; see her "Family Strategies and Medical Power: 'Voluntary' Committal in a Parisian Asylum, 1876–1914," in Porter and Wright, eds., *The Confinement of the Insane*, 79–99.

5

"Loaded Revolvers"

Ontario's First Forensic Psychiatrists

ALLISON KIRK-MONTGOMERY

In November 1869 Joseph Workman, the medical superintendent of the Provincial Lunatic Asylum in Toronto, Ontario, explained to members of the Canadian Institute his views on the position of medical witnesses in court. The medical expert, he bragged, "is a loaded revolver, very dangerous to be toyed with, and still more so to be roughly handled ... [lawyers] can not tell on which side it may kill; and here, and here only, lies the safety of our profession in the witness box."[1] Yet less than a decade after his exultant speech, he lamented that "we have in Canada, arrived at times in which the competency of medical experts to testify to mental condition, is declared to be no greater, or more reliable, than that of ordinary men."[2] In 1898 Daniel Clark, Workman's successor at the Toronto Asylum, spoke for the first generation of Canadian psychiatrists when he bitterly compared giving evidence in courts of law to "wasting his sweetness on the desert air."[3]

This chapter will examine the first three decades of forensic psychiatry in Ontario, Canada through the careers of the three men who dominated the specialty: Joseph Workman (1805–94), Daniel Clark (1830–1912), and to a lesser extent, their more controversial colleague Richard Maurice Bucke (1837–1902).[4] Together and separately these asylum doctors appeared in the witness box in over two dozen trials and hearings, almost all for murder; the main sources are trial and other justice system documents, newspaper reports, and the professional texts they wrote. The goal of this chapter is to address an enduring historiographical concern in a specific time and place through two questions: To what extent and in what ways did forensic psychiatry "medicalize" the criminal justice system of late-century Ontario? And conversely, what factors determined psychiatrists' forensic role and the content of expert psychiatric testimony in this period?[5]

For the twentieth century, psychiatrists' participation in capital cases has received some attention, as has the expansion of psychiatry into pre-trial clinics and other quasi-judicial bodies.[6] But for the beginnings of the field in Ontario, from about 1870 to 1900, there has been little examination of how the psychiatric expert-witness role or content of the insanity defence changed over time.[7]

The related and larger issue is the power of psychiatrists to shape not only outcomes in particular criminal cases but the legal and cultural meanings of insanity, guilt, and innocence. It is received wisdom that alienists, as early psychiatrists called themselves, have helped to shape gender, class, and race identities, in and out of asylums. And historians have noted the limited power of ordinary witnesses, family and community, and criminal lunatics themselves to offset official and medical narratives of deviance.[8] Yet when Canadian scholars have reconstructed particular court cases featuring insanity defences, alienists are depicted as frustrated in their professional and medical ambitions. Martin Friedland's study of the Valentine Shortis murder trial in 1895 also underlined the marginal status of medical knowledge in the face of political and social factors.[9] In the most famous trial in Canadian history, the treason trial of Louis Riel, Daniel Clark's expert testimony for the defence is usually depicted as irrelevant to the outcome.[10] In general, the law was gathering strength as the profession that provided the administrative and cultural framework for the management of deviance. But was it the law versus medicine, as alienists themselves claimed?[11]

This chapter argues, first, that alienists were formidable actors in Ontario's criminal justice system, in and out of the courtroom. They did not wield power through any fixed authority as expert witnesses; instead, by pre- and post-trial services to the state, both formal and informal, they established their superior status as experts in insanity over other types of medical witnesses. With lawyers and other justice officials, they negotiated the reception of medico-legal constructs on a foundation of common professional cause. By the end of the nineteenth century, psychiatrists had earned a secure role in the justice system.

Secondly, the early psychiatrists were powerful shapers of the meanings of crime and insanity, perhaps more so in Ontario than in other jurisdictions. Despite their position on the defence side of the courtrooms, Ontario alienists like Joseph Workman, Daniel Clark, and Richard M. Bucke were forensic conservatives who helped to curtail the use of the insanity defence, and even of mental disorder as a mitigating factor, in trials for murder. Their testimony and their silences confirm that the province's first forensic psychiatrists applied medical and criminological theory to further personal, professional, and class interests.

Under English common law, on which Canadian common and statute law is based, a person legally insane at the time of commission of an act prohibited by law cannot be held responsible.[12] This is because the law insists on "moral guilt," *mens rea*, as a necessary element of culpability: only wrong actions that are freely chosen deserve punishment. In general, in the nineteenth century in Britain and its colonies, common law defined the mental state of intent as a function of intellect. As in the famous McNaughton rules of 1843, the usual question for the jury was "did the defendant 'know the nature and quality of the act he was doing,' and if he did know it, did he 'know he was doing what was wrong?'"[13]

However, in English practice at mid-century in criminal courtrooms, the principle of *mens rea* was freshly subject to varying interpretations; this openness was a consequence of reforms in punishment and criminal justice procedures.[14] Doctors, juries, lay witnesses, and particularly lawyers, in their expanded role as counsel for the defence from 1836,[15] pushed to enlarge what constituted legal insanity by adding temporary madness and partial insanities, particularly delusions and disorders of the emotions and the will.[16] Controversy about what tests could be used to determine capacity and responsibility travelled from the United States and Britain to the colony, and by the 1840s the issue of insanity as a medico-legal problem appeared in a small but significant and growing number of criminal trials.[17]

In early Ontario[18] as elsewhere, doctors were called on to assist the courts in establishing the mental status of a person accused of crime, and as their authority grew, medical testimony became indispensable in support of an insanity plea by about 1870. However, mid-century medical witnesses were rarely asylum doctors, despite their experience with the insane, in contrast to the pattern in England and the United States.[19] Alienists from the asylums in Toronto (opened 1841) and London (1859) appeared in criminal trials infrequently and only late in the century – the 1870s – relative to the history of their institutions.[20] Even the medical men of Rockwood Asylum, Kingston (1855), which housed a larger proportion of criminal lunatics than any other provincial asylum into the 1880s, almost never testified. Instead, the prosecution (and defence until the mid-1870s) relied on local jail doctors, who were both cheaply available to the courts and experienced in the identification of the insane (jails being the institutions of first and sometimes only resort for the mentally disturbed).[21]

At first, this absence suited asylum doctors. As illustrated by the attitudes of Joseph Workman, Canada's most famous alienist of the nineteenth century,[22] early psychiatrists were interested more in therapeutics than in medical jurisprudence, and they were fearful of losing hard-earned public support for their young asylums through contamination with prisoners. Workman forced the government to make separate institutional arrangements for criminal lunatics from 1855,[23] as juries were acquitting defendants on the grounds of insanity in small but significant numbers.[24]

Further, there was not much professional incentive for alienists to appear in criminal courtrooms. They enjoyed a state-endorsed monopoly over the care of the insane: in Ontario there was no competition from either the religious sector, as in Quebec[25] and France,[26] or from doctors operating private asylums, as in England and the United States, until 1884. On the contrary, Ontario asylum men were determined to avoid the experience of their American colleagues in the 1860s, where on the stand and in the press, medical experts were subjected to withering criticism of their personal and professional ethics for defending rich killers.[27] In the 1860s Workman himself may have been put off criminal court work by his civil court experience of judges unimpressed by his claims to special knowledge in cases over contested wills.[28] A rash of malpractice cases in Ontario in the same years did not improve relations between the professions.[29]

The asylum doctors had other responsibilities in criminal justice that may have predisposed them to keep out of criminal courtrooms. Alienists were consulted by the justice system in less-publicized pre- and post-trial assessments as often as they appeared in public, usually to establish whether an accused was mentally fit to stand trial or to undergo punishment. The federal Cabinet sometimes requested expert opinion on the state of mind of a person convicted of a capital offence when it decided either to commute a death sentence or to allow it to stand. Post-trial work for the federal Department of Justice paid well compared to testifying: $100 plus expenses for a few hours' interviews, reviews of trial transcripts, and a report on the sanity or insanity of a prisoner at the time of the interview.[30] This was a very large sum when compared to the $300 annually that a junior asylum doctor earned at that time, and possibly ten times the going per diem rate for defence witnesses.[31] Appearing in trials seems to have disqualified an alienist from lucrative official post-trial work in any given case. It is most important, of course, to remember that each of these asylum superintendents held his appointment at the discretion of the provincial government, the same government that managed the court system.

Workman's expert-witness career began in 1873, two years before his retirement, when he was at the peak of his reputation and power. His timing and written explanations suggest a mix of selflessness and self-interest. He may finally have felt free to intervene at the trial stage to prevent the conviction and unjust punishment of lunatics.[32] In a few cases in our period, alienists petitioned Department of Justice officials and gave newspaper interviews in the hope of preventing the execution of killers they considered severely disordered, though as we will see, they also fought to have the full weight of the law imposed on other convicts.[33]

Workman was hoping to duplicate in Ontario the role that some European specialists attained, that of "friend and helper of the Court, and not of either of the litigants before it."[34] The impartial and well-compensated "friend" would enjoy an exclusive and mandated status, comparable to the relatively unfettered power Workman enjoyed as medical superintendent of the Toronto Asylum. He probably hoped to gain financially rewarding work as an expert witness and to promote his new career as consulting psychiatrist in private practice, an ambition that excited leading English alienists at the time.[35] Lastly, as we will see, he wished to fight the spread of certain medico-legal constructs that were beginning to appear in Ontario courtrooms.

When Workman and other alienists appeared in trials, nearly eight times out of ten between 1873 and 1900 they were called by the defence. The Crown was not often motivated to pay for expert opinion because defendants were tried under a presumption of sanity. Despite this lopsided burden, the defence market was meagre, and not only because of competition from local doctors. Most defendants, especially those whose mental disorder had interfered with their earning abilities, could afford expert testimony only in homicide cases, where the expense could be weighed against a possible trip to the gallows.[36] For lesser offences, defendants and their families often preferred to risk a fixed sentence in jail or prison, rather than the shame and uncertainty of an indeterminate incarceration in an asylum or jail, the likely outcome of a successful insanity plea. Alienists almost never appeared for female defendants, partly because women rarely committed serious crimes of violence except for infanticide. Further, because juries were famously reluctant to convict mothers in infant and child murders, there was little need to resort to the insanity defence.[37] In sum, when Workman, Clark, and Bucke testified as experts, it was usually in homicides, where the accused were almost always men and where the stakes were high for both the Crown and the defendant.

Though they appeared for defendants, their desire to be "friends of the court" led them to assist the prosecution's case, indirectly and directly, as several lawyers and their accused clients learned to their cost. Alienist ambitions in the nineteenth century were not at first constrained by the modern notion of privileged communication between doctor and patient, especially where crime was involved. Legal and medical tracts on professional ethics were more concerned with duty to the court than to the client or patient,[38] an indication of the importance of the state in the development of professional authority. In perhaps his first appearance as a defence witness, and without being asked by either side, Workman volunteered evidence that helped to convict that defendant of murder.[39]

A few years later, in the 1873 trial of James Carruthers, who killed his wife, Workman was the only medical witness for the defence, but the defendant could not have fared worse had there been no insanity defence. The doctor's ambivalence was plain in his testimony: "He may have delusions and yet be sound in other matters ... [in cross-examination] I do not say that he is insane now, but his mental capacity is low ... I can hardly express a decided opinion in his state."[40] In his private diary, Workman wrote that hanging was a "proper" fate for Carruthers, whom he suspected of feigning.[41] Indeed, Carruthers died on the scaffold.

Alienists' testimony provides many examples of qualifying phrases that diluted their testimony for the defence. They justified these responses, first, as the proper answer to the inadequacies of questions. Workman and most alienists argued that the legal test, based on intellectual functioning, reflected a metaphysical and outmoded notion of behaviour as the willed and voluntary product of reason alone.[42] Many residents of the asylum could distinguish right and wrong, he and other alienists testified. Further, responsibility, like disorder, existed on a continuum and should be matched to degrees of punishment. The arbitrary nature of homicide law in particular – that disordered defendants were either completely innocent by reason of insanity or guilty and condemned to death – seemed to fly in the face of medical knowledge that the body affected the mind.[43]

But incomplete and obfuscating testimony may also have been a strategy aimed at the legal audience in order to raise the level of compensation for expert witnesses. Workman considered himself poorly paid for his knowledge.[44] In 1873 he fumed that all he received for his seven days spent examining an accused murderer, attending his trial, and testifying, at the state's request, was "my Railway fares and hotel disbursements, and not a farthing for my professional opinion or evidence, or for the inflictions of a myriad of bugs in the Peterboro hotel."[45] It was both a common-law tradition and cost-conscious practice that witnesses (including experts) were not paid for their testimony by the Crown.[46] When they were subpoenaed by the defence, though the consensus in medico-legal texts was that they were required to sit in court and take the stand, medical writers advised doctors that they could not be compelled to provide their *expert*, considered opinion if unpaid. Instead, American medico-legal rhetoric advised that they give "impromptu answers" or refuse to commit to a position.[47]

Hesitation was sometimes an admission that science and medicine could not penetrate the mind's secrets. To the key question "could the defendant distinguish between right or wrong?" at the time of the offence, psychiatrists occasionally responded that they could not project backwards into the past or that they needed more observation of the defendant. Yet when an alienist did express a strong opinion, it was not necessarily the product of clinical signs or mainly medical theory. For example, Workman applied class-based criteria to separate lunatics from feigners. In 1873 James Fox was arrested minutes after he slit the throat of his ex-employer's wife. There had been a dispute about wages, but no comforting, rational explanation of the crime could be sustained because Fox had also killed a small boy who happened to be present. In response to rumours about the defendant's strangeness and paranoid delusions, the Crown called on Workman to examine the accused before the trial. The interview went badly. Fox ignored some of the alienist's questions, and when he did respond, it was with insolence. He called Workman "Dr Blackleg" (swindler) and "Impostor" and suggested Workman look in the jail chamber pot for his fees.[48]

Fox had insulted the alienist's professional as well as his personal authority. The therapeutics of psychiatry in the nineteenth century required an imbalance of power between patient and doctor, constituted most obviously in alienists' control over treatment in the asylum. Clinicians were to discipline and dominate by the force of their personalities.[49] Workman was proud of his professional, charismatic bearing and piercing eye.[50] It is not surprising, then, that Fox's small mutiny cost him everything. On the basis of two interviews lasting less than fifteen minutes each, Workman testified that "the tenor of his manner & language led me to the conclusion he was simulating ... he was a humbug throughout."[51] Other medical witnesses, one with a "great deal of anxiety," agreed. Fox was found guilty, and despite the judge's and Crown attorney's support for commutation and an invitation from the federal government to Workman to reconsider his opinion, he was hanged.

One expression of Workman's moral and legal conservatism, similar to that of the first generation of asylum superintendents in England and in the United States,[52] was his opposition to the lawyer-led defence of moral insanity. For its proponents, it was a disease that affected the parts of the mind that governed moral behaviour but left other faculties intact; Workman attacked it in medical journal articles as a vaguely defined construct associated with the junk science of phrenology.[53] According to him, it incorrectly medicalized "moral abnormality, or utter disregard of the proprieties and conventionalities of social life."[54] Though the term appeared in asylum documents in Ontario from at least 1848, unlike in the United States, it was rarely used in the courts until the 1870s, the first decade in which the majority of Ontario insanity defendants were represented by lawyers.[55]

Further, the construct brought the threat of non-asylum medical witnesses claiming special expertise.[56] In the trial of wealthy farmer Christopher Ward for the murder of his wife in 1876, Workman and two other defence experts emphasized Ward's paranoid delusions as the proof of his insanity and as the engine of his frenzied violence. However, the defendant's attending physician, also called by the defence, testified that Ward suffered not merely from intellectual impairment but also from moral insanity. As a defence witness in a Toronto murder trial in 1880, Charles Berryman, a professor of medical jurisprudence, described moral insanity as "a moral perversion ... the brain or appendages might be so diseased, that a man might know the difference between right and wrong."[57] Both these trials resulted in guilty verdicts. Workman was probably referring to the Ward trial among others when he wrote a few years later that the diagnosis of moral insanity was "death-bearing": its mention earned the wrath of judges, encouraged juries to convict, and allowed politicians to hang those convicted of capital crimes.[58] But he also used his criticism of moral insanity to affirm the forensic expertise of alienists above other kinds of medical men.

In the Alden murder trial of 1876, Workman's same-side opponent was Richard Bucke, the freshly appointed medical superintendent of the asylum in Hamilton, Ontario. Bucke was the first Ontario alienist to offer mental deficiency, rather than disorder, as a defence against a murder charge. All the defence medical men involved in the trial accepted that Francis Alden, the son of a wealthy American family, functioned at a low intellectual level, and they testified that his ability to know right from wrong was limited. Both Workman and Bucke were obviously influenced by the Italian criminologists (Lombroso's *L'uomo delinquente* had just been published), who claimed that deviant tendencies could be detected in morphological signs such as asymmetry of head and chest.[59] On the stand, Workman said that Alden's body and particularly heart abnormalities could be physical signs of insanity. However, Bucke undercut Workman by stating that these same "imperfections" spoke not to insanity but to congenital defect. The younger man may have been influenced by expert testimony in a notorious Italian multiple murder case of that year.[60] "I think," Bucke proclaimed, "that intellectually he is almost an idiot, and that morally he is an idiot."[61] However, Workman understood what Bucke did not: courts accepted only the most severely intellectually impaired under the defence of natural imbecility, and moral idiocy (like moral insanity and other "lesions of the will") rarely impressed courts. Alden was found guilty, although the alienists' testimony and recommendations to mercy from jury and judge led to a commutation.

In the Ward and Alden trials, the defence faced the problem of its own witnesses disagreeing. However, early courtroom battles more often pitted alienists for the defence against jail doctors for the prosecution, and the skirmishes could continue outside the courtroom. During the McConnell murder trial in 1876, Workman directed the jury's attention to a scar on the defendant's head, saying, "Every man who has had his skull fractured is on the high road to insanity."[62] The jury found the defendant guilty, and he was hanged. After the execution, Workman was incensed to learn that "a certain chatty medical gentleman," probably the Hamilton jail surgeon, had been telling all who were interested that Workman's opinion in the case had been disproved by the post-mortem. Workman tried to refute the story during a presentation to other doctors. While waving a cross-section of McConnell's skull before his audience, he claimed that a plaster cast taken immediately after the execution "showed not a trace of the fracture," and he asked his audience to "guess how the one exhibited to me became so nicely smoothed down."[63]

Workman saw skulduggery everywhere, not only among his medical confreres. Especially, he resented the "odium" cast upon him "by a rabid and bloodthirsty Press"[64] (the Toronto *Globe* retaliated by accusing him of dosing society with "sickly drivel ... under the shallow disguise of science, falsely so-called").[65] Yet the transcripts show that he was usually treated with respect on the witness stand.[66] Despite his satisfaction with the hangings of Fox and Carruthers, after disappointing verdicts in the Ward, Alden, and McConnell trials of 1876, he effectively left forensic psychiatry.[67]

Daniel Clark succeeded Workman as medical superintendent of the Toronto Asylum (he held the post from 1875 to 1905) and assumed his place as Canada's foremost forensic psychiatrist of his generation.[68] Clark was noted for his critical forensic writings and teaching and his long expert-witness career, which covered three decades, activities that both shaped forensic psychiatry in Canada and illustrate the forces that shaped it. Like Workman, Daniel Clark aimed for independence from lawyers and tried to stay above the adversarial system. In his early work he refused to divulge his opinion before the trial to counsel that hired him, a policy that usually benefited the Crown because of his moral and legal conservatism.[69] His initial strategy was defensive: he advised doctors to keep to the narrow role that the courts imposed for expert witnesses, that of providing a medical opinion only. It was the job of the jury to determine the legal fact of responsibility. "'Is there insanity?' asks the Court of the medical witness [but] 'Is he responsible?' is an enigma for the judge and jury to solve."[70]

For Clark, the alienist's role was not to prevent every injustice. In one early case he "was subpoenaed by the Crown, but the Queen's council [sic] knowing that my opinion would be that this man showed evidence of insanity, I was not put in the witness box." Clark sat in the courtroom without testifying, and he later scorned the defendant's lawyer for not having "sufficient acumen to see that this refusal to examine me by the prosecution was presumptive evidence of my opinion being inimical to the case of the Crown counsel."[71] Yet in another case in which the defence lawyer risked calling Clark without knowing his opinion, it cost the defendant his life. This was the trial of Clark Brown for murder in 1879.[72] After complaining for weeks of head pain and of hearing voices, Brown killed his father and sister with an axe. The defendant's lawyer called Clark to the stand, hoping that he would support the insanity defence – Clark had been subpoenaed but not called by the Crown – but Clark testified that he was sane.

Brown's lawyer offered the jury a defence of temporary insanity brought on in part by "self-abuse." The strategy was reasonable: well-known psychiatric ideas linked masturbation to mental disorder, and temporary insanity defences occasionally succeeded in the middle decades of the century for alcohol-induced homicide or for infanticide and, later, for lesser offences.[73] However, Clark rejected the existence of a temporary insanity that left no symptoms in the body or the mind. His view typified the growing emphasis in medicine of somatic origins and physical signs of disease. Probably more important, it was the defendant's habit of masturbation that disqualified him from psychiatric support. Clark confirmed that Brown was a masturbator (diagnosed immediately from his "unmanly" shyness and desire for solitude).[74] Whereas Workman's age cohort was relatively unexcited about the habit,[75] Clark and many late-century doctors (and other Canadians) believed that "onanism" was a badge of vice, a self-imposed addiction.[76] Other doctors called by the defence agreed with Clark's diagnosis of sanity, and some backed off their earlier opinions of insanity. As Clark proudly told the court during another murder trial three years later, "I discovered the assimulation [in Brown] and pronounced it as such and he was executed."[77]

Clark increasingly feared being "foxed" by defendants, and the resulting repercussions on his professional status and on public support for his asylum.[78] He told courtrooms and medical students that very often the insanity plea was attempted by "people with gross natures – who belong to the criminal classes, in which a sense of right and wrong is very much blunted,"[79] but not enough to earn Clark's support in the courtroom. Consequently, he typically qualified his testimony in support of insanity by stating, "assuming ... that the prisoner ... is not a malingerer." (This response usually triggered an enthusiastic pursuit of the possibility by the prosecution.[80])

Clark's caution intensified in the early 1880s in the aftermath of two notorious trials outside Ontario that generated a backlash against the insanity defence.[81] In October 1881 Quebec asylum doctor Henry Howard testified for the defence in the trial of Hugh Hayvern, who had killed a fellow prisoner. Influenced by French criminology and American neurology, Howard favoured a "criminal hereditary neurosis"[82] that generally explained and, more radically, excused crime. He argued that Hayvern had killed out of "epileptic impulse and not reason," and he regarded the defendant's criminal history and inebriety as more signs of his poisoned heredity.[83] Howard's radical testimony compromised his career,[84] although he wrote and presented extensively, trying to justify his position.[85] Despite the attention the case received in American medical journals[86] and a lengthy critical editorial in the Montreal medical press,[87] his diagnosis was met with resounding silence by most of his Ontario colleagues.

Alienists were sensitive to response to the Hayvern trial because it took place in the months after the assassination of American president James Garfield by the alleged lunatic Charles Guiteau.[88] Throughout this spectacular trial, Canadian asylum doctors – and newspaper editors – generally agreed with the prosecution asylum experts that Guiteau was sane.[89] They followed the acrimonious battle of experts and the ridicule that expert witnesses faced in the American courtrooms. In a dramatic newspaper interview, Bucke commented that Charles Guiteau was a "moral idiot ... totally destitute of moral qualities." In statements that illustrate that adherence to

a Lombrosian determinism did not lead to a soft stance on deviants, he proclaimed that Guiteau should be "killed as a protection to society – killed
just as you would kill a wild beast or a rattlesnake."[90] Bucke's animal
metaphors show that Lombrosian atavism – the concept that criminal man
was a throwback to an earlier stage of human development – had arrived
in Ontario, in its harshest expression.[91]

One year later, when Frederick Mann murderously attacked the Cooke
family in January 1883, the embarrassments and dangers of professional
discord must have been fresh in the minds of Daniel Clark and Richard
Bucke. The young hired hand had killed his employers and two of their
children by strangulation and with an axe, and had attacked another three
members of the Cooke family.[92] Doctors Clark and Bucke were called in by
the defence before the trial. The lawyer's detailed notes for a defence of
"uncontrollable irresistible impulse," with sample questions addressed to
Bucke, is strong evidence that Bucke originally agreed to testify for the
defence.[93] Yet according to Clark, neither doctor ever saw any evidence of
unsoundness: Mann displayed his sanity by chatting amiably with the
alienists on social philosophy and "good naturedly criticized" Richard
Bucke's own work, *Man's Moral Nature*.[94] Thereafter Clark informed both
sides that they would testify to sanity if called to the stand. The defence
lawyer advised his young client to withdraw his plea of not guilty. The
nineteen-year-old, whom the press called "the boy-murderer," was consequently hanged without any evidence being heard.[95]

In the Mann case Clark and Bucke placed professional solidarity ahead
of the defendant's right to a public trial of his innocence by reason of insanity. Under Daniel Clark's personal authority, boosted by the small number
of alienists and the hierarchical asylum structure in Ontario, alienists never
sat on opposite sides of the courtroom from each other in murder trials
from the Mann trial until at least 1900.[96] This strategy was meant to safeguard claims to objective, scientific knowledge, though it left doctors vulnerable to cross-examination on collusion.

The Mann case also illustrates that alienists had strong powers over the
fate of defendants even without testifying; they could and did prevent the
issue of insanity from coming into the courtroom in this and several other
cases.[97] Further, by so doing, they could prevent insanity from becoming a
reason for commutation of a death sentence (medical commissions to investigate the state of mind of a convict were struck only where the matter
became part of the evidence). Despite increases in Ontario's population and
prosecutions, the absolute number of murder trials in which the defendant's sanity was an issue declined by more than a third from the 1870s to

the 1880s.[98] (This drop no doubt reflects defence disillusionment with its success rate.)

The practice of forensic psychiatry was conducted not only in the court-rooms and in examining rooms of prisons and jails but in the newspapers, as Clark and Bucke promoted their public hygiene function.[99] The press reported that Mann had flown into a passion in "revenge for a fancied insult" after he was reminded that he was only a servant and not a family member.[100] With the help of journalists, Clark confirmed this motive. Mann was a person with "keen intelligence ... but low moral nature ... [the] type of man found everyday," he warned.[101] The message was clear: dangerous insurgents try to abuse the insanity defence, but alienists can detect the frauds.

It is probable that a political crisis closer to home had also been chilling the reception of insanity defendants in Ontario courts from at least 1876. In that year Louis Riel, the French Canadian leader of the Red River uprising and a murderer in the eyes of many Ontarians, had entered Beauport Asylum in Quebec. Ontario newspaper editors rumbled about false claims of insanity used to forestall criminal charges.[102] In 1885, after leading an armed rebellion, Riel was captured and tried for treason, in the most notorious trial and most famous insanity defence in Canadian history.[103] Daniel Clark was the main defence witness, and two aspects of his testimony are significant.[104] First, Clark, as usual, kept to a conservative definition of legal insanity as intellectual defect. He stated that Riel's acts of treason were rooted in "egotistic" delusions ("no sane man would have imagined that he could come into the Saskatchewan, and that he could gather around him such a force as would enable him to become monarch of this country").[105] Here and in other trials Clark advocated the "product test" as an improvement on the right-wrong knowledge test.[106] Formulated by the American alienist Isaac Ray but also a part of juridical discourse on insanity in England, this was a careful and limiting standard.[107] Its reassuring thrust was that the presence of severe mental disorder alone did not justify an acquittal: only if the crime was an outcome, a direct product, of the insanity should it be excused. However, in lukewarm testimony, Clark admitted that Riel was sane according to the present law and, typically, refused to provide an opinion on the accused's legal responsibility.[108]

Clark's testimony also demonstrates the importance of germ theory in his thinking on psychopathology; he used it to narrow what would qualify as insanity and assigned other disorder to vice.[109] True insanity, a disease, was the product of an external force or agent, such as a germ or bacterium, with a predictable course of symptoms. The "real" insane person could be detected by the mental normalcy that preceded the crime and often appeared at lucid intervals. For Clark, Riel was a recurrent maniac who moved in and out of states of delusional unsoundness: "these peculiarities come and go with the invasion of disease and departure of the corporeal abnormal condition," he told the court.[110] Only when his illness was active could it exempt a defendant from punishment, and Clark argued that lunatics who committed crimes during lucid intervals should be punished as sane.[111] Insanity, then, was not to be confused with an inherited, permanent condition. In newspaper interviews, Clark contrasted Riel, the insane delusionary, with Charles Guiteau, the sane "crank," a man with a long and continuous history of peculiarity, who had assassinated President Garfield in 1881 in order to "save the Republic," as instructed by God.[112] Riel, of course, was hanged, against the protests of all of French Canada and many other citizens and international observers. Always a civics lesson and often narrowly political, the Cabinet decision to withhold or bestow mercy on convicted murderers for many years after the Riel trial had to be weighed for its potential impact on French-English politics and national unity.[113]

The core of Clark's and Bucke's etiological thinking, and therefore of their forensic logic, was a mix of moralism, social Darwinism, atavism, and degeneration, with heredity the dark connecting thread.[114] English doctors had used heredity to explain criminal insanity at least from the Oxford trial of 1840,[115] and Canadian medical men were writing heredity into medicolegal topics by the 1850s.[116] However, it gained a stranglehold on causal explanations with degeneration and later with Lombrosian atavism.[117] Clark believed in a Lamarckian transmission down generations of a general or constitutional weakness, whose toxic products included most individual and social pathology.[118] For him, degeneration explained but did not excuse criminality (or insanity or epilepsy).[119] His courtroom work to the 1890s reflects the French alienist Valentin Magnan's views and Cesare Lombroso's early doctrine that it was possible, through vigilance over one's base instincts, thoughts, and actions, to overcome defective heredity. Delusions, Clark believed, could be either resisted or "indulged,"[120] and mental disorder therefore was at root a moral defect and a desertion of public duty. Accordingly, he at first valued punishment as a deterrent and considered that rehabilitation could be achieved in institutions, whether they be asylums, industrial schools, or workhouses for drunkards.[121]

Addiction to vice, sexual "excess," and drunkenness, thought to switch on the degeneration process,[122] disqualified some defendants from insanity defences. Neither Clark nor any other Ontario alienist testified for the defence, as far as I am aware, in any case of sexual violence, no matter how deranged the accused.[123] Alienists' opinions varied where accused killers were also were condemned for alcoholism or drunkenness. Across the Western medical world, doctors debated whether inebriety was a medical or moral defect, and in Quebec alienists were willing to consider it a mitigating factor.[124] In 1873 Joseph Workman had been willing to testify that alcohol-induced homicide could be a product of functional or temporary insanity.[125] But the temperance movement was gaining strength; by the 1890s much of Ontario was "dry." In the province, Richard Bucke took the hardest line. He led the campaign against alcohol use in asylums, and testified only for the prosecution in trials for alcohol-related homicides, one of which ended in a hanging.[126]

For Clark, inebriety magnified guilt where the defendant belonged to the lowest social classes. In the case of Benjamin Parrott, who killed his elderly mother with an axe on a Hamilton street in 1899, Clark insisted on the full force of punishment. He and another doctor examined Parrott before the trial at the request of the attorney general and pronounced him sane. Although lay testimony revealed that the defendant was known as a "nutter" and "Crazy Parrott," no medical evidence of his state of mind was introduced at the brief trial. He was found guilty and sentenced to death. When Clark learned of a petition asking for Parrott's sentence to be commuted to life imprisonment on the grounds of his mental state, the alienist informed the minister of justice that he did not support it. He concluded, "Both Dr. Russell [another asylum superintendent] and myself could find no insanity in the man and no evidence that he is otherwise than a drunken human brute."[127] Two other asylum doctors, appointed to a medical commission, soon concurred that Parrott was sane.[128] Not surprisingly, he was hanged on schedule, one month later.

Clark's observations in the Parrott reports suggest how completely atavism justified his class-based moralism.[129] Though he wrote that idiots, imbeciles, epileptics, and the feeble-minded should not be held fully responsible because they lacked higher types of reasoning, few alleged lunatics that Clark met in the dock were members of categories that deserved to be excused from crime.[130] Thus in 1886, when John Rivennes was on trial for killing a fellow transient, Clark warned his lawyer that he would testify against the accused. For Clark, Rivennes was a type "saturated with laziness and cupidity, because of which a living is procured at the expense of the honest workers of society": he was morally guilty as well as medically sane.[131]

Clark's stern medico-moral judgments expressed and probably boosted an anxiety about deviants shared by many elements of society. During the second half of the nineteenth century, the early Victorian optimistic belief in the curative asylum and the reforming prison faded in the face of the recidivism of crime and the chronic nature of much mental disorder. Clark's prime, the 1870s through the 1890s, coincided with a period of anti-professional popular sentiment in Ontario.[132] If in elite discourse in Anglo-American jurisdictions, criminal man was also reconstructed as a creature of stunted heredity and toxic environments, in Ontario this view did not translate into milder treatment for deviants.[133] A relatively high proportion of Ontario's convicted murderers were hanged, and penitentiary regimes for criminal lunatics may have been crueller than in other jurisdictions.[134] In England, criminal justice regulations made medical examination mandatory in suspect cases, and a new verdict of "guilty but insane," introduced in 1883, had the effect of encouraging English jurists to be receptive to the insanity defence.[135] In Scotland and in various states of the United States, judges were willing to entertain broader definitions of insanity than McNaughtan.[136] In Canada, however, the Criminal Code of 1892 retained the standard verdicts and its insanity provisions were interpreted by an increasingly hostile Ontario judiciary.[137] Judges applied stringent procedural rules, tighter standards of proof, and a reverential and narrow reading of the McNaughten test: the jury was sometimes told that if the defendant knew only that he was breaking the law, he was legally sane.[138] The provincial justice system's harsh response may have arisen in fears aroused by working-class unrest worsened by the late-century depression, rural depopulation, and national insecurity; but surely the alienists' mix of moralism and scientific determinism offered a medical imprimatur for those who urged tighter sanctions on the marginal classes.

If one purpose of alienists' forensic work was to block access to the insanity defence to certain social types, another was to mitigate the sanctions that threatened deserving defendants through the use of parallel constructs differently applied. Clark considered that alcoholism was a true disease among respectable citizens only.[139] In 1896 he testified for well-off defendant V.R. Lapointe that his drinking "sprees" were probably unconnected with his paranoia and, indeed, with the deadly shooting spree he had conducted on the streets of Brockville.[140] In place of the discredited disease entity called temporary insanity, Clark preferred impulsive insanity, a disease of the will that erupted without warning into a fit of homicidal mania. The victim of irresistible impulse was an automaton, driven to an act despite full knowledge that it was wrong. British alienist Henry Maudsley's concept was controversial and his name was not cited, though the concept was used on the stand.[141] To diagnose impulsive insanity, Clark advocated the "control test":[142] the relevant question was "could the defendant have controlled his behaviour?" When the defendant belonged to the respectable classes, Clark's answer was no. Like other late-century alienists, he argued that when crime was triggered by a "sudden impulse to deviate from the well-beaten track of a life-long rectitude" as opposed to "an ingrained vicious nature," guilt was mitigated or removed.[143] This stress on change in character as a symptom of disease was not new, but it was emphasized in current Anglo-American and European criminological and psychiatric discourse.[144]

Domestic killers who were motivated by deep grief and anxiety were also considered to be in the grip of irresistible impulse. Such a man was the well-connected William Harvey, who killed his wife and daughters in a fit of despair in 1889, though alienists' participation in the Harvey trial may also have been driven by their desire to support an embarrassed colleague.[145] A phalanx of Ontario's top asylum men – Clark, Workman, C.K. Clarke of the Kingston Asylum, and Stephen Lett from the private Homewood Retreat near Guelph[146] – testified that Harvey was sane at the time of his trial but insane during the triple killing. However, the psychiatrists' alliance wobbled over the type of insanity that Harvey suffered from. Lett said that Harvey erupted in "an explosion of nerve force" but returned to normal immediately after the slayings, a classic Maudsleyan impulsive insanity. Clark (and Clarke) believed that the symptoms of a homicidal mania should have lasted beyond the killing: how else to distinguish legitimate disease from a sudden dethronement of reason by passion?

The disagreement also reflected that Harvey was a less-than-ideal candidate for an insanity defence: though he had once been respectable, he was always peculiar (a masturbator according to the local jail doctor), and at the time of the killings he was facing bankruptcy and an embezzling charge. Stephen Lett, the local asylum doctor, had a personal involvement that made his diagnosis of fleeting insanity seem self-serving. The doctor had posted bail for Harvey on an embezzling charge the night before the killings, and he insisted Harvey had been sane at that time; but within a few hours he had apparently gone mad, killed his family, and recovered again. As a local newspaper opined, "rot!!!"[147] The jury rejected the opinions of the top alienists in Canada, as did the Cabinet. Neither Lett nor Workman testified in a murder trail again. Harvey was hanged, though thousands signed a petition for commutation.

Creative medical defences against murder charges were possible – and beginning in the 1890s, more often successful – where the defendant's family could afford them.[148] Albert Wilson was tried in 1893 for the

murder four years earlier of his sweetheart, Mary Jane Marshall. Daniel
Clark was the star defence witness who applied a modified temporary
insanity diagnosis and tapped into the late-century acceptance of unconscious acts to reconfigure the homicide as the fruit of disease. He testified
that Wilson had inherited a strong family weakness towards insanity, a
"want of inhibiting power" that broke out into full-blown physical disease
– homicidal mania – when Marshall told Wilson that she would not marry
him. This medical narrative stripped all malice and intent from the story,
though Wilson had earlier threatened to kill the girl. For Clark, Wilson's
ingenious escape immediately after the killing may have been an act, not
of criminality, but of the cunning of a "fixed physical" disease, impulsive
insanity. Tapping into the growing popular and medical concept of the
unconscious, Clark stated that there was no doubt that Wilson was "not
himself" at the time of the crime: the alienist considered that Wilson's four
years of evading the law while living under an assumed name in the United
States were markers of an absence state.[149] Though Clark stated that
Wilson "must have known he was breaking the law of the land if he
intended to take life ... taking all the facts sworn to be true – there is no
doubt in my own mind he was insane."[150] This was Clark's first trial
victory: Wilson was found not guilty by reason of insanity, with the help
of the persuasive defence counsel B.B. Osler. The verdict enraged many
observers. One woman wrote to an editor that "now it would be open
season on girls." [151] Clark himself may have had second thoughts about
his part in the trial; he never wrote up the Wilson case for presentation or
publication.

These better orchestrated defences of the 1890s indicate that the role of
the expert psychiatric witness was changing. Lawyers were more firmly in
charge of defence strategies, and Ontario alienists adjusted to their subor-
dinate role in the adversarial courtroom as friend of the defence, if not of
the court. Clark had reconsidered the responsibilities of witnesses to their
clients; he regularly informed lawyers or prosecutors of his opinion before
court, and he advised his students to do the same.[152] On the stand, he ven-
tured beyond his medical opinion to give judges and juries his legal opinion
on responsibility. By the 1880s alienists had crowded out jail doctors,
medical school teachers, and private practitioners as competent defence
experts in murder trials.[153] The domination of services to the insane by
public officials based in segregative institutions meant that no competition
to forensic psychiatry arose in Ontario to speak for the criminally insane.
Environmental ideas of the causation of crime – poverty, maltreatment,
poor nutrition – had begun to circulate in medical and official networks.

But it was prison inspectors, not psychiatrists or jail doctors, who worried that the spectacle of a ravaged "brain-softened" murderer, convicted with the help of Bucke's expert testimony, could damage the image of justice.[154]

There were, of course, many factors relating to the crime, victim, place of trial, and presiding judge that influenced the verdict and outcome of murder trials other than the expert-witness evidence. But alienists were indeed "loaded revolvers," in Workman's phrase. Subject to the very real constraints of the legal system, they employed lethal power – more than they acknowledged, as the example of Daniel Clark shows. When Clark told defence lawyers that he would not support an insanity defence, no such defence was attempted.[155] Where he testified or reported that an accused was sane, that man was hanged.[156] Where he testified strongly for the defence in homicides, in four of nine cases the defendants were found not guilty on the grounds of insanity;[157] where the jury found guilt, it was usually moderated with a recommendation to mercy. Of more than two dozen trials in which alienists testified, where they strongly argued the insanity of the defendant in trials, only one convicted murderer (William Harvey) and one traitor (Louis Riel) suffered the full force of the law. Psychiatrists learned to confine their criticism of the justice system to lawyers and juries, and they were careful to exonerate Cabinet, the dispensers of royal mercy, for any miscarriages of justice that occurred.[158] After a hiatus of a dozen years when prison doctors did most of the post-trial reports, Clark's name began to appear again on medical commissions on convicted murderers.[159] In sum, most insanity defences failed, but insanity was an effective mitigating factor, and that state of affairs was as alienists preferred.

A drift away from rancorous interprofessional debate both signalled and promoted this new tolerance for forensic psychiatry. Canadian justice system officials also subscribed to medico-sociological philosophies of risk and segregation.[160] The certainty that long-term confinement would follow encouraged Clark and Bucke to support a few non-insane medical defences for epileptics and young "degenerates."[161] C.K. Clarke, who followed Daniel Clark as head of the Asylum for the Insane in Toronto, lost interest in matters of guilt and innocence. What fascinated him instead was prevention, by which he meant how to minimize the risk to society presented by groups such as immigrants and degenerate juveniles.[162] Forensic psychiatrists, therefore, continued to define themselves as doctors of the public health working in the service of the state.[163] The history of the insanity defence is about the maintenance of order rather than the recognition of human frailty.[164]

The defence of his profession, coupled with his self-assigned duty to protect the social body, first propelled Joseph Workman to appear as an expert witness in murder trials in the 1870s. Imported medical and criminological theories hardened the attitudes of his colleagues Daniel Clark and Richard Bucke to deviance, and the structure of medicine and the justice system in the province encouraged all three men in their conservative practice. In Ontario the first forensic psychiatrists supported the idea of criminal responsibility by unlinking mental disorder from innocence in explanations for serious criminal behaviour, by whittling away the medical bases of insanity defences, and by limiting the social groups that could access these defences. Alienists occasionally provided justification for defences of diminished responsibility, but mainly for the respectable. By rejecting constructs of criminal insanity that spoke to innocence and by enlisting medical theory in the service of full, individual responsibility for the "dangerous classes," Joseph Workman, Daniel Clark, and Richard Bucke led psychiatry in Ontario into a safer place in the criminal justice system of the new century.

NOTES

1 Joseph Workman, "On the Position of Medical Witnesses, Chiefly in Cases of Questionable Insanity" (synopsis of a paper read before members of the Medical Section of the Canadian Institute on 19 November 1869), *Canada Medical Journal and Monthly Record* 6 (1869–70): 289–95.
2 Joseph Workman, "Insanity and Crime," *Canada Lancet* 9, no. 1 (September 1876): 18.
3 Daniel Clark, "A Few Canadian Cases in Criminal Courts in Which the Plea of Insanity Was Presented," *Transactions of the American Medico-Psychological Association* 2 (1896): 178; and "Another Chapter in the History of Canadian Jurisprudence of Insanity," *Transactions of the American Medico-Psychological Association* 4 (1898): 348.
4 S.E.D. Shortt, *Victorian Lunacy: Richard M. Bucke and the Practice of Late Nineteenth-Century Psychiatry* (New York: Cambridge University Press, 1986); Wendy Mitchinson, *The Nature of Their Bodies: Women and Their Doctors in Victorian Canada* (Toronto: University of Toronto Press, 1991), 335–55; Ramsay Cook, *The Regenerators: Social Criticism in Late Victorian Canada* (Toronto: University of Toronto Press, 1985), 85–104; Ian Dowbiggin, "'Keeping This Young Country Sane': C.K. Clarke, Immigration Restriction, and Canadian Psychiatry, 1890–1925," *Canadian Historical Review* 76 (1995): 598–627.

5 The major contributions include Nigel Walker, *Crime and Insanity in England*, vol. 1, *The Historical Perspective* (Edinburgh: Edinburgh University Press, 1968); Charles Rosenberg, *The Trial of the Assassin Guiteau: Psychiatry and the Law in the Gilded Age* (Chicago: University of Chicago Press, 1968); Roger Smith, *Trial by Medicine: Insanity and Responsibility in Victorian Trials* (Edinburgh: Edinburgh University Press, 1981); Ruth Harris, *Murders and Madness: Medicine, Law, and Society in the Fin de Siècle* (Oxford: Clarendon Press, 1989); James Mohr, *Doctors and the Law: Medical Jurisprudence in Nineteenth Century America* (New York: Oxford University Press, 1993); Joel Eigen, *Witnessing Insanity: Madness and Mad-Doctors in the English Court* (New Haven: Yale University Press, 1995).

6 Kimberley White-Mair, "Negotiating Responsibility: Representations of Criminality and Mind-state in Canadian Law, Medicine and Society, 1920–1950" (PhD thesis, University of Toronto, 2001); Jennifer Stephen, "The 'Incorrigible,' the 'Bad,' and the 'Immoral': Toronto's 'Factory Girls' and the Work of the Toronto Psychiatric Clinic," in *Law, Society, and the State: Essays in Modern Legal History*, ed. Louis A. Knafla and Susan W.S. Binnie (Toronto: University of Toronto Press, 1995), 405–42. Robert Menzies, *Survival of the Sanest: Order and Disorder in a Pre-Trial Psychiatric Clinic* (Toronto: University of Toronto Press, 1989); Dorothy E. Chunn and R. Menzies, "Gender, Madness, and Crime: The Reproduction of Patriarchal and Class Relations in a Psychiatric Court Clinic," *Journal of Human Justice* 1 (1990): 33–58; Dowbiggin, "'Keeping This Young Country Sane'"; Guy Grenier, *Les monstres, les fous et les autres: la folie criminelle au Québec* (Montréal: Éditions Trait d'Union, 1999).

7 For Ontario, see Allison Kirk-Montgomery, "Courting Madness: Insanity and Testimony in the Criminal Justice System of Victorian Ontario" (PhD thesis, University of Toronto, 2001). For the history of expert medical testimony, see Thomas Forbes, *Surgeons at the Bailey: English Forensic Medicine to 1878* (New Haven and London: Yale University Press, 1985); M. Clark and C. Crawford, eds., *Legal Medicine in History* (Cambridge: Cambridge University Press, 1994); C.A.G. Jones, *Expert Witnesses: Science, Medicine and the Practice of Law* (Oxford: Clarendon Press, 1995); Mohr, *Doctors and the Law*. For Newfoundland, see Jerry Bannister, "Surgeons and Criminal Justice in Eighteenth-Century Newfoundland," in *Criminal Justice in the Old World and the New: Essays in Honour of J.M. Beattie*, ed. Greg T. Smith, Allyson N. May, and Simon Devereaux (Toronto: Centre of Criminology, 1998).

8 James E. Moran, *Committed to the State Asylum: Insanity and Society in Nineteenth-Century Quebec and Ontario* (Montreal and Kingston: McGill-Queen's University Press, 2000), 141–66; Robert Menzies, "The Making of Criminal Insanity in British Columbia: Granby Farrant and the Provincial Mental Home,

Colquitz, 1919–1933," in *Essays in the History of Canadian Law*, vol. 6, ed. Hamara Foster and John McLaren; Robert Menzies, "Historical Profiles of Criminal Insanity," *International Journal of Law and Psychiatry* 25 (2002): 379–404; Kathleen Kendall, "Criminal Lunatic Women in Nineteenth Century Canada," *Forum on Corrections Research* 11 (September 1999): 46–9. See also Robert Peter Bartlett, "Introduction: New Approaches to Established Themes in the History of Psychiatry," *International Journal of Law and Psychiatry* 25 (2002): 299–302.

9 Martin L. Friedland, *The Case of Valentine Shortis: A True Story of Crime and Politics in Canada* (Toronto: University of Toronto Press, 1986).

10 Simon N. Verdun-Jones, "'Not Guilty by Reason of Insanity': The Historical Roots of the Canadian Insanity Defence, 1843–1920," in *Crime and Criminal Justice in Europe and Canada*, ed. Louis A. Knafla (Waterloo: Wilfrid Laurier Press, 1981), 179–218. For the trial transcript, see *The Queen vs. Louis Riel ... Report of Trial at Regina ...* (Ottawa: Queen's Printer, 1886; CIHM microfiche series no. 30472). Among other works, see Desmond Morton, ed., *The Queen v Louis Riel* (Toronto: University of Toronto Press, 1974); Thomas Flanagan, *Louis "David" Riel: "Prophet of the New World"* (Toronto: University of Toronto Press, 1996); Cyril Greenland, "The Life and Death of Louis Riel. Part II: Surrender, Trial, Appeal and Execution," *Canadian Psychiatric Association Journal* 10, 4 (August 1965): 253–65.

11 Smith, *Trial by Medicine*; Mohr, *Doctors and the Law*; Rosenberg, *Trial of the Assassin Guiteau*; Janet A. Tighe, "The Legal Art of Psychiatric Diagnosis: Searching for Reliability," in *Framing Disease: Studies in Cultural History*, ed. Charles E. Roseberg and Janet Golden (New Brunswick, NJ: Rutgers University Press, 1992), 206–28.

12 For the history of the formal law of insanity, see Verdun-Jones, "'Not Guilty by Reason of Insanity,'" 179–218, and many of the works cited previously.

13 *M'Naghten's Case* [1843] 10 Cl. & Fin. 200, 8 E.R. 718, [1843–60] all E.R., 233. See Richard Moran, *Knowing Right from Wrong: The Insanity Defense of Daniel McNaughtan* (New York: Free Press, 1981).

14 Joel Eigen, *Unconscious Crime: Mental Absence and Criminal Responsibility in Victorian London* (Baltimore: Johns Hopkins University Press, 2003), 158–60.

15 6 William 4, c.44, known as the Felon's Counsel Act. On the rise of defence counsel in England, see J.M. Beattie, "Scales of Justice: Defense Counsel and the English Criminal Trial in the Eighteenth and Nineteenth Centuries," *Law and History Review* 9 (1991): 221–67.

16 For an introduction, see Smith, *Trial by Medicine*, chap. 3. For the mid-century insanity defence as a replacement for provocation defences, see Martin Wiener, "Judges v. Jurors: Courtroom Tensions in Murder Trials and the Law of Criminal

Responsibility in Nineteenth-Century England," *Law and History Review* 17, no. 3 (Fall 1999): 467–505.

17 In the 1850s and 1860s the issue of insanity arose in at least fifteen murder trials per decade. See Kirk-Montgomery, "Courting Madness," chap. 4; also table 7.5: "Jury Verdicts in Murder Cases by Decade, Insanity Trials, Ontario, 19th Century."

18 I use "Ontario" to refer to the jurisdiction that was successively Great Britain's colony of Upper Canada, then Canada West, and from 1867 the province of Ontario in the Dominion of Canada.

19 Eigen, *Witnessing Insanity*, 130–2; Mohr, *Doctors and the Law,* 100.

20 Of the more than two hundred criminal justice events (trials and insanity hearings in Ontario) in the nineteenth century that my research has turned up, alienists testified in only about 10 per cent.

21 Moran, *Committed to the State Asylum,* 79.

22 On Workman, see *Dictionary of Canadian Biography*, vol. 12, s.v. Thomas E. Brown, "Workman, Joseph"; Rainer Baehre, "'The Ill-Regulated Mind': A Study in the Making of Psychiatry in Ontario, 1830–1921" (PhD diss., York University, 1985), 193–287; Christine I.M. Johnston, *Father of Canadian Psychiatry* (Victoria: Ogden Press, 2000).

23 Moran, *Committed to the State Asylum,* 141–66, 150–3.

24 Kirk-Montgomery, "Courting Madness," 227.

25 Moran, *Committed to the State Asylum,* 46–7.

26 Janet Goldstein, *Console and Classify: The French Psychiatric Profession in the Nineteenth Century* (Cambridge: Cambridge University Press, 1987), chap. 5.

27 Mohr, *Doctors and the Law,* 140–53.

28 Workman, "On the Position of Medical Witnesses," 294–5.

29 Ibid., 289.

30 Library and Archives Canada (hereafter LAC) RG 13 vol. 1410, file 67A, H. Bernard to minister of justice, 31 December 1873; LAC, RG 13, vol. 1413, file 91A. Though sources are scant, one prominent American doctor testified in a Canadian court in 1873 that he usually received as a defence witness $30 to $40 per day; see Archives of Ontario (hereafter AO) RG 22-452-2-7, 229–54.

31 For medical income and wealth in the second half of the century in Canada, see R.D. Gidney and W.P.J. Millar, *Professional Gentlemen: The Professions in Nineteenth-Century Ontario* (Toronto: University of Toronto Press, 1994), 189–92.

32 In 1873 the government ignored Workman's recommendation for a temporary respite of the death sentence of the murderer John Tryon. See "Extracts from the Diary of Joseph Workman," ed. Alfred E. Lavell, vol. 1, 1867–82, entry for 9

December 1873, in Academy of Medicine Collection, Thomas Fisher Rare Book Library, University of Toronto.

33 Workman's report resulted in commutation in Hotchkiss 1875; Order-in-Council of 30 November 1875, Privy Council 1192; see Joseph Workman, "Case of Erastus Hotchkiss," *American Journal of Insanity*, January 1876, 405–18. See LAC, RG 13, vol. 1419, file 165A; LAC, RG 13 C-1, vol. 1411, file 77A; and other cases mentioned elsewhere in this paper.

34 Workman, "On the Position of Medical Witnesses," 289.

35 Andrew Scull, Charlotte MacKenzie, and Nicholas Hervey, *Masters of Bedlam: The Transformation of the Mad-Doctoring Trade* (Princeton, NJ: Princeton University Press, 1996), 244–5, 261–2.

36 All twenty-six Ontario trials studied in which alienists gave testimony from 1870 to 1900 were homicides, twenty-four for murder and two for manslaughter. The alienists also appeared in two special hearings to determine the fitness of an accused to stand trial.

37 Constance Backhouse, "Desperate Women and Compassionate Courts: Infanticide in Nineteenth Century Canada," *University of Toronto Law Journal* 34 (1984): 462–4; Mark Jackson, ed., *Historical Perspectives on Child Murder and Concealment, 1550–2000* (Aldershot, UK: Ashgate, 2002); Tony Ward, "The Sad Subject of Infanticide: Law, Medicine and Child Murder, 1860–1938," *Social & Legal Studies* 8, no. 2 (1999): 163–80. Smith, *Trial by Medicine*, 146–85. On juries' gender bias in cases of child killing, see Clark, "A Few Canadian Cases," 183. See also Kirk-Montgomery, "Courting Madness," chap. 6.

38 On lawyers, see W. Wesley Pue, "Becoming 'Ethical': Lawyers' Professional Ethics in Early Twentieth Century Canada," in *Glimpses of Canadian Legal History*, ed. Dale Gibson and W. Wesley Pue (Winnipeg: University of Manitoba Legal Research Institute, 1991), 258.

39 Workman testified on cause of death, not the question of insanity; see Workman, "On the Position of Medical Witnesses," 289–95.

40 LAC, RG 13, vol. 1410, file 65A, transcript 14–5.

41 Workman, "Diary," 182.

42 Workman, "On Crime and Insanity," *Transactions of the Canada Medical Association*, 1877, 5.

43 For other Canadian psychiatrists' complaints on medico-legal relations, see Daniel Clark, "A Psycho-Medical History of Louis Riel," *American Journal of Insanity*, July 1887, 11,15; Daniel Clark, "Medical Evidence in Courts of Law," *Canada Lancet* 11, no. 4 (1 December 1878): 5–6, also published in *American Journal of Insanity*, January 1879; Henry Landor, "Insanity in Relation to Law" (paper read before the Association of Officers of Asylums for the Insane of the United States and Canada, at Toronto, 8 June 1871; London: Daily Free Press,

1871), 22; John H. Arton, "Insanity and Its Medico-legal Aspects," *Canada Lancet* 18, no. 5 (January 1886): 129–31; Henry Howard, "Fools and Their Folly," *Alienist & Neurologist* 6 (1885): 248–61; W.J. McGuigan, "The Criminal Insane – A Change in the Law Required," *Dominion Medical Monthly* 6 (May 1896): 481–5; C.K. Clarke, "Canadian Law in Regard to Responsibility," *Queen's Quarterly* 6 (1898): 279–80.

44 As did English and American medical witnesses. See Mohr, *Doctors and the Law*, 169–79 and elsewhere; James Mohr, "The Origins of Forensic Psychiatry in the United States and the Great Nineteenth-Century Crisis over the Adjudication of Wills," *Journal of the American Academy of Psychiatry and the Law* 25, no. 3 (1997): 280–2. Roger Chadwick, *Bureaucratic Mercy: The Home Office and the Treatment of Capital Cases in Victorian Britain* (New York and London: Garland Publishing, 1992), 97–8. The *Canada Lancet* carried news of the American doctors' battle for just compensation in the courts; see vol. 11, no. 2 (October 1878): 64. See also William Bayard, "Medical Evidence before the Law Courts," *Maritime Medical News* 10 (1898): 269.

45 LAC, RG 13, vol. 1410, file 67A, J. Workman to H. Bernard, deputy minister of justice, 20 December 1873. See also Workman, "Diary," 16 December 1873, 224.

46 R. Vashon Rogers Jr, *Law and Medical Men* (Toronto and Edinburgh: Carswell, 1884), 27; Chadwick, *Bureaucratic Mercy*, 97–8.

47 Ibid., 29–30.

48 LAC, RG 13, vol. 1411, file 73A.

49 Anne Digby, *Madness, Morality and Medicine: A Study of the York Retreat, 1796–1914* (Cambridge: Cambridge University Press, 1985), 61.

50 Obituary, "Joseph Workman," *American Journal of Insanity* 51 (July 1894): 133.

51 LAC, RG 13, vol. 1411, file 73A.

52 This is a major theme of Rosenberg, *The Trial of the Assassin Guiteau*; see also Mohr, *Doctors and the Law*, 145–8.

53 Joseph Workman, "Moral Mania," *American Journal of Insanity*, April 1863, 406–16; "On Crime and Insanity," 10–1; "Moral Insanity – What Is It?" *American Journal of Insanity*, January 1883, 334–41. For Daniel Clark's identical view, see LAC, RG 13, vol. 1430, file 282A, trial transcript, 252–3, and also Daniel Clark, *Mental Diseases: A Synopsis of Twelve Lectures Delivered at the Hospital for the Insane, Toronto* (Toronto: W: Briggs: Montreal: C.W. Coates, 1895), 301. See also Scull et al., *Masters of Bedlam*, 98–9; Roger Cooter, "Phrenology and British Alienists," in *Madhouses, Mad-Doctors and Madmen: The Social History of Psychiatry in the Victorian Era*, ed. Andrew Scull (Philadelphia: University of Pennsylvania Press, 1981).

54 Workman, "Moral Insanity," 335.

55 G.E. Berrios, "J.C. Prichard and the Concept of 'Moral Insanity,'" *History of*

Psychiatry 10 (1999): 112; K. Joliffe, *Penitentiary Medical Services, 1835–1983* (Ottawa: Ministry of the Solicitor-General, 1984), 60–7. For the United States, Tighe, "The Legal Art of Psychiatric Diagnosis."

56 AO, RG 22-452-2-7, 229–54.

57 LAC, RG 13, vol. 1417, file 142, 48.

58 Workman, "Moral Insanity," 338. For moral insanity in a Manitoba murder case, see Richard Kramer and Tom Mitchell, *Walk towards the Gallows: The Tragedy of Hilda Blake, Hanged 1899* (Toronto: Oxford University Press, 2002), 177–82.

59 Robert Nye, *Crime, Madness, and Politics in Modern France: The Medical Concept of National Decline* (Princeton, NJ: Princeton University Press, 1984), 99.

60 On the impact of the infamous trial in 1876 of a mentally deficient child killer, see Patrizia Guarnieri, *A Case of Child Murder: Law and Science in Nineteenth-Century Tuscany*; trans. Claudia Miéville (Cambridge: Polity Press, 1993), 139, 153.

61 LAC, RG 13, vol. 1415, file 116A.

62 LAC, RG 13, vol. 1414, file 108A, Workman in cross-examination.

63 Workman, "On Crime and Insanity," 6.

64 LAC, RG 13, vol. 1414, file 108A, letter to the minister of justice, 28 May 1876.

65 Editorial, "Dr. Workman on Criminal Insanity," Toronto *Globe*, 4 August 1876, 2.

66 *Guelph Weekly Herald*, 14 November 1889, n.p., LAC, RG 13, vol. 1426 (1,2), file 235A. See also LAC, RG 13, vol. 1410 file 65A.

67 As far as I can determine, his only other appearances in murder trials were in LAC, RG 13, vol. 1416, file 133A, and in LAC, RG 13, vol. 1426 (1,2), file 235A.

68 On Clark, see *Dictionary of Canadian Biography*, vol. 14, s.v. Barbara L. Craig, "Clark, Daniel."

69 Clark, "Another Chapter," 351.

70 Clark, "Medical Evidence," 97.

71 Ibid., 100.

72 LAC, RG 13, vol. 1417, file 139A.

73 For Bucke on masturbatory insanity, see Shortt, *Victorian Lunacy*, 125–7; also Henry Howard, *Mental and Moral Science; with Some Remarks upon Hysterical Mania* (Read before the Medico-Chirurgical Society of Montreal; [Montreal] 1878; CIHM microfiche series no. 08781), 5. The plea of masturbatory insanity was attempted and again failed in the murder trial of Brown (LAC, RG 13, vol. 1435, file 303A), but resulted in an insanity acquittal for theft in 1895 (AO, RG 22-451-5-3, 242–5). For mid-century temporary insanity defences in Ontario, see Kirk-Montgomery, "Courting Madness," chap. 3. For the United States, see Wiener, "Judges v. Jurors."

74 See also Mitchinson, *The Nature of Their Bodies*, 295–6.

75 LAC, RG 13, vol. 1413, file 91A, 28 May 1875, Workman et al., Medical Report.

76 LAC, RG 13, vol. 1417, file 139A. Clark wrote about this case in "A Few Canadian Cases," 190–1; and *Mental Diseases*, 149–56.

77 LAC, RG 13, vol. 1419, file 165A, 244.

78 Ontario, *Report of the Commissioners Appointed to Enquire into the Prison and Reformatory System of Ontario* (Toronto, 1891) (hereafter OPRC), 645.

79 LAC, RG 13, vol. 1419, file 165A, 246.

80 For example, the cross-examination in *The Queen vs. Louis Riel*, 130.

81 For England, see Smith, *Trial by Medicine*, 125–8; for the United States, Mohr, *Doctors and the Law*, 148.

82 Howard, *Mental and Moral Science*, 13.

83 RG 13, C1, vol. 1418, notes of evidence, 16. For an overview of epilepsy as a defence, see Eigen, *Unconscious Crime*, 139–52.

84 Grenier, *Les monstres, les fous et les autres*, 183–92.

85 Among other works, see Henry Howard, "The Queen versus Hugh Hayvern for the Murder of John Salter. Second Paper," *Canada Medical Record* 10 (1881–82), 58–62; and "Criminal Responsibility," *Alienist & Neurologist* 7 (1886): 376–88.

86 James Kiernan, "Medico-Legal Relations of Epilepsy: A Study of the Hayvren[sic]-Salter Homicide," *Chicago Medical Review* 5 (1882): 61–7.

87 Francis W. Campbell, R.A. Kennedy, and James C. Cameron, "The Hayvern Murder Case," *Canada Medical Record* 10 (1881–82): 37–42.

88 Rosenberg, *The Trial of the Assassin Guiteau*.

89 For an example of Canadian press coverage, see "The Doomed Assassin," Toronto *Globe*, 27 January 1882, 2.

90 "A Moral Idiot," *London Advertiser* (London, Ont.) 8 July 1881, 2.

91 Shortt, *Victorian Lunacy*, 98–109.

92 LAC, RG 13, vol. 1419, file 173A.

93 Law Society of Upper Canada Archives, John Maxwell fonds, PF40, "Notebook of John Maxwell."

94 Clark, "A Few Canadian Cases," 175; on Bucke's work *Man's Moral Nature: An Essay* (Toronto and New York, 1879), see Shortt, *Victorian Lunacy*, 85–91.

95 "What the Insanity Plea Is Founded On," *Cornwall Freeholder* (Cornwall, Ont.), 11 May 1883; *Ottawa Free Press*, 18 September 1883.

96 Alienists never opposed each other in twenty-six trials for murder and manslaughter.

97 See also AO, RG 22-441-1-10, 140–56; with others written up by Clark in "A Few Canadian Cases," 180–1.

98 Kirk-Montgomery, "Courting Madness," table 7.5: "Jury Verdicts in Murder Cases by Decade, Insanity Trials, Ontario, 19th Century."

99 The significance of mass journalism in late-century perceptions of the criminal is a central theme of Marie-Christine Leps, *Apprehending the Criminal: The Production of Deviance in Nineteenth-Century Discourse* (Durham: Duke University Press, 1992).

100 "The Hawkesbury Tragedy," Toronto *Globe*, 5 January 1883, 1.

101 "Mann, the Murderer: Dr. Clarke [*sic*] Predicts that He Will Die Calmly Tomorrow," *Toronto Globe*, 11 October 1883, 5.

102 Editorial, "The *Globe* and the *Nouveau Monde*," Toronto *Globe*, 31 May 1876, 2.

103 See note 10 above. For contemporary medical comment, see Clark, "A Psycho-Medical History of Louis Riel"; Arton, "Insanity and Its Medico-legal Aspects"; C.K. Clarke, "A Critical Study of the Case of Louis Riel," parts 1 and 2, *Queen's Quarterly* 13 (April 1905), and 14 (July 1905): 14–26.

104 *The Queen vs. Louis Riel*, 128–32.

105 Ibid., 129.

106 LAC, RG 13, vol. 1430, file 282A; and also in 1896, the trial of LePointe, described in Clark, "Another Chapter," 338–40; see also "Lapointe's Trial," Toronto *Globe*, 23 May 1896, 12; and "Lapointe's Insanity," *Perth Courier* (Perth, Ont.), 29 May 1896, 7.

107 Walker, *Crime and Insanity in England*, 1: 104–5; Mohr, *Doctors and the Law*, 146 et passim.

108 Clark could have supported the defence more strongly, particularly in cross-examination, where experts were allowed more latitude in their answers.

109 Nye, *Crime, Madness, and Politics*, 85.

110 Clark, "A Psycho-Medical History of Louis Riel," 18. Clark also wrote about Riel in "A Few Canadian Cases," 183–90.

111 Clark, "Medical Evidence," 14.

112 Clark, "A Psycho-Medical History of Louis Riel," 18. Toronto *Globe*, 18 November 1885, cited in Morton, ed., *The Queen v Louis Riel*, xxix–xxx. For Guiteau's delusions, see Rosenberg, *The Trial of the Assassin Guiteau*, 29–31.

113 Friedland, *The Case of Valentine Shortis*, 150, 182–3. For commutation decisions in the case of allegedly mentally disturbed offenders, see Jonathan Swainger, "A Distant Edge of Authority: Capital Punishment and the Prerogative of Mercy in British Columbia, 1872–1880," in *Essays in the History of Canadian Law*, vol. 6, *British Columbia and the Yukon*, ed. Hamar Foster and John McLaren (Toronto: University of Toronto Press, 1995), 218–21; also Carolyn Strange, "The Lottery of Death: Capital Punishment in Canada, 1867–1976," *Manitoba Law Journal* 23 (1996): 594–619; Jonathan Swainger, *The Canadian Department of Justice and the Completion of Confederation* (Vancouver: UBC Press, 2000), 66–7.

114 Shortt, *Victorian Lunacy*, 103–4.

115 Smith, *Trial by Medicine*, 125.

116 George D. Gibb, "Hereditary Insanity, Characterized by Periodical Attacks, Sudden Death, and Coroner's Inquest," *Canada Medical Journal* 1 (January 1853): 648–53.

117 Degeneration theory was one of the most powerful intellectual themes of the later century. See Edward Shorter, *A History of Psychiatry: From the Era of the Asylum to the Age of Prozac* (Toronto: John Wiley & Sons, 1997), 93–9; Harris, *Murders and Madness*, chap. 2; Shortt, *Victorian Lunacy*, 98–109; Janet Oppenheim, *Shattered Nerves: Doctors, Patients, and Depression in Victorian England* (New York: Oxford University Press, 1991), 265–92; Rafael Huertas, "Madness and Degeneration, III: Degeneration and Criminality," *History of Psychiatry* 4 (1993), 141–58.

118 Clark credited "Lamarck, Beale, Spencer, Darwin, Romanes and Weismann" in *Mental Diseases*, 237, but not the French originators of degeneration theory, B.-A. Morel and V. Magnan, nor Henry Maudsley, who popularized degeneration for English readers.

119 Clark, *Mental Diseases*, 241.

120 LAC, RG 13, vol. 1430, trial transcript, 249.

121 OPRC, 638–48.

122 Clark, "A Few Canadian Cases," 181.

123 As in the case of the murderer Almeda Chatelle: LAC, RG 13, vol. 1832, file 273A (0249).

124 Mariana Valverde, *Diseases of the Will: Alcohol and the Dilemmas of Freedom* (Cambridge: Cambridge University Press, 1998); for a Quebec alcoholic insanity defence, see LAC, RG 13, vol. 1439 (1) and vol. 1440 (2,3), file 321A. Montreal doctors petitioned for the commutation of one labourer's death sentence on the grounds of dipsomania: LAC, RG 13, vol. 1425, file 229A. See also Georges Villeneuve, "Alcoholism and Responsibility," *Montreal Medical Journal* 27 (1898): 928–33.

125 AO, RG 22-452-2-7, trial testimony, 229–54.

126 Shortt, *Victorian Lunacy*, 129–30; LAC, RG 13, vol. 1415, file 117A, trial transcript, 15; see also AO, RG 22-452-2-7, 229–54.

127 LAC, RG 13, vol. 1438, file 311A, Daniel Clark to David Mills, minister of justice, 9 May 1899. Doctors Lett and Phelan also examined Parrott after this date, but their reports are missing.

128 "Case of Benjamin Parrott," Toronto *Globe*, 16 June 1899, 2.

129 Clark, "Another Chapter," 345; "Crime and Responsibility," *American Journal of Insanity* 47 (April 1891): 501–2; "A Few Canadian Cases," 175; and *Mental Diseases*, 314; AO, RG 22-443-4-4, 315–36.

130 Clark expressed the somaticism of Charles Mercier; see Michael Clark, "Rejection

of Psychological Approaches to Mental Disorder in Late Nineteenth-Century British Psychiatry," in *Madhouses, Mad-Doctors and Madmen*, ed. Scull, 284.

131 Clark, *Mental Diseases*, 299–300; "A Few Canadian Cases," 182. Rivennes was found not guilty because of weak evidence, according to Clark.

132 Gidney and Millar, *Professional Gentlemen*, 310–13.

133 Martin Wiener, *Reconstructing the Criminal: Culture, Law, and Policy in England, 1830–1914* (Cambridge: Cambridge University Press, 1990), 217.

134 Carolyn Strange, "Discretionary Justice: Political Culture and the Death Penalty in New South Wales and Ontario, 1890–1920," in *Qualities of Mercy: Justice, Punishment, and Discretion*, ed. Carolyn Strange (Vancouver: UBC Press, 1996), 130–65; Daniel Hack Tuke, *The Insane in the United States and Canada* (London 1885), 237–8; Peter Oliver, *'Terror to Evil-Doers': Prisons and Punishments in Nineteenth-Century Ontario* (Toronto: University of Toronto Press, 1998), chap. 8.

135 For the Trial of Lunatics Act, 46 & 47 Vict., c. 38, see Walker, *Crime and Insanity in England*, 1, 188–92. See also Tony Ward, "Law, Common Sense, and the Authority of Science: Expert Witnesses and Criminal Insanity in England, ca. 1840–1940," *Social & Legal Studies* 6, no. 3 (1997): 343–62).

136 For Scotland, see Tony Ward, "Observers, Advisers, or Authorities? Experts, Juries and Criminal Responsibility in Historical Perspective," *Journal of Forensic Psychiatry* 12, no. 1 (April 2001): 115–6; for the United States, Rosenberg, *The Trial of the Assassin Guiteau*, 103.

137 Criminal Code (1892), 55–56 Vict., c. 29, s. 11.

138 LAC, RG 13, vol. 1430 file 279; LAC, RG 13, vol. 1428, file 259A; Kirk-Montgomery, "Courting Madness," chap. 3. On the Criminal Code, see Simon Verdun-Jones, "The Evolution of the Defences of Insanity and Automatism in Canada from 1843 to 1979: A Saga of Judicial Reluctance to Sever the Umbilical Cord to the Mother Country?" *University of British Columbia Law Review* 14 (1979): 1–73, and Friedland, *The Case of Valentine Shortis*, 38–41.

139 OPRC, 642; Clark, *Mental Diseases*, 306, 291; "The Public and the Doctor in Relation to the Dipsomaniac," *Canadian Practitioner* 13 (April 1888): 110–11.

140 "LaPointe's Trial," Toronto *Globe*, 23 May 1896, 12.

141 Trevor Turner, "Henry Maudsley: Psychiatrist, Philosopher, and Entrepreneur," in *The Anatomy of Madness: Essays in the History of Psychiatry*, vol. 3, *The Asylum and Its Psychiatry*, ed. W.F. Bynum, Roy Porter, and Michael Shepherd (London: Routledge, 1988).

142 Clark, *Mental Diseases*, 294. Landor also subscribed to a control test: see "Insanity," 20. The same criticisms were made by C.K. Clarke in "Canadian Law in Regard to Responsibility," 279–80.

143 Clark, *Mental Diseases*, 307.

144 See C.K. Clarke on the "accidental" criminal in "Canadian Law in Regard to Responsibility," 275; also Nye, *Crime, Madness, and Politics*, 84.

145 LAC, RG 13, vol. 1426 (1,2), file 235A.

146 Lett appeared in a few trials; see Cheryl Krasnick Warsh, *Moments of Unreason: The Practice of Canadian Psychiatry and the Homewood Retreat, 1883–1923* (Montreal and Kingston: McGill-Queen's University Press, 1991), 21–36.

147 *Palmerston Telegraph* (Palmerston, Ont.), 7 November 1887, clipping in LAC, RG 13, vol. 1426 (1,2), file 235A.

148 See also the Shortis trial: Friedland, *The Case of Valentine Shortis*, chap. 5.

149 For English examples of absence states as defences to murder, see Eigen, *Unconscious Crime*.

150 AO, RG 22-443-4-4, 315-36.

151 Letter to editor, *Sarnia Observer* (Sarnia, Ont.), 16 September 1893, page number missing.

152 Clark, *Mental Diseases*, 318.

153 Only testimony derived from examinations made expressly for the purpose became admissible evidence on the question of insanity; some judges challenged the value of family history of insanity and previous bouts of disorder, as lay witness testimony became less relevant. See Kirk-Montgomery, "Courting Madness," chap. 2.

154 LAC, RG 13, vol. 1428, file 259A, "Murderer's Brain Soften's [sic]," clipping of interview with Dr Chamberlain, inspector of prisons, [newspaper unknown], 29 April 1893, n.p.

155 AO, RG 22-441-1-10, 140-56; LAC, RG 13, vol. 1419, file 173A; the Rivennes case of 1886, described in Clark, "A Few Canadian Cases," 180-1.

156 LAC, RG 13, vol. 1438, file 311A; LAC, RG 13, vol. 1417, file 139A.

157 AO, RG 22-443-4-4; the cases of Burrell and Saxton, noted in AO, RG 22-443-4-6, 188-9; see also "LaPointe's Trial," Toronto *Globe*, 23 May 1896, 12.

158 Clark, "Another Chapter," 348; see also Clarke, "Canadian Law in Regard to Responsibility," 283.

159 LAC, RG 13, vol. 1430, file 280; LAC, RG 13, vol. 1432, file 287.

160 Robert Vipond and Georgina Feldberg, "The Law of Evolution and the Evolution of the Law: Mills, Darwin, and Late-Nineteenth-Century Legal Thought," in *Essays in the History of Canadian Law*, vol. 8, *In Honour of R.C.B. Risk* (Toronto: University of Toronto Press, 1999), 561-82.

161 Clark and Clarke testified for the "boy-killer" Kearney in 1896; see LAC, RG 13, vol. 1430, file 279; Bucke found "larvated epilepsy" in the case recorded in AO, RG 22-392-0-1193.

162 C.K. Clarke, "The Care and Treatment of the Criminal," *Canadian Journal of Medicine and Surgery* 15, no. 1 (January 1904): 9-14. Ian Dowbiggin, *Keeping*

America Sane: Psychiatry and Eugenics in the United States and Canada, 1880–1940 (Ithaca: Cornell University Press, 1997), 140.

163 Mariana Valverde, *The Age of Light, Soap, and Water: Moral Reform in English Canada, 1885–1925* (Toronto: McClelland & Stewart, 1991), 44.

164 As Richard Moran concluded for nineteenth-century England in "The Origin of Insanity as a Special Verdict: The Trial for Treason of James Hadfield (1800)," *Law and Society Review* 19 (1985): 487–519; and "The Punitive Uses of the Insanity Defense: The Trial for Treason of Edward Oxford (1840)," *International Journal of Law and Psychiatry* 9 (1986): 171–90.

6

Turbulent Spirits

Aboriginal Patients in the British Columbia Psychiatric System, 1879–1950

ROBERT MENZIES AND TED PALYS

REMEMBERING CHARLEY WOLVERINE

In the late fall of 1941, sixty-two-year-old Charley Wolverine,[1] a member of the Dakelh (formerly Carrier) First Nation of west-central British Columbia, was becoming increasingly erratic and confused. He had been wandering aimlessly around his home reserve at night for several weeks when the village chief at last decided to summon the local British Columbia Provincial Police (BCPP) constable. The latter promptly jailed Charley and called in two white general physicians from a nearby town. Although Charley was deaf, non-English-speaking, disoriented, and nearly blind, the two medical men quickly determined that he was an insanity case who needed immediate institutionalization. They filed the necessary involuntary certification forms under the provincial *Mental Hospitals Act*,[2] to which they appended an application for admission completed by the BCPP constable and legal authorization from the presiding stipendiary magistrate for the district.

Following a train journey south, Charley was shepherded into the admission unit at Essondale, the province's flagship psychiatric facility in the Vancouver suburb of Coquitlam, eight hundred kilometres from his home, where he was bathed, photographed, and given a preliminary examination. The admitting physician noted, "He is very dull and seclusive in his manner ... He takes no interest in his surroundings. He is quite deaf and it is difficult to talk to him. He is markedly confused in his conversation, and his memory is faulty for past events."[3] Thereupon the doctor ushered Charley Wolverine first onto the Centre Lawn wards and from there a few dozen metres westward to the Male Chronic (West Lawn) Building.

Through that winter and into the spring and summer months of 1942, Charley Wolverine's family members and friends mustered what few resources availed them in a fruitless campaign to bring Charley home. With assistance from village members who enjoyed some fluency in written English, his wife, Martha, directed letter after letter to institutional authorities, variously imploring and reasoning with them, appealing to their sense of humanity, and relentlessly insisting on his immediate release back to his home and community. Various other relatives (including his married daughter) also wrote, generating through the term of Charley's confinement a formidable body of correspondence that survives to the present day in his clinical dossier, stored at the British Columbia Archives in Victoria.

A prophetic note that Martha sent in February to Medical Superintendent E.J. Ryan consisted of "a few lines to say we want you to send Charley Wolverine back to [the village], we all want him to come back, if he will not get better, then we would like him to come home and die here at his own home ... His [three teenaged] children want to talk to him before he has to die." Two months later Martha tried again, begging for the railway fare to come visit him in hospital:

I have not seen him for a long time now, and Im[4] not too well. My husband he has never written me a letter ... Lots of people get pass on the train, Indian Agent give one to them, so please you send me one ... Ive not got any money or I would pay my own fare to Essondale ... Two hospital here both for Indians we don't want Charley to stay such a long way, his [people] want him, seems there is no straight talk ... I want to talk to him. I got your letter and everybody is sorry and cry. I walk all the time please send Charley back, I ask you please, or send me a pass to come down to him.

In a penultimate note, composed in mid-July, Martha tried in desperation to invoke the influence of the federal Indian Affairs Branch and the provincial police:

The Indian Agent is at Vancouver just now so I cannot see him about Charley. May be you will see the Indian Agent and the Police man say Charley is alright and he can come back soon. I see the police on Sat night. Ruth [her daughter] is home from [residential] school and she is sorry her father is not in [the village] and she cry all the time ... The house I have to live in has no window and its too cold I want my

husband to come back and fis it so I can live in my own hous. I am sorry every day
... Soon I go to Vancouver. Ruth says good bye and I say good bye to Charley.
Cheers to you all, thanks a lot.

But all was for naught. When he did respond to Martha and her relatives,
Superintendent Ryan's communications recurrently underscored the superior medical treatment that Charley was enjoying, his supposed satisfaction
with hospital life, and above all else, the manifest hopelessness of his case.
In December 1941 Ryan wrote to Martha, "[Charley] is still rather dull and
confused and takes no interest in his surroundings ... He shows considerable mental failure, but is no active trouble on the ward ... He is in no condition mentally to carry on outside the hospital." Early in the new year
Ryan added, "It is impossible to discuss his past difficulties on account of
his poor knowledge of English" and "[h]e ... seems quite content and satisfied in his present surroundings, but spends most of his time in bed ... He
seems pleasant and happy in his surroundings but does not make any effort
to talk at all, even with other Indians on the ward and has shown little
improvement physically." On the subject of Charley's possible return to his
village, Ryan's assertion of March 1942 was typical: "We do not feel that
he is in any condition to be outside the hospital at the present time ...
Should his condition improve ... your wishes will certainly be born in
mind."

When the Indian agent for Charley's district sought out Ryan later that
spring, the latter responded more favourably to this white voice of state
authority than he had to Martha, while continuing to stress that strict conditions would necessarily adhere to any contemplated discharge from
Essondale. "In reference to the above, he is in bed most of the time. He has
an old tubercular condition of the chest which is not very active at the
present time, but he is dull, simple and shows considerable mental deterio-
ration ... His wife and friends are agitating constantly for his release, and
we would be agreeable to his returning if conditions are such that he could
be properly supervised, and he would need an escort. It might be advisable
to place him in the hospital for a time before returning home." As it turned
out, such measures were not needed. The tuberculosis to which Ryan
referred entered an acute phase just two months after that exchange. At
around 10:30 on a late summer weekday morning, nine months after his
admission, Charley Wolverine died, far from his family, on the wards of the
Essondale West Lawn Building. The presiding physician called in the
Roman Catholic priest and wired the Indian agent to contact the next of
kin. Charley's parting psychiatric diagnosis (doubtless influenced by an

Indian Affairs Branch nurse's report that he had suffered "a slight stroke" a month prior to admission) was "arteriosclerotic dementia." Two days later Charley Wolverine at last began his journey home in the hold of the Vancouver–Prince Rupert steamer, encased in an institutional casket bound for burial near the village where he had spent all but nine months of a too-brief life. In one affectingly understated, encapsulating coda, Superintendent Ryan penned a final missive to Martha in mid-September of 1942: "In reply to your letter of the 6th inst., in reference to your late husband, I am enclosing herewith cheque for $6.65 which is in the amount of cash he had on admission to the Hospital, and also a small black purse. Kindly acknowledge receipt of these. I am obtaining a copy of his picture and will forward it to you."

INTERROGATING PUBLIC PSYCHIATRY
AND ABORIGINALITY

Charley Wolverine's story is one of thousands of human dramas that populate the pages of the clinical records assembled, over the past 130 years, under the auspices of the British Columbia mental health system. What distinguishes his narrative is that Charley Wolverine was a man of First Nations heritage. His journey from the village of his ancestors to the wards of Essondale therefore extends beyond information about asylum patient life in the province during the World War II era to mine a previously untapped vein of information regarding Indigenous experience in British Columbia. Charley's commitment, hospitalization, and ultimate demise, and the roles of British Columbia's medical and policing communities, the federal Indian agent, and Charley's family in the creation of that experience, raise important questions about the recursive relations of race, ethnicity, Aboriginality, and psychiatry across the province and nation that have not yet been addressed in the literature.

Apart from a few sporadic references and singular "case studies" (such as that of the Canadian Métis leader Louis Riel),[5] the psychiatric historical record is peculiarly silent on the important subject of Aboriginality. We attempt to address that deficiency by exploring the attributes and experiences of a hundred Native patients who entered British Columbia's public mental hospital system under the provisions of the province's Mental Hospitals Act between 1879 and 1950. In doing so, we add to a wealth of patient-centred research that has emerged over the past two decades.[6] At its best, this body of work powerfully depicts the range of human experience that has left its imprint on psychiatric settings, historical and current;

the intrinsically contested and contradictory nature of ideas about, and policies and practices aimed at containing, madness; the complex interplay of power relations that shape encounters between psychiatrized people, medical professionals, community, and state; and above all else, the resolute capacity of human beings to challenge affliction, segregation, and stigma in the face of sometimes unfathomable odds.

Our sample was drawn from the 193 registered Aboriginal clinical files stored in the British Columbia Archives and Riverview East Lawn Records facilities. We selected every second case from a list of cases ordered chronologically (substituting randomly ahead or back for 12 files that were unavailable in the databases or accession groups) and then randomly added three cases to reach our final sample size of 100.[7] The records in each file include a diverse collection of legal documents, personal and family histories, clinical, social service, and psychological reports, ward notes, patient interviews, and correspondence. Together they afford an illuminating historical window into the administration, operations, organizational culture, and daily life of the provincial psychiatric machinery. Even more important, they open a revealing portal into the lived experiences of patients and their families through their own speech and writings, as preserved in the files, and through observations compiled by medical professionals and line staff.

While the files must be recognized as second-order artifacts that are far from mimetic renderings of the human record, and while the earlier files (through to about 1910) are sometimes threadbare, the collection constitutes a rich and compelling archive of hospital life during the late nineteenth and early twentieth centuries.[8] As in jurisdictions elsewhere, these hospital case files have come to offer an absorbing and potent resource for students of madness, psychiatry, and public health history. Read in the context of the sweeping systemic, ideological and human developments against which their lives played out, these patient biographies figure prominently in the exciting new psychiatric histories that have flourished in the wake of the 1980s pioneering work of Dale Peterson and the late Roy Porter[9] and, more recently, of various other writers from around the world.[10]

We base our analysis and discussion in this chapter on our detailed transcriptions of the 100 sample files (totalling 462 single-spaced pages of text), supplemented by other primary documents, including government reports, institutional correspondence, and media clippings. Our analysis layers in the institutional, cultural, and human environments that framed Indigenous patient biographies; considers how ideas about Aboriginality, pathology, and reason figured into the medico-legal management of "insane" Native people; and illustrates some of the efforts that patients and their advocates made to resist and transcend official imputations of pathology, identity, and race.

INSTITUTIONALIZING NATIVE PEOPLE IN BRITISH COLUMBIA

Understanding the experiences of Charley Wolverine and his Indigenous compatriots in British Columbia's mental health complex requires an appreciation of who these people were and where they came from, as well as of the changing institutional context in which they were held and the broader social relations between Aboriginal and non-Aboriginal people of which their institutional confinement formed a part.

Table 6.1 shows demographic information available to us through the patient files. There were slightly more males than females, with an average age at admission (for those for whom we know it) of thirty-seven years (the range was from eight to eighty-five). The sample was about evenly divided between those categorized as married (38) and as single (37), with smaller numbers widowed, separated, or living common law. While most individuals were childless, the 37 patients who were known to be parents had a total of 119 children among them (or 3.2 per parent patient). Formal education levels were low: most (46) had experienced no formal education; 31 had received a primary level of instruction at most, with at least 13 of these having been sent to residential school.

The deep penetration of European religion and missionary work – as well as European definitions of what practices constituted "religion" – were plainly evident in the files, with most patients identified as Roman Catholic (53) or Church of England (19). Employment records revealed the diversity of Aboriginal labour experience in the province. Of the 96 women, men and children for whom information was available, the largest number (33) were considered to have no employment; job categories for the others included (in decreasing order of frequency) "housewives," fishers, general labourers, hunters and trappers, ranch workers, farmers, domestics, students, band chief, boat builder, cannery worker, and "prostitute."

Among those patients so identified, 82 were status Indians and thus under the jurisdiction of the federal Indian Act, with the consequence that the federal Indian Affairs Department and Branch paid their hospital maintenance fees as wards of the dominion.[11] Another 3 originated in the

Table 6.1   Attributes of selected Aboriginal patients in British Columbia, 1879–1950

	Number	Percentage[a]		Number	Percentage[a]
Gender			Religion		
Male	57	57	Roman Catholic	53	58
Female	43	43	Church of England	19	21
			United Church	8	9
			Methodist	4	4
Marital status			Salvation Army	4	4
Single	38	40	Presbyterian	1	1
Married	37	40	Protestant (unspec'd)	1	1
Widowed	15	16	None	1	1
Separated	3	4			
Common law	2	2			
			Occupation		
			None	33	34
Number of children			Housewife	28	19
None	55	60	Fisher	12	13
1	10	11	Hunter-trapper	7	7
2	6	7	Labourer	8	8
3	6	7	Ranch worker	5	5
4	5	5	Farmer	4	4
5	6	7	Domestic	3	3
6	2	2	Student	2	2
7	1	1	Band chief	1	1
10	1	1	Boat builder	1	1
			Cannery worker	1	1
			Prostitute	1	1
Years of education					
None	46	46			
Primary (1-7 yrs)	31	31	First Nations standing		
No mention[b]	23	23	BC status Indian	82	90
			Yukon transfer patient	3	3
			Enfranchised/		
			Non-status	6	7

[a] Cases with missing information were excluded from the percentage calculations.
[b] In most of these cases, there was probably no educational background.

Yukon Territory,[12] and 6 were enfranchised (through their acquisition of Canadian citizenship, mixed-blood heritage, or, in the case of some women, via marriage to non-Aboriginals). Map 6.1 shows that these women, men, and children originated from virtually every region of the province (and, in the case of the three Yukon patients, from beyond), spoke many different languages and dialects, and hailed from bands, tribes, localities and nations representing a diverse cultural and geopolitical heritage.[13] By the time period canvassed in this study, few traditional territories were beyond the reach of medico-legal administration and intervention.

THE INSTITUTIONAL CONTEXT

Compared to its counterparts in central and eastern Canada, the British Columbia mental health system is of relatively recent origin. The province's public asylum operations officially began with the opening in 1872 of the Victoria Lunatic Asylum in traditional Songhees First Nations territory on the north shore of the city's inner harbour.[14] For the next eight decades, institutional psychiatry in British Columbia would parallel other Canadian and international jurisdictions in experiencing an explosion in physical facilities, organizational structures, professional and frontline personnel, and patient populations.

By 1950 the provincial mental health apparatus had become an expansive enterprise. Along with Essondale, it comprised the Provincial Mental Hospital, New Westminster (which opened in 1878 and specialized, from the mid-1930s, in the care of the cognitively disabled); the Colquitz Mental Home, on the fringes of Victoria (with its cohort of "criminally insane" or otherwise "difficult to manage" men); and branch facilities around the province. In their annual report for fiscal year 1949–50, hospital administrators enumerated 4,602 patients in residence, 53 medical staff on payroll, and gross operating costs of $4.8 million per annum.[15] From those first tentative overtures of the Victoria asylum through to mid-twentieth century, a total of 28,100 women, men, and children would pass through the doors of one or more of these psychiatric edifices.[16]

ABORIGINAL/NON-ABORIGINAL RELATIONS

As historians have recounted, the nineteenth century represented an era of profound devastation for the First Peoples of the province. Complex, sophisticated, and diverse societies that had occupied the entirety of the northern Cordillera for at least ten millennia soon faced the intrusive politics, economies, religions, and languages of successive waves of encroaching Europeans. Cultures that were flourishing at first contact and through the early years of the fur trade became increasingly vulnerable, as the century unfolded, to the combined impacts of disease, depopulation, assimilation, dispossession, and poverty. Missionaries covered the territory in an effort to "Christianize" its "heathen" inhabitants and later administered residential schools that allegedly would "modernize" their children.[17] Pan-

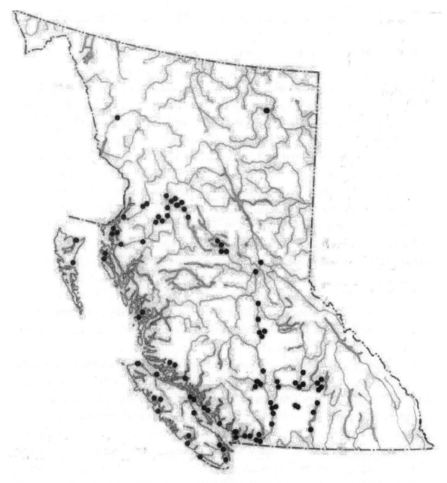

Map 6.1   Geographic origins of Aboriginal psychiatric patients in British Columbia

demics of measles, smallpox, tuberculosis, and other infectious diseases unleashed a decades-long reign of misery and death.[18]

As British Columbia's Aboriginal population fell, non-Aboriginals arrived en masse and multiplied: the Native proportion of the provincial population fell from 71 per cent at Confederation to 2.4 per cent in the 1951 census.[19] Colonial and Westernized political, legal, labour, health, education, family, and social institutions further reinforced Aboriginal marginalization and displacement.[20] A fragmented "Indian" reserve system that evolved through the later nineteenth century served, temporarily at least, to "legalize" the expropriation of Aboriginal land; by the early

1900s, First Peoples occupied just one-third of 1 per cent of the province's land mass.[21]

Aboriginal peoples' post-fur-trade experiences with the European colonizers ranged from over-attention and intrusiveness when it came to imposed efforts at assimilation and the criminalization of Aboriginal culture and practices (e.g., required attendance at residential schools; banning of the potlatch) to rejection and neglect (e.g., exclusion of Aboriginals from the commercial fishery; making it illegal for Aboriginal people to hire lawyers to assert land rights). The psychiatric establishment, at least during the years canvassed by our research, appears closer to the latter than the former. Our scouring of the hospital registries[22] located only 193 patients whom medical authorities identified as "Indian" or "Native" on hospital admission between 1879[23] and the end of calendar year 1950. While this figure is almost certainly an underestimate (at least with respect to non-status Indians), based as it is on frequently incomplete information, and on documents and impressions assembled by white male professionals who were often indifferent to Aboriginals' own concepts of identity, the relative dearth of First Peoples in these mental health settings (a scant 0.7 per cent of the total admissions) remains a graphic and consistent pattern throughout the time period.[24]

Of course, "out of sight, out of mind" would have been consistent with other policies of the day. Although the phenomenon of "over-representation" in contemporary times is well known[25] – the imprisonment rate for Aboriginal people far exceeds their representational proportion in the general population – Don McCaskill suggests that this phenomenon is relatively recent: "Perhaps the most serious consequence of the colonial experience in human terms has been the disproportionately large number of native people coming into conflict with the law and their subsequent incarceration in correctional institutions in this country. It is interesting to note that the high incidence of conflicts with the law have occurred only within the last twenty years since native people have begun to extend their participation beyond the boundaries of the reserve and compete within the structures of the dominant society."[26] It is thus important to note that our records date to a time when the reserve system and federal intervention were at their strongest and when, from the 1920s onward, an oppressive system of Indian agent–administered "location tickets" restricted movement, required full-time residential school attendance, and – combined with other exclusionary policies – kept Aboriginal populations in isolated surveillance. The police, medical authorities, and the provincial and federal governments all had mechanisms to remove those who were trouble for themselves or others. When Aboriginal people did turn up on the hospital rolls, it was often as a regulatory response to social conflict or individual disturbance, more than as a therapeutic measure aimed at dispensing medical treatment to people in need.

THE INSTITUTIONAL EXPERIENCE

Even a surface scanning of the Aboriginal patient files succeeds in evoking the breadth of human endurance, affliction, conflict, and resolution that they collectively harbour. In what follows, we consider the social forces that propelled Aboriginal patients into hospital settings and effected their characterization as "insane," and we examine Native peoples' own recorded understandings of their racial and medical identities, their imputed pathologies, and their relationship to the state's therapeutic and legal order.

Table 6.2 outlines the main categories of patient deployment, official decision-making, and psychiatric labelling that structured the institutional careers of this "insane" Aboriginal cohort. At first glance, the synopsis suggests that the Indigenous patient experience was not entirely different from that of other inmates, as exhibited by Native pathways taken to the asylum, their lives on the hospital wards, and their depictions by legal and medical authorities.[27]

However, a closer examination of these patterns, combined with a qualitative probing of the clinical files, sharply exposes the pervasive and frequently determinative presence of racialized ideas about health and madness. Isaiah Coventry, for example, was a Shuswap Lake area band chief in 1921 who, while characterized as "an Indian of the very best type," had increasingly deteriorated over time and became "careless in his personal appearance." Another patient, Julia Friendly, originally from the upper Fraser Valley, had been widowed when her husband died violently while working for the Canadian Pacific Railway. This "small Indian woman of middle life and an imbecile" was living on relief during the Great Depression in a ramshackle hut on the Burnaby waterfront when municipal authorities, citing her "demented" behaviour and financial burden to the community, mobilized to have her certified.

The records also reveal that Aboriginal people made claims of their own upon medical authorities and were sometimes able to enlist the psychiatric apparatus to serve their purposes. For example, Philip,[28] the very first "Indian" to enter psychiatric facilities in the province, was admitted to the New Westminster Asylum from Yale (at the south end of the Fraser

Table 6.2   Institutional experiences of BC Aboriginal patients[a]

	Number	Percentage[a]		Number	Percentage[a]
Which hospital					
PHI[b]	19	19	Epilepsy	6	6
Essondale	64	64	Paranoia	4	4
PHI/Essondale	16	16	Melancholia/depression	3	3
Essondale / Colquitz	1	1	Chronic brain syndrome	2	2
			Toxic psychosis	1	1
Status on admission					
Certified from community	89	89	Treatment in hospital		
Certified from GIS/BIS[c]	4	4	None stated	68	68
Deported from USA	2	2	Medication for paresis	11	11
Oakalla Gaol transfer	2	2	Sedatives for epilepsy	6	6
NGRI[d]	2	2	ECT	3	3
Certified from Coqualeetza	1	1	ECT psychotropic drugs	2	2
			Malaria for paresis	2	2
Who initiated admission[e]			Psychotropic drugs	2	2
Indian agent/Supt	25	27	Mercury for paresis	1	1
Physician	23	25	Metrazol	1	1
Constable/police	13	14	Dilantin for epilepsy	1	1
Family members	10	11	Anti-Parkinsonism drugs	1	1
Jailer or warden	4	4	Sterilization	1	1
GIS or BIS supt	4	4	Vitamins/penicillin	1	1
Community members	3	3			
Local band nurse	2	2		Yes	No
Band reserve chief	2	2	Reasons for admission[f]		
Priest	1	1	General psychosis	58	42
Indian Dept teacher	1	1	Unmanageable/destructive	18	82
Immigration officials	1	1	Violent	13	87
Provincial Welfare Dept	1	1	Senile dementia	12	88
Division of VD Control	1	1	Wandered off	10	90
Criminal court (NGRI)	1	1	Suicidal/att'd suicide	10	90
			Threatening	8	92
Diagnosis			Mentally "defective"	6	94
Mental deficiency	21	26	Epileptic seizures	5	95
Dementia/schizophrenia	19	20	Killed someone	2	98
Senile/terminal dementia	17	18	Sexual assaults	2	98
Paresis/neurosyphilis	13	14	Escaped from GIS	1	99
Manic depressive	7	8			

[a] Cases with missing information were excluded from the percentage calculations.
[b] Public Hospital for the Insane (formerly the New Westminster Asylum).
[c] Girls' and Boys' Industrial Schools.
[d] Not guilty by reason of insanity.
[e] Who signed admission application (in practice, several people were often involved).
[f] Cases received multiple codings where more than one category applied.

canyon) in February 1879, on the urging of other Aboriginals in the area who, according to the medical certificate, reported that he was "insane and that they are afraid of him."

The social regulatory function of psychiatric commitment is by far the most resounding theme in the historical mental health literature,[29] and that function is evident here in official reactions to Aboriginal persons seen as troublesome, obdurate, wild, abusive, resistive, or otherwise indecipherable. A common thread linking these diverse cases of Aboriginal certification was the perceived unruliness and intractability of Native persons earmarked for psychiatric intervention. At least as pivotal as their mental disturbance – and often the apparent basis for concluding one existed – was the fact that such people were breaching social and racial conventions through their recalcitrant, transgressive, destructive, and generally incomprehensible conduct. For a constellation of reasons, their relations and communities, or the government agents who oversaw their lives, or the educational, health or correctional institutions into which they had gravitated, could no longer manage them in accustomed ways.[30]

The Aboriginal certification process was governed in large part by the ubiquitous presence of state and civil institutions in the lives of these 100 individuals and in the wider management of their villages, bands, tribes, and nations. Again and again, as the statistics in table 6.2 show, it was largely the individual and collective interventions of federal Indian agents, provincial police constables, and medical professionals that marked Native routes to the asylum. These interlocking networks of government and expert scrutiny operated in concert with the activities of missionaries, priests and pastors, nurses, teachers, and, increasingly by the 1930s, social workers practising in the field service of the provincial Welfare Branch.

Sometimes Indian agents would assume the primary responsibility for committal, as with agent W.E. Collison of Prince Rupert, who decided in 1929 that a delusional Winston Murphy had become an imminent risk to his wife and five children and accordingly secured the Tsimshian fisher's removal to Essondale, where he contracted tuberculosis and died two years later. On other occasions, medical practitioners took the lead. Three years prior to Winston Murphy's hospitalization and in a village located farther down the province's mainland coast, a physician on the regional hospital staff took it upon himself to contact Essondale medical superintendent H.C. Steeves about one of his patients, eighteen-year-old Johnson Longstreet, who reportedly "has struck his father a couple of times and has the family pretty well scared." Receiving the needed documents by return mail, the medical man coordinated Longstreet's certification to the Coquitlam hospital, where he would spend the next thirty-eight years until he finally died from pulmonary edema in the mid-1960s.

Tallulah Bill was a transfer patient from the Coqualeetza Indian Hospital who had been working with her husband and five children in the hops harvest near Agassiz. It was the Coqualeetza medical staff who in the early fall of 1943 certified Tallulah. They first admitted her to the Sardis institution in the throes of an apparent acute psychotic episode, and then – describing her as "[m]uttering in her Indian language ... running around the ward in the nude [and] fighting to get out of her bed" while in hospital – arranged for her relocation down the Fraser valley to Essondale. Tallulah too died there, four years later, having contracted a particularly gruesome strain of tuberculosis of the bone.

Beyond the grim prospects of displacement, illness, and death, life on the wards of Essondale and, earlier, the New Westminster Public Hospital for the Insane (PHI), must have been a profoundly alienating cultural experience for these Aboriginal patients. Once committed, an individual often would discover that she or he was the only Native person on the floor or, at times, in the entire institution. Unilingual patients frequently had no one with whom to carry on a simple conversation, no translators who might mediate their encounters with hospital staff, and until the latter half of the twentieth century, no cultural resources available to connect them with the Aboriginal world beyond the asylum walls.

British Columbia is the province with the greatest diversity in its Aboriginal peoples: one-third of Canada's First Nations are in the province, and five of the country's eleven Aboriginal language systems are indigenous to British Columbia. Even if another Aboriginal patient was in the institution, the two might not speak the same language, particularly in the early years of the residential schools, before English became the common provincial language. This fact only highlights the racism and ignorance of Aboriginal diversity embodied in Superintendent Ryan's letter regarding Charley Wolverine, in which he noted that Charley "does not make any effort to talk at all, even with other Indians on the ward."

Opportunities for labour, especially among women, who were generally denied outdoor work, were limited and banal. As noted in table 6.2 above, the majority of Indigenous patients (68 of 100) received absolutely no form of psychiatric treatment during an era when mental hospitalization could be described at its best as a benevolent warehousing and at its worst as an alternative form of imprisonment. It was not insignificant that police and medical authorities played cooperative roles in the institutionalization of Charley Wolverine, with whose story we opened this chapter; nor was that a rare event. As Edward Staples's Dakelh father commented in a handwritten note in 1951: "Edward he has nothing going and Police send him out. You know your self, all u know he joke too much and when he work – he always doing good ... Let me know why you hold him so long. I think Police was mistake."

Isolated, impoverished, far distant, and frequently illiterate in English, relations could usually ill afford the train or steamer passage needed to visit the hospital and were forced to enlist others who could draft or transcribe correspondence to patients on their behalf. For the latter, failing a fortuitous recovery or some other timely intervention, hospital life soon devolved into a lonely, grinding, monotonic repetition of gloomy institutional routine – and for too many, a slow decline toward death.

Compounding the tribulations of Native patients were the racializing thoughts, words and deeds of some mental hospital staff. In 1924 the attending PHI physician described eighteen-year-old Sliammon youth Wilbert Roper as being of "very low mental gauge," declaring that it was "very difficult to elicit anything from him, except the occasional grunt, typical of his race." Similarly, upon administering an intelligence test in the early 1940s, the resident Essondale psychometrist observed of Pauline Boone that "she does not show much interest and makes no effort to respond, remarks in Indian fashion 'I don't know.'" Corresponding with a Department of Indian Affairs official during the winter of 1926, Essondale medical superintendent H.C. Steeves wrote of Lucy David, a "dementia praecox case" from the Yukon who would be dead four months later of nephritis, that "she takes no interest in her appearance whatever as is customary with the persuasion to which she belongs." Ten years later, Secwepemc patient Randall Winfree gained a rather more favourable appraisal from his ward physician, who allowed that "for an Indian" he had "not too bad a mentality."

According to some staff reports – for example, a psychometrist's 1950 evaluation of Peace River Slavey (Dene-thah) trapper Donald Napier – a "deficient" Native mind state might not prove to be as detrimental to rehabilitation as for whites, as perhaps "detailed knowledge of the patient's environmental situation would reveal that its demands are not great ... [and] ... his intellectual status would not render him inadequate to cope with simple requirements of everyday living."

In other instances, a demonstration of willingness to assimilate could become an indicator of recovery and a passport to liberty, as with Edna Paul, another Aboriginal woman from the Yukon, who won her release in the summer of 1955 after seven years spent on the Essondale East Lawn wards. On her discharge, the physician in charge reported authoritatively: "It is interesting to note that when the patient was severely ill she could not speak English and in spite of being in an English environment she did not learn even a few simple words, but during the last 3 or 4 months she started to show good progress and ... at the same time developed a need to learn the language and in the last few weeks she could express herself quite relevantly in short sentences. She was therefore discharged ... to the care of [the] Indian Commissioner for BC."

That said, the medico-legal powers circulating through British Columbia's therapeutic confines were not unitary, totalizing, or unchallenged. As illustrated by Martha Wolverine's letters, which began this chapter, conflict over the inherent meanings of mental disorder and what to do about it infused these historical clinical files. Aboriginals and whites often harboured very disparate conceptions of what constituted insane and normal.[32] It is clear from the medical files we reviewed that, consistent with Loo's discussion of Indigenous invocations of legal discourse, doctrine, and subjecthood in late nineteenth- and early twentieth-century British Columbia, Aboriginal people often assertively challenged state medical apparatus inertia, as, for example, did the brothers of Catherine Jamieson and Andrew Napoleon. Both steadfastly rebuffed medical requests that they add their signatures to treatment permission forms, the latter brother asserting: "I'm sorry can't sign this paper you sent unless we find out what is wrong with Andrew. If you'd explain in an easier way that we can understand ... I will sign the paper."

While the racial hierarchies of governing institutions remained firmly in place throughout the period, and while these recurring life tragedies showed that individual resistance was often futile, one need scarcely be a devout Foucauldian to acknowledge the formidable potential for Aboriginal identity to assert itself through power struggles with white medico-legal authority.

As was true of asylum inmates more generally,[32] Aboriginal patient resistance was everywhere in evidence. It took many forms. Some patients refused to eat, to work, to communicate with professionals and attendants, or to conform to the daily hospital routine. A few people lashed out at others,[33] and three women undertook nine suicide attempts (one successfully, as chronicled below). Others endeavoured to recruit allies from outside the hospital – for example, the earlier-mentioned Edward Staples, who during the early 1950s tried to solicit help in his release from Canadian Legion officials and from his Indian agent.[34]

Eleven of 100 patients effected a total of 41 escapes from Essondale and the PHI. Jack Calhoun, originating from the Skeena River district, ran off four times between his transfer to the PHI from Oakalla Prison in 1915 (where he was awaiting trial for breaking and entering) and his death in 1925 from tuberculosis. Wilbert Roper's death from the same disease was no doubt hastened by a broken back suffered when the Sliammon youth removed a pane of glass and leapt some thirty feet from a dormitory bathroom window in a failed effort to take flight. His father had complained bitterly to his Indian agent that Wilbert was being abused in hospital and had endeavoured at one point personally to spirit his son via motor launch away from hospital. In another exploit prior to their TB-induced deaths in 1944, Lydia Tom and Pauline Boone bolted from a women patients' spring "walking party," rowed down the Fraser River, hitched a ride from Steveston to Vancouver, and "entertained several men" during a week of partying in a downtown hotel room before authorities caught up with them.

Especially affecting were the interventions of relations, community members, and other advocates who peppered Essondale and PHI physicians from all regions of the province with their inquiries, supplications, and importuning. The loss of their institutionalized parents, spouses, siblings, and children could have a devastating impact on Aboriginal families who were already grappling with a liminal existence at the margins of a growingly prevalent and imposing Eurocentric social order. For example, through the late 1920s and into the following decades, we encounter countless dispatches from the family of long-term patient Johnson Longstreet; his father wrote in early 1927 that Johnson's "mother cannot eat and some times when she thinking for Johnson because he is only one boy we get," and his mother added five months later, "I got a baby boy [in] march and he die on last week I am very sorry."

Notwithstanding vast distances, barriers of language, and the imperviousness of white authority, correspondents could show extraordinary eloquence and fortitude in their myriad efforts to secure information about their relatives' welfare in hospital and better the circumstances of their detention. As Olive Kirk's sister pleaded to doctors in a 1950 missive, "I don't think she needs to be there much longer. I need her very desperately here. I will also take good care of her … The children miss her very much … I will do anything if you'd let her come home."

And finally, the bonds of kinship survive even the institutional deaths of departed members: Timothy Fergus's family, although utterly destitute, expended borrowed funds on a box and coffin, which they freighted to Essondale from their Vancouver Island village in 1937, along with instructions (conveyed by the local Indian agent) that physicians "have the body shipped home with as little expense as possible," and Jennie Flinders's mother, on learning of the young Gitxsan woman's death from TB in the early fall of 1950, forwarded one last list of appeals: "We sure want her clothes all of them and her picture which we've told you to take and develop and we'll now be expecting it in a few days. We want her picture which they took on her burial day. We want to ask you whether there something wrong in her brain or her head, some day we'll go down there and see her grave yards perhaps October. We'll be expect your welcome answers."[35]

CONCLUSIONS

As this initial, fleeting glance at the world of British Columbia's Aboriginal psychiatric patients draws to a close, we outline the manifold ways in which these assembled institutional and human narratives variously ended, and we offer a final reflection on the enduring meanings of these turbulent lives, both within the times and spaces they collectively inhabited, and for the present.

Table 6.3 summarizes details of the outcomes of these Native people's asylum encounters. First, and arguably the most lacerating finding of this entire study, was the discovery that, for the majority of Aboriginal people who entered the British Columbia mental health system, their committal was effectively a sentence of death. Of the 97 individuals whose fate we know, 62 died on the wards and infirmaries of Essondale and the PHI. Only 35 left hospital alive: 20 of these were released on "probation,"[36] 5 were discharged in full, 5 escaped, 3 received "special probation,"[37] and 2 gained transfer to a home for the aged. Physicians characterized only 9 of these discharged patients as "recovered" and another 16 as "improved."

Among those who died, nearly half (26 in all)[38] yielded to the ravages of tuberculosis. In all, 36 of the 100 Aboriginal inmates contracted this infectious and lethal bacillus either before or during their hospital confinement.[39] The average age of demise for the 65 patients whose death record appeared on file was forty-seven years (one child expired at age eight, and 16 people failed to reach age thirty). Their appallingly high mortality rate no doubt contributed to the Aboriginal patients' relatively brief average length of hospitalization (four years and seven months), although 9 people were institutionalized for more than ten consecutive years, and one man remained on the wards one year short of four decades. And for 6 of the 35 patients who survived the asylum, there would be further involvement with the state psychiatric enterprise.

In the final analysis, about a third of the Aboriginal patients succeeded, at least temporarily and to a partial degree, in breaking free of the gravitational forces that the British Columbia mental health apparatus exerted over them. These included Sarah Loveless, a married Nisga'a woman diagnosed with "melancholia" (following a suicide attempt by hanging), who won her probation in the fall of 1912 on the strength of interventions by

Table 6.3   Outcomes of Aboriginal psychiatric encounters[a]

	Number	Percentage[a]		Number	Percentage[a]
Status on discharge			Age of death[d]		
Deceased	62	64	LT 10	1	2
Probation	20	21	10–19	2	3
Discharge in full	5	5	20–29	13	20
Escape	5	5	30–39	5	8
Special probation[b]	3	3	40–49	16	25
Home for the aged	2	2	50–59	7	11
			60–69	13	20
			70–79	5	8
Condition on discharge			80–89	3	5
Deceased	62	65			
Improved	16	17			
Recovered	9	9	Length of hospitalization[e]		
Unimproved	8	8	LT 1 mth	6	6
			GE 1 mth, LT 6 mths	19	19
			GE 6 mths, LT 1 yr	11	11
Cause of death[c]			GE 1 yr, LT 2 yrs	17	17
Tuberculosis	26	43	GT 2 yrs, LT 5 yrs	23	23
Bronchopneumonia	9	15	GT 5 yrs, LT 10 yrs	13	13
Exhaustion: senile dementia	5	8	GT 10 yrs, LT 20 yrs	2	2
Chronic Heart failure	4	7	GT 30 yrs, LT 40 yrs	5	5
Cerebral hemorrhage	3	5			
Pulmonary edema	2	3			
Nephritis (kidneys)	2	3	Subsequent admissions		
Exhaustion: schizophrenia	1	2	None mentioned	94	94
Exhaustion: epilepsy	1	2	One	3	3
Bright's disease	1	2	Two	2	2
Suicide by hanging	1	2	Seventeen	1	1

[a] Cases with missing information were excluded from the percentage calculations.

[b] Under the BC Mental Hospitals Act, these cases received a six-month probationary leave from hospital into the care of a relative or other guardian, against the advice of physicians.

[c] Thirty-six patients did not die in hospital; in one case of death the cause was unspecified; and the institutional fate of two people is unknown.

[d] Mean age at death = 46.6 years (range = 8–86). Included are 8 patients with medical indications of "approximate" ages.

[e] Mean length of hospitalization = 4 years and 7 months (range = 3 days to 38 years, 11 months and 2 days).

the local Indian agent and Anglican archdeacon; Zelda Braithwaite, a sixty-five-year-old woman from the northern mainland coast suffering from "senile dementia," whose children secured her release in early 1923 after just two months in the Public Hospital for the Insane; the irrepressible Randall Winfree, who walked away from Essondale several times before an exasperated medical staff discharged him "on escape" in late 1944; and

Sam Ketchum, Kamloops-born and a long-time fixture on the Essondale and Riverview Hospital[40] chronic wards, whose thirty-nine–year institutional history of multiple diagnoses, somatic "treatments," and abortive escapes finally came full circle when he vanished for good one week prior to Christmas in 1979.

As these statistics show, however, far more emblematic were those women, men, and children who, once institutionalized, never left the hospital wards alive. Their numbers included Mabel, a blind, elderly Vancouver Island Kwakiutl (Kwakwaka'wakw) woman showing the terrible, advancing effects of chronic tertiary syphilis, who survived detention at the PHI for scarcely five months in 1900 before succumbing to a cerebral hemorrhage in early July. There was also eleven-year-old Len Moon, a "mentally deficient" boy from the Nicola valley, certified for recurrently wandering off his reserve, who died from tuberculosis in midsummer 1922 after barely a year of confinement, and who received an institutional burial despite his impoverished mother's pleas to have his body sent back home. Hugh Tugwell, of the Secwepemc nation, passed away at Essondale of chronic pulmonary edema in late spring of 1962 after a thirty-seven-year career in the provincial hospital system, a career initially prompted by his recurrent epileptic seizures and general unmanageability as a Boys' Industrial School inmate, and which featured a thirty-four-year consecutive stretch of incarceration in the prison-like milieu of the Colquitz Mental Home.

Vancouver-born Agnes Reid died at her own hand. Her twenty-one-year life in many ways epitomized the Aboriginal experience with Canadian and provincial state institutions, as she graduated successively from four years of residential school in the province's interior, to the Girls' Industrial School in the Lower Mainland, to the secure wards of Essondale a few kilometres distant. Described by one hospital physician as "the most dangerous patient we had in the hospital," Agnes was in her eighth year of psychiatric detention in the late fall of 1951 when, alone at night in the locked side-room of the "J" ward for recalcitrant patients in the East Lawn (Chronic Women's) Building, she managed to slip out of the straitjacket in which the staff had encased her. Slightly after 11:00 pm, nurses found Agnes Reid hanging lifeless from the window screening, with the five-foot-long straitjacket cord and a strip torn from her nightgown taut around her neck. Her final note, scrawled with a pencil on the cell wall in total darkness, read in part: "hope you all be happy now I've made up my mind ... love to you ... now that it is done ... can't see but [h]ope you can read it."

In a subsequent coroner's inquest, the jurors determined that "no blame [is] to be attached to anyone on this Institution."

So absolved, the medical authorities closed the books on Agnes Reid's case and bundled her terminated file, the accumulated digest of a broken life, off to the Essondale clinical records stackroom. The documents languished there (almost certainly unread) for nearly half a century until their transfer across the Strait of Georgia to the provincial archives in Victoria. But after all these years, we now find ourselves in the unforeseen (and daunting) position of being able to ponder the relevancies of Agnes Reid's melancholy life journey – and that of the similarly fated pathways taken by Hugh Tugwell and little Len Moon and Mabel (whose Aboriginal name, and English surname, we will probably never know) and, of course, the ill-fated Charley Wolverine, with whose story this chapter began.

These accumulated human and institutional narratives, to be sure, register at myriad levels, and they invite alternative ethical readings and historical interpretations. Without question, the files chronicle with disconcerting frequency examples of lives ruined, power abused, professional arrogance, and racial intolerance inscribed into the very foundations of our public health institutions. Yet these 100 accounts of affliction, segregation, and death are also vivid reminders that madness is a complex and contested cultural phenomenon, and its impact is never preordained. In this sense, the documents speak volumes as much about the limitations as about the effects of state and psychiatric power. They show that historical actors are capable of resisting, and sometimes even transcending, the "insanity" and death that surround them on every side. If the remarkable stories of Charley Wolverine, Agnes Reid, and their many Aboriginal counterparts in the British Columbia asylum system can tell us anything, it is that the miracle of human identity can survive even the darkest of institutional spaces and the corrosive passage of time. With Indigenous people and all others, this is the key historical lesson – and the abiding moral implication – of "patient-centred" research on psychiatry, sanity, and madness.

NOTES

We gratefully acknowledge the generous funding support provided by Simon Fraser University (through its President's Research Grant and SSHRC Small Grant programs) and by Associated Medical Services Inc. (for a Hannah Grant-in-Aid awarded in 2001). This project has benefited enormously from the wonderful research assistance contributed by Kathy McKay, Jenny Clayton, Jeffie Roberts, and Joel Freedman. Thanks as well to James E. Moran and David Wright for their detailed editorial input; to Wenona Victor, Georges Sioui, Renisa Mawani, Dorothy E. Chunn, and two anonymous reviewers for McGill-Queen's University Press for their critical commentary; and to the professionals and staff at the British Columbia Archives and the Riverview Hospital Research Advisory Committee and East Lawn Clinical Records Service (especially Paul Anderson, Diane Carter, Laurie Chaplin, Mac Culham, William Honer, Michelle Purcell, Pauline Verral, and Kathy Zomar). Portions of this chapter were presented in June 2004 at the annual meetings of the Canadian Law and Society Association held in Winnipeg, Manitoba.

1 We pseudonymize patient names throughout the chapter, and we alter or generalize locations and other potentially identifying details wherever needed to safeguard confidentiality.
2 The original BC Insane Asylums Act of 1873 (36 Vict., no. 28, amended 1893) was the principal mental health law in the province until the enactment of the 1897 Hospitals for the Insane Act (61 Vict., c.101). Retitled the Mental Hospitals Act in 1912, the legislation remained in place (with revisions in 1940, including the establishment of appeal boards) until the Mental Health Act came into force in 1964.
3 All direct quotations, if not otherwise referenced, derive from the patient clinical files.
4 We retain without comment all original spelling, grammatical, and other errors from the patient file documents.
5 Thomas Flanagan, *Louis Riel* (Ottawa: Canadian Historical Association, 1992); George R.D. Goulet, *The Trial of Louis Riel: Justice and Mercy Denied: A Critical, Legal and Political Analysis* (Calgary: Tellwell, 1999).
6 Thomas E. Brown, "'Living with God's Afflicted': A History of the Provincial Lunatic Asylum at Toronto, 1830–1911" (PhD thesis, Queen's University, 1980); Dorothy E. Chunn and Robert Menzies, "Out of Mind, Out of Law: The Regulation of 'Criminally Insane' Women inside British Columbia's Public Mental Hospitals, 1888–1973," *Canadian Journal of Women and the Law* 10 (1998): 1–32; Megan J. Davies, "The Patient's World: British Columbia's Mental Health Facilities, 1920–1935" (MA thesis, University of Waterloo 1987); Mary-Ellen Kelm, "Women, Families and the Provincial Hospital for the Insane, British Columbia, 1905–1915," *Journal of Family History* 19 (1994): 177–93; James E. Moran, *Committed to the Asylum: Insanity and Society in Nineteenth-Century Quebec and Ontario* (Montreal and Kingston: McGill-Queen's University Press, 2000); Geoffrey Reaume, *Remembrance of Patients Past: Patient Life at the Toronto*

Hospital for the Insane, 1870–1940 (Toronto: Oxford University Press, 2000); Cheryl Krasnick Warsh, *Moments of Unreason: The Practice of Canadian Psychiatry and the Homewood Retreat, 1883–1923* (Montreal and Kingston: McGill-Queen's University Press, 1989).

7 Of these 100 files, 97 were available in the British Columbia Archives (44 in the GR 2880 collection, "British Columbia, Mental Health Services, Originals, 1872–1942," and 53 in the 93-5683 accessions group, "Riverview Hospital Client Clinical Files, 1946–1969"). The remaining 3 files, all closed during the 1970s, are under the auspices of the Riverview East Lawn Clinical Records Service and are held at the Iron Mountain storage facility.

8 The canonical source on historical case file research is Franca Iacovetta and Wendy Mitchinson, eds., *On the Case: Explorations in Social History* (Toronto: University of Toronto Press, 1998).

9 Dale Peterson, *A Mad People's History of Madness* (Pittsburgh: University of Pittsburgh Press, 1982); Roy Porter, *A Social History of Madness* (New York: E.P. Dutton, 1989).

10 See, among many others, Jonathan Andrews and Anne Digby, eds., *Sex and Seclusion, Class and Custody: Perspectives on Gender and Class in the Historiography of British and Irish Psychiatry* (Amsterdam: Rodopi, 2002); Ellen Dwyer, *Homes for the Mad: Life inside Two Nineteenth-Century Asylums* (New Brunswick, NJ: Rutgers University Press, 1987); Jeffrey L. Geller and Maxine Harris, eds., *Women of the Asylum: Voices from Behind the Walls, 1840–1945* (New York: Anchor Doubleday, 1994); Bronwyn Labrum, "Looking beyond the Asylum: Gender and the Process of Committal in Auckland, 1870–1910," *New Zealand Journal of History* 26, 2 (1992): 125–45; and Yannick Ripa, *Women and Madness: The Incarceration of Women in Nineteenth-Century France* (Minneapolis: University of Minnesota Press, 1990).

11 The fees, amounting to $1.00 daily per patient, rose to $1.35 in the mid-1930s. See British Columbia Archives, GR 542, box 23, file 8, H.W. McGill, deputy superintendent general of Indian Affairs, Dominion of Canada, to H.M. Cassidy, director of social welfare, Province of British Columbia, 24 November 1936.

12 In 1899 the British Columbia and dominion governments struck an agreement for the transfer at federal expense of Yukon psychiatric patients (both Aboriginal and non-Aboriginal) to the Provincial Hospital for the Insane. See British Columbia Archives, GR 2880, box 7, file 953.

13 We use contemporary names and spellings of Aboriginal bands and nations and include original names where needed for purposes of comparison. A comprehensive listing of current First Nations in British Columbia is available from the Union of BC Indian Chiefs Web site at <http://www.ubcic.bc.ca>. See also Robert J. Muckle,

The First Nations of British Columbia (Vancouver: University of British Columbia Press, 1998).

14 Gerry Ferguson, "Control of the Insane in British Columbia, 1849–78,"in John McLaren, Robert Menzies, and Dorothy E. Chunn, eds., *Regulating Lives: Historical Essays on the State, Society, the Individual and the Law* (Vancouver: University of British Columbia Press, 2002), 63–96.

15 "Annual Report for Twelve Months Ended March 31st, 1950." Mental Health Services, Province of British Columbia. Department of Provincial Secretary, BC *Sessional Papers*, 1951 9: 10, 15, 72 (Victoria: Queen's Printer, 1951).

16 For general accounts of the British Columbia psychiatric hospital system and its patients, see Davies, "The Patients' World"; Kelm, "Women, Families and the Provincial Hospital for the Insane, British Columbia, 1905–1915"; Robert Menzies, "'I Do Not Care for a Lunatic's Role': Modes of Regulation and Resistance inside the Colquitz Mental Home, British Columbia, 1919–33," *Canadian Bulletin of Medical History* 16 (1999): 181–213; Robert Menzies and Dorothy E. Chunn, "The Gender Politics of Criminal Insanity: 'Order-in-Council' Women in British Columbia, 1888–1950," *Histoire sociale/Social History* 31 (1999): 241–79.

17 Brett Christophers, *Positioning the Missionary: John Booth Good and the Confluence of Cultures in Nineteenth-Century British Columbia* (Vancouver: University of British Columbia Press, 1998); Elizabeth Furniss, *Victims of Benevolence: Discipline and Death at the Williams Lake Indian Residential School, 1891–1920* (Williams Lake: Cariboo Tribal Council, 1992); J.R. Miller, *Shingwauk's Vision: A History of Native Residential Schools* (Toronto: University of Toronto Press, 1996); John S. Milloy, *A National Crime: The Canadian Government and the Residential School System, 1879–1986* (Winnipeg: University of Manitoba Press, 1999); Peter Murray, *The Devil and Mr. Duncan* (Victoria: Sono Nis Press, 1985).

18 Mary-Ellen Kelm, *Colonizing Bodies: Aboriginal Health and Healing in British Columbia, 1900–50* (Vancouver: University of British Columbia Press, 1998). See also Robert Boyd, *The Coming of the Spirit of Pestilence: Introduced Infectious Diseases and Population Decline among Northwest Coast Indians, 1774–1874* (Vancouver: University of British Columbia Press 1999); Robert M. Galois, "Measles, 1847–1850: The First Modern Epidemic in British Columbia," BC *Studies* 109 (1996): 31–43.

19 See Jean Barman, *The West beyond the West: A History of British Columbia*, 2nd Ed. (Toronto: University of Toronto Press, 1996), 363.

20 Among other British Columbia sources, see Jean Barman, "Taming Aboriginal Sexuality: Gender, Power, and Race in British Columbia, 1850–1900," BC *Studies* 115/116 (1997–98): 237–66; Douglas Cole and Ira Chaikin, *An Iron Hand upon*

the People: The Law against the Potlatch on the Northwest Coast (Vancouver: Douglas & McIntyre, 1990); Robin Fisher, *Contact and Conflict: Indian-European Relations in British Columbia, 1774–1890* (Vancouver: University of British Columbia Press, 1977); Douglas Harris, *Fish, Law, and Colonialism: The Legal Capture of the Aboriginal Fishery in British Columbia* (Toronto: University of Toronto Press, 2001); Rolf Knight, *Indians at Work: An Informal History of Native Indian Labour in British Columbia, 1858–1930* (Vancouver: New Star Books, 1978); John Lutz, "After the Fur Trade: The Aboriginal Labouring Class of British Columbia, 1849–1890," *Journal of the Canadian Historical Association,* n.s. 2 (1992): 69–94; Paul Tennant, *Aboriginal Peoples and Politics: The Indian Land Question in British Columbia, 1849–1989* (Vancouver: University of British Columbia Press, 1990); *Tina Loo, Making Law, Order, and Authority in British Columbia, 1821–1871* (Toronto: University of Toronto Press, 1994).

21 Cole Harris, *Making Native Space: Colonialism, Resistance, and Reserves in British Columbia* (Vancouver: University of British Columbia Press, 2002).

22 British Columbia Archives, GR 1754, boxes 1–2, vols. 1–6, "Provincial Mental Hospital, Essondale, Originals. Admission Books 1872–1947"; and GR 3019, box 89-941-1, vol. 1, "Riverview Hospital, Originals, 1934–1971. Admission Book 1947–51."

23 Evidently, no Aboriginal person spent time at the Victoria Lunatic Asylum during its brief existence as the province's first psychiatric establishment between 1872 and 1878.

24 Overall hospital patient admissions, Aboriginal admissions, and study sample numbers by decade were as follows (the statistics in the first two columns derive from the Mental Health Services 1951 annual report (see note 15 above):

Years	Total general admissions	Total aboriginal admissions	Study sample
1872–79	144	1	1
1880–89	205	2	1
1890–99	659	3	2
1900–09	1,559	7	3
1910–19	3,774	25	13
1920–29	4,963	39	22
1930–39	6,264	46	24
1940–49	9,117	59	29
1950–	1,415	11	5

25 Ross Gordon Green, *Justice in Aboriginal Communities: Sentencing Alternatives* (Saskatoon: Purich, 1998); Kayleen M. Hazlehurst, ed., *Legal Pluralism and the Colonial Legacy: Indigenous Experiences of Justice in Canada, Australia, and*

New Zealand (Brookfield VT: Aldershot, 1995); Marianne O. Nielsen and Robert A. Silverman, eds., *Native Americans, Crime, and Justice* (Boulder: Westview Press, 1996); *Royal Commission on Aboriginal Peoples, Aboriginal Peoples and the Justice System: Report of the National Round Table on Aboriginal Justice Issues* (Ottawa: Royal Commission on Aboriginal Peoples, 1993).

26 Don McCaskill, "Native People and the Justice System," in Ian A.L. Getty and Antoine S. Lussier, eds., *As Long as the Sun Shines and Water Flows: A Reader in Canadian Native Studies* (Vancouver: University of British Columbia Press, 1983), 288–98.

27 Summaries of BC patient attributes are available in Davies, "The Patients' World"; Mary-Ellen Kelm, "Women and Families in the Asylum Practice of Charles Edward Doherty at the Provincial Hospital for the Insane, 1905–1915" (MA thesis, Department of History, Simon Fraser University); Robert Menzies, "Historical Profiles of Criminal Insanity," *International Journal of Law and Psychiatry* 25 (2002): 379–404; Menzies, "'I Do Not Care for a Lunatic's Role.'" See also the annual reports of the provincial asylums and mental hospitals, published from Confederation onward in the BC *Sessional Papers* (see note 15 above).

28 Philip, like many BC Aboriginal people of the era, had an English given name, but no known surname.

29 See notes 6, 9, 10, and 16 above.

30 Frantz Fanon observes how, for racialized peoples, the personal experience of madness is intertwined with the historical processes of colonialism. "A normal Negro child," Fanon writes in *Black Skins, White Masks* (New York: Grove, 1967 [1952], 147), "having grown up within a normal family, will become abnormal on the slightest contact with the white world." Our thanks to Renisa Mawani for bringing this quotation to our attention.

31 On general Aboriginal understandings of health and illness, see Kelm, *Colonizing Bodies*. For a recent account of ideas about insanity and violence among the Tununirmiut of North Baffin Island during the early twentieth century, see Shelagh D. Grant, *Arctic Justice: On Trial for Murder, Pond Inlet, 1923* (Montreal and Kingston: McGill-Queen's University Press, 2002).

32 Mark Finnane, "Asylums, Families and the State," *History Workshop Journal* 20 (1985): 134–48; Kelm, "Women, Families and the Provincial Hospital for the Insane, British Columbia, 1905–1915"; Labrum, "Looking beyond the Asylum"; Patricia E. Prestwich, "Family Strategies and Medical Power: 'Voluntary' Committal in a Parisian Asylum, 1876–1914," *Journal of Social History* 27 (1994): 799–818; Reaume, *Remembrance of Patients Past*.

33 The ward progress notes and incident reports describe 9 of the 100 Aboriginal patients as having committed some act of violence while in hospital. Four people recorded one assault each. Two committed two assaults apiece, and 3 were

involved in "several" or "many" incidents (not all of which physicians deemed worthy of documenting).

34 The agent described Edward Staples's letter as being "quite intelligent for a patient of a Mental Hospital."

35 Medical Superintendent Ryan's reply, addressed not to Mrs Flinders but to her husband, read as follows: "In reference to your late daughter, she had no clothes except a coat which was forwarded to you at the time of her death. In reference to the picture there are no pictures as your letter arrived too late for pictures to be taken of the coffin. It was suggested that a picture of the grave be taken later as at the present time it would simply show a mound."

36 Most involuntarily certified people released from Essondale or the Public Hospital for the Insane were granted six-month periods of "probation" in the community under s. 21 of the provincial Mental Hospitals Act. On the successful completion of the probationary term, a patient would typically receive a discharge in full, and hospital administrators would close her or his file. Authorities could revoke probation and recommit the patient in the event of mental relapse or other apprehended problem.

37 Under the Mental Hospitals Act, ss. 33 and 36, hospital physicians were empowered to grant six-month terms of "special probation" to patients when the latter were discharged against medical advice (usually on the insistence of family members).

38 Of the others, 9 were victims of pneumonia, while 6 died from the effects of advanced syphilis (paresis), 5 died of "exhaustion of senile dementia," 4 of chronic cardiac failure, 3 of stroke or hemorrhage, 2 each of kidney failure and edema of the lung, and 1 each of exhaustion of schizophrenia, exhaustion of epilepsy, Bright's disease, and suicide by hanging.

39 See note 18 above.

40 With the passage of a revised BC *Mental Health Act* in 1964, the Provincial Mental Hospital, Essondale, became Riverview Hospital. See generally Ministry of Health and Ministry Responsible for Seniors, Province of British Columbia, "Guide to the Mental Health Act," 15 November 1999, <https://www.healthservices.gov.bc.ca/mhd/pdf/MentalHealthGuide.pdf>.

7

"Prescription for Survival"

Brock Chisholm, Sterilization, and Mental Health in the Cold War Era

IAN DOWBIGGIN

Few Canadians in the twentieth century enjoyed the international eminence of psychiatrist Brock Chisholm (1896–1971). Chisholm was Canada's deputy minister of health during World War II and the first director-general of the World Health Organization (1948–53). Throughout the early decades of the Cold War, he spoke out repeatedly on a wide range of social, political, economic, and cultural issues, one of those rare public figures whose opinions were heeded by influential policy-makers the world over. In his many utterances on matters of public health, Chisholm consistently gave the impression that he was urging novel solutions to pressing problems that faced the twentieth-century world. The perception that he was an iconoclast and ahead of his time has led his biographer to call him Canada's "first postmodern thinker."[1]

Yet such an interpretation ignores the wider historical context surrounding Chisholm's life and career as a pivotal international figure. Certain aspects of his career placed him squarely within the broad twentieth-century population control movement, which peaked in the 1950s and 1960s, a movement with roots that date back to the theories of Thomas Malthus in the early nineteenth century and, more recently, to the eugenics and mental hygiene movements of the early twentieth century, with their advocacy of sterilization as a method of contraception.[2] Chisholm, like so many others in the population control field, believed that population growth was a sign of irrational fertility, itself a source of global instability, triggering rising rates of emotional and physical illness and breeding the conditions that led to war and revolution at a time in world history when atomic weapons threatened the future of humankind itself. As John Rock, co-discoverer of the first oral contraceptive, or "pill," put it in 1963, "the greatest menace to world peace and decent standards of life today is not atomic energy but sexual energy."[3] Chisholm agreed and shared the belief common among demographers that, even with the arrival of "the pill," sterilization (vasectomy for men and tubal ligation for women) was the most effective contraceptive method for avoiding the global catastrophe that uncontrolled "sexual energy" would likely spark. In other words, world peace and security rested on the ability of families to free themselves of the distress, poverty, and bad health generated by unwanted children, and access to sterilization services was a key to achieving this goal.

Thus, from the perspective of the early twenty-first century, Chisholm, though he often invoked the spectre of future disasters to justify his policy recommendations, was very much a product of his own time. By the time he died in 1971, his vision of population control, rather than adumbrating coming trends, was actually being overtaken by new and different interpretations of reproductive rights that rejected his authoritarian proposals and stressed instead women's freedom to choose.

Virtually from the beginning of his career as a psychiatrist, Chisholm believed that the goal of psychiatry was to show how human beings could "take the tension out of sexual development" and thus pave the way for "effective social development." For Chisholm (taking a page out of Sigmund Freud's theories), modern civilization was increasingly becoming neurotic because religious taboos about contraception and sexual expression made people unhappy and frustrated, rendering them unable to function as responsible human beings in a world that demanded higher standards of citizenship than ever before. At the same time, he became convinced that world peace and stability were being challenged by runaway population growth among the least intelligent groups of society and in the least developed regions of the world. By the outbreak of World War II, Chisholm had concluded that what the world needed most of all was "proper methods of birth control" that would make the lives of the civilized, intelligent classes happier and curtail the fertility of the relatively uncivilized and less intelligent groups around the world.

Chisholm was born in Oakville, Ontario, on 18 May 1896, into a straitlaced Presbyterian family. Much of his life was spent rebelling against what he called the "poisonous" value systems of his religious parents and like-minded people.[4] In 1915, at the age of nineteen, he enlisted in the Canadian army and served with distinction on the Western Front, winning the Military Cross twice. Wounded in September 1918, Chisholm achieved the rank of captain by the time he left the service the following year.

His exposure to the grim conditions of trench warfare during World War I left him with vivid and indelible convictions about the seemingly fine line between mental health and psychiatric illness. Chisholm was not alone in coming to these conclusions. At the same time, physicians in other armies were developing the first theories about "shell shock," the condition of psychological breakdown that they claimed was a result of the traumatizing effects of modern warfare.[5] Military intelligence testing, introduced during World War I, also revealed the startling news that the mental age of the average US soldier was only thirteen. Robert Yerkes, head of the US military's mental testing program, concluded that almost one out of every two American inductees was a mental defective.[6] For Chisholm, like other psychiatrists of his day, the war taught that the challenges of peacetime lay in devising health strategies that would prevent the many "mental weaklings" in society from succumbing to the aggression, guilt, fear, and anxiety that he alleged were the root causes of war in the first place. The task facing psychiatry after World War I was to develop "mental hygiene" approaches to curb the rate of mental and nervous disease.[7] Chisholm would return to this theme of psychiatry winning the peace by treating society's "mental weaklings" during and after World War II.

In the meantime, he entered medical school in 1919 at the University of Toronto where he enrolled in two courses on psychiatry, taught by C.K. Clarke. By the early 1920s Clarke, dean of medicine at the University of Toronto and medical director of the Canadian National Committee for Mental Hygiene (CNCMH), was Canada's pre-eminent psychiatrist. He disdainfully rejected many of the neo-Freudian theories of sexuality that Chisholm would later entertain, but Clarke's own views on public health and preventive psychiatry clearly influenced the young medical student. Right up to his death in 1924, Clarke taught that modern health care systems were useless without the diagnostic and therapeutic expertise of psychiatrists, an opinion Chisholm quickly adopted.[8]

Following his graduation from medical school in 1924, Chisholm spent a year doing postgraduate studies at the Middlesex Hospital in London, England, and then returned to set up a private medical practice in Oakville.

Six years of general practice reinforced his burgeoning interest in psychiatry. Many of his patients were what might be called "the worried well," those persons whose emotional troubles seemed severe enough to warrant psychiatric treatment but not serious enough to require institutionalization in a mental hospital. The emotional troubles about which these patients tended to complain were frequently sexual in nature and pointed to the conjugal unhappiness of numerous married couples.

Armed with this clinical experience, Chisholm was like so many psychiatrists in Canada and the United States who gravitated towards the mental hygiene movement after stints in private practice. By the early 1930s he was part of this growing group within Canadian psychiatry. Chisholm became good friends with Clarence Hincks, who became the medical director of the CNCMH in 1924 and the US-based National Committee for Mental Hygiene in 1930, and he shared with Hincks a belief in the necessity of creating a firm place for psychiatry within the public health field. Hincks would later describe Chisholm as being "twenty years ahead of his time ... He was more than a psychiatrist. He was the greatest humanist I ever met."[9]

Chisholm's connections to Hincks, Clarke, and the mental hygiene movement not only signalled his resolve to promote psychiatry as an indispensable medical specialty in the struggle to prevent disease. They also indicate his indebtedness to the eugenics movement of the early twentieth century. Eugenics, a term coined by Charles Darwin's cousin Francis Galton in 1883, was normally defined as the scientific study of human breeding. The most glaring example of eugenics was the sterilization law introduced by Adolf Hitler's Third Reich in 1933, a program that ultimately led to the sterilization of roughly 400,000 Germans by 1939. The two high points for the eugenics movement in Canada occurred in 1928 and 1933 when Alberta and British Columbia respectively became the only two provinces to pass sterilization laws that approved involuntary vasectomies for men and tubal ligations for women.[10]

Many of the spokespersons for eugenics in Canada were also active in the mental hygiene movement. Clarke had been a leading crusader in Canada against the eugenic threats posed by mass immigration to Canada between the 1890s and World War I. C.B. Farrar, head of the Toronto Psychiatric Hospital and member of the Eugenics Society of Canada (ESC), also warned about the need for sterilization programs as a means of contraception for those unable to control their own fertility. Clarence Hincks too played a crucial role in the evolution of Canadian eugenics by providing expert advice to the Alberta government when it was develop-

ing its 1928 Sexual Sterilization law.[11] By the 1930s most advocates of
sterilization, like Hincks, rejected justifications of the operation that
stressed how it could seriously reduce the incidence of hereditary mental
illness from one generation to the next. Instead, they tended to endorse
sterilization as a means of relieving mental patients of the duties and
stress of raising children and preventing their offspring from being
exposed to poor methods of parenting. Advocates also favoured sterilization because it enabled them to discharge hospitalized patients into the
community, an appealing policy for cash-strapped governments in the
midst of the Great Depression. Sterilizing inmates freed up beds for more
severely disabled patients, providing opportunities for the handicapped to
enjoy a better quality of life outside institutional settings. Chisholm was
from a younger generation than figures such as Hincks and Farrar, and
thus was not as wedded to the earlier eugenic ideas underlying their
support for sterilization. But his later emphasis on sterilization as a birth
control and population control method betrayed the deep influence they
had exerted on him at an early stage in his career when his own ideas
about mental health were still forming.

Chisholm's theories about the links between birth control and mental
health first gained notoriety in 1937 when he served as an expert witness
for the defence at the trial of Dorothea Palmer. Palmer was a nurse
employed by the Parents' Information Bureau (PIB) in Kitchener, Ontario.
She had been arrested for distributing birth control information to a
French-speaking Roman Catholic family in a suburb outside Ottawa. After
nineteen days of testimony and four of argument, during which forty
expert witnesses (including Chisholm) testified amid intense press scrutiny,
Palmer was acquitted.

While from a strictly legal standpoint the trial was about the Canadian
Criminal Code's prohibition of the sale or advertisement of contraceptives,
much of the testimony in Palmer's defence had a distinctly eugenic flavour.
The PIB was headed by A.R. Kaufman, a Kitchener, Ontario, manufacturer
and owner of the Kaufman Rubber Company. Kaufman was also treasurer
of the ESC, someone who was convinced that the birth rate of the lower
classes was far too high and threatened to swamp the fertility of the fit,
"intelligent" classes of society. Through the PIB, he offered contraceptive
services to both his employees and unemployed families. In particular, he
endorsed sterilization as a birth control method and backed the ESC-led
campaign to pressure Ontario into passing a sterilization law (it never did).
Along with the ESC, Kaufman worried that if the dependent classes were
allowed to breed as they wished, there would be so many destitute and

unhappy people that they might launch a political revolution someday. He chose as Palmer's defence attorney F.W. Wegenast, a fellow member of the ESC. Wegenast summoned like-minded eugenicists, including ESC president William Hutton, an ardent proponent of sterilization laws for the handicapped, to testify on Palmer's behalf.[12]

Chisholm was chosen as a defence witness because of his expertise in intelligence testing and his studies into the effect of sexuality on psychological development. But on the stand Chisholm defended Hutton's theory that the country was facing a "biological crisis" triggered by the fertility of the less intelligent groups in society. The intelligent classes were also in dire need of birth control information, he added, because their reliance on contraceptive techniques such as withdrawal, or coitus interruptus, was leading to unhappy marriages, dysfunctional children, and unhealthy family psychological conditions. For Chisholm, intelligent people were paying a steep emotional price for obeying their "social conscience" and limiting the size of their families through these unsatisfying methods. What emerged from his testimony was his mounting belief that the prohibitions against birth control needed to be dismantled for *all* Canadians in order both to serve eugenic purposes and to free human beings from the emotional troubles that he thought were due to frustrated sexuality.[13]

Kaufman's and Chisholm's paths would cross again later in the 1960s when they were both members of the Association for Voluntary Sterilization. In the meantime, the arrival of World War II meant the federal government was looking for professionals such as Chisholm to help with the process of selecting the best servicemen, and in 1941 he was appointed director of Personnel Selection for the Canadian army. Thrilled that the army had decided to use psychological screening of all recruits, Chisholm went hard to work creating a system for determining which serviceman fit what job in the armed services. In September 1942 he was promoted to the post of director-general of Medical Services for the Canadian army, a clear signal that the military establishment believed that the mental health of men and women in the armed forces was as important as their physical health.

Yet Chisholm viewed his task as something grander and more ambitious than simply screening out the sort of misfits who had made it into the ranks in wars gone by. He also sought to exploit military training as a way of moulding personality and character in order to rectify the mistakes of upbringing made by parents in peacetime. Typically, he refused to keep his opinions to himself. As the conflict overseas wore on,

Chisholm began speaking out and soon gained the reputation of outspo-
kenness that would follow him for the rest of his life. Whatever the topic,
in the final analysis he revealed his inveterate fondness for broad schemes
of social engineering, a taste that dated back to his early years in the
mental hygiene movement, when he was surrounded by other physicians
with pro-eugenic opinions.

Wartime proved to be the setting that made Chisholm into an international opinion-maker. In a few short years he became renowned as an
expert on mental health, and his tendency to say contentious things, rather
than ruining his career, only accelerated his meteoric rise as a world-
famous doctor, culminating in July 1948 when he was voted the first director-general of the World Health Organization (WHO). Perhaps the two
biggest controversies he created occurred in 1944 and 1945. The first was
sparked by a speech in which he blamed Canadian mothers for spoiling
their sons and unfitting them for military life and the emotional strain of
combat. This trend in upbringing, Chisholm contended, accounted for the
close to 25 per cent rate of mental breakdown in the Canadian armed
forces, not shell shock.[14] The heated public reaction to his speech suggested
that he was the first to broach this topic, but appearances were deceptive.
Chisholm's views were symptomatic of the theory of "momism," a concept
that gained popularity among psychiatrists with experience dealing with
men in uniform during World War II. Edward Strecker, chair of the Department of Psychiatry at the University of Pennsylvania medical school and
former president of the American Psychiatric Association, claimed that
mothers made their sons immature when they failed to "untie the emotional apron string." By producing psychoneurotic young men for the
armed forces, Strecker and Chisholm maintained, mothers put the nation's
very survival at risk.[15]

The second controversy (1945) stemmed from another speech, with
Chisholm this time holding Canadian parents accountable for damaging
their children's cognitive and emotional development by encouraging
their youngsters to believe in Santa Claus. According to him, the social
danger of this form of parenting lay in its capacity to create people who
could not think for themselves and who thus were "easy meat for dema-
gogues and mob orators."[16] In both controversies, Chisholm showed his
visceral tendency to make parents – not the social, political, or cultural
environment – responsible for the troubles of the world in the twentieth
century. For him, the root cause of war, poverty, hatred, intolerance, and
injustice was the way traditions, customs, and unquestioned religious
faith governed the family and produced generation after generation of

neurotic individuals who could not adapt to the threatening world of the atomic age. Under the wise professional guidance of experts like himself, people could be weaned away from these vestiges of days gone by, and the entire world would be a better place. In Chisholm's opinion, what was chiefly needed was improved access to modern methods of birth control, such as sterilization.

His growing belief that it was psychiatry's job to help train a new generation of world citizens made him an inspired choice as the WHO's first director-general. During his five years in the post he maintained a breakneck pace, travelling around the world and consulting with countless health care officials from various countries. In these travels he learned of the tremendous toll diseases such as tuberculosis, smallpox, cholera, and malaria exacted on the world's population, and he worked indefatigably to try to reduce the incidence of these afflictions. But he kept coming back to the view that had earlier crystallized in his mind, his belief that to combat disease and disability, it was necessary to construct an entirely new world order based on a revolutionary interpretation of citizenship that stressed emancipation from traditional mores and primary loyalty to humankind in general, rather than to family, tribe, or country. Nothing less than the survival of the entire world appeared to hang in the balance. And no issue was more fundamental to the survival of the world than the control of fertility.

As Chisholm concluded in the 1950s, in order to save the world from disastrous overpopulation, the value systems surrounding sex, marriage, fertility, and reproduction were in particular need of reform. In voicing this opinion, he was following a current in American social science that drew attention to the severe crisis the world would face if drastic measures to stem population growth were not taken right away. Demographers cited the fact that it had taken all of human history to reach a world population of 1 billion by 1800, but that another 1½ billion people had been added since then. The problem was especially acute in developing countries such as India, where the nation's population had grown by almost 25 million in only five years after World War II, chiefly as a result of the way modern medicine had dramatically cut the death rate. Optimists argued that population increases such as these were temporary. They cited the example of Europe, where, they contended, overpopulation had convinced people to reduce the size of their families voluntarily when it became obvious that children were no longer economically necessary. Thus the birth rate would decline until the population stabilized again. In the short term, however, population data were following disturbing patterns.

From his vantage point at the WHO, Chisholm was as aware of these trends as anyone. He did not agree with everything each demographer alarmed over population growth said during the 1950s, but he certainly shared their belief that political and environmental catastrophes were in store for the planet if prevailing fertility patterns did not change radically. He also believed that the only obstacle to changing these patterns was organized religion, notably the Roman Catholic Church. This lesson was driven home during his four-year stint at the WHO when an attempt to get the organization to support population control through the provision of contraceptives in developing countries was scuttled by opposition from Catholic countries as well as the Canadian government, which feared the political clout of the Catholic Church in Quebec.[17] In a basic sense, Chisholm's views in the 1950s had not altered since the Dorothea Palmer trial of 1937, when he warned that a "biological crisis" resulting from uncontrolled fertility might explode any day into violent revolution or war.

Alarm over global population growth in the Cold War era had been voiced most strongly by William Vogt, whose runaway international best-seller *Road to Survival* (1948) urged nations to undertake "vigorous birth control campaigns." Vogt warned that if this were not done, another, more destructive world war lay in the future. Population growth, he argued, put unsustainable pressure on natural resources such as water and food supply. War resulted when nations sought to acquire these critical resources from neighbouring countries. Vogt applauded ideas such as H.L. Mencken's proposal of "sterilization bonuses," which governments could use to entice "permanently indigent individuals, many of whom would be physically and psychologically marginal," to permanently end their fertility and prevent "their hordes of offspring" from begetting their own kind.[18] Other prominent Americans who also wanted to slow population growth, such as John D. Rockefeller III, founder of the Population Council in 1952, were wary about endorsing sterilization as a contraceptive method and were more concerned about controlling population quantity than biological quality. But others felt no hesitation about proposing coercive (if necessary) sterilization of the over-fertile or expressing their worries about the differential birth rate between the so-called fit and unfit classes.[19]

One population control advocate who backed sterilization as a form of birth control was business tycoon Hugh Moore. Rockefeller was the most respectable figure associated with the population control movement in the 1950s, but Moore was its most outspoken and dynamic. The wealthy inventor of the Dixie Cup, the first disposable sanitary paper drinking cup, Moore turned his formidable attention to world population in the late 1940s after reading Vogt's *Road to Survival*. From that point to his death in 1972 he devoted his considerable wealth and energy to the cause of population control. Moore coined the phrase "the population bomb" in the mid-1950s, years before environmentalist Paul Ehrlich made it famous in his 1968 best-seller of the same name. For Moore, overpopulation, especially in the developing "Third World," created the social and economic conditions that attracted people to communism. His tendency to draw links between overpopulation and the threat of communism constituted a powerful message to policy-makers in the 1950s and was highly similar to Chisholm's own thinking. Moore's message also enabled him to launch international organizations dedicated to providing foreign aid to developing countries in the form of access to birth control programs and services.

Less interested in research than activism on the population front, and often accused by moderates such as Rockefeller of scaremongering, Moore had concluded by the late 1950s that voluntary sterilization held the key to limiting global fertility. His preference for sterilization led him in 1964 to become president of the Human Betterment Association of America (HBAA), a small activist organization headquartered in New York City. Neither influential nor well funded, the HBAA was ripe for Moore's leadership. It had been founded in 1937 as the Sterilization League of New Jersey (SLNJ), a tiny, socially elite group originally dedicated to pressuring New Jersey's state legislature into passing a eugenic sterilization law. This attempt failed, and when the respectability of eugenic sterilization faded as a social reform after World War II because of the stigma of Nazism, the SLNJ (renamed Birthright in 1943 and the HBAA in 1950) barely managed to survive until the 1960s.[20]

Yet gradually Moore was able to re-energize the group after he joined it in 1953. Under his guidance the HBAA became the Human Betterment Association for Voluntary Sterilization in 1962 and then the Association for Voluntary Sterilization (AVS) three years later. Thanks to Moore's leadership, the AVS steadily shifted its focus from widening sterilization access in the United States to helping promote mass sterilization programs in overpopulated and underdeveloped countries such as India. AVS officials always maintained that they advocated voluntary sterilization for consenting men and women, but that argument met resistance from the Roman Catholic Church, which condemned sterilization as a form of contraception; from the medical profession, which worried about lawsuits against surgeons for performing the operation; and from the public, which often associated sterilization with the Nazi experiment with eugenic sterilization in the 1930s. AVS officials continually had to defend their intentions in the face of accusations from various interest groups that popularizing sterilization as a method of birth control could lead to horrendous, Nazi-like abuses. Indeed, when it came to defending access to sterilization services for minorities, disadvantaged groups, and the handicapped, it was difficult to know precisely where AVS representatives imagined voluntarism ended and coercion began. Moore's attitude was fairly typical of the people who belonged to the AVS: he believed that unless elective sterilization was widespread, especially among those classes and in those countries that most needed it, then broad programs of compulsory sterilization would be urgently required.[21] His attitude toward population control could best be summed up as: Enact voluntary sterilization laws now, or else!

Moore's leadership of the AVS in the 1960s made it more high-profile, if not immediately more respectable. By the time he became president, the association's membership already included prominent Americans such as John Rock, William Vogt, the bioethicist Joseph Fletcher, and Planned Parenthood Federation of America president Alan Guttmacher, second only to Margaret Sanger as a birth control campaigner in American history. Chisholm joined the AVS in 1960, when he readily accepted Guttmacher's nomination to the organization's Medical and Scientific Committee. By then, Canada's A.R. Kaufman and George W. Cadbury were also AVS members.

Relations between the AVS and Chisholm grew so cordial that he was invited to be the keynote speaker at its annual conference in 1962. One year later he agreed to serve as AVS honorary president. In 1966 he joined Margaret Sanger as an honorary chairman of the AVS International Advisory Committee. If Chisholm dissented from any of the cardinal principles of the association or Hugh Moore's work in the population field, he kept his disagreements to himself. As he told the AVS, he was "proud" of his affiliation with "[your] very worthy cause."[22]

Chisholm's association with the AVS dovetailed with his steadily growing interest in radical approaches to population control. As he increasingly became alarmed over the threat of global overpopulation in the 1950s, he expressed admiration for Japan's draconian 1948 eugenic laws, which had been passed in the wake of World War II in an effort to ease the overcrowding that some observers (such as Vogt) believed was the reason for the country's imperialist aggression before and during the war. Chisholm applauded the "dramatic reduction" in Japan's birth rate as a result of the extensive use of abortion and sterilization as contraceptive methods. "Unfortunately," he wrote in *Maclean's* magazine in 1959, "Japan is the only country taking really effective steps in this direction," and he enjoined other countries to "mak[e] responsible family planning possible for our hundreds of millions of hungry people." One nation whose efforts filled him with hope was India, where he noted that the government was paying men to undergo sterilization.[23] Otherwise, echoing Hugh Moore's gloomy forecasts, Chisholm warned that "the great increase in population pressure" would breed "hopelessness," paving the way for the "present flight to authoritarianism" in the form of communism and other totalitarian systems of government.[24]

Chisholm, like his allies in the AVS, tended to stress the social and political benefits of family planning. But they also viewed sterilization and other birth control measures as means for realizing the WHO's definition of health as not merely "the absence of illness, but a state of complete physical, mental, and social well-being."[25] The AVS position was that "education, service and research in the field of voluntary sterilization enhances this 'well-being' for many couples distressed by anxieties and tensions caused by fear of repeated unwanted pregnancies." Chisholm elaborated on this theme when he addressed AVS members at their annual meeting on 8 February 1962. Repeating the article of faith of the population control movement, he asserted that hunger and nuclear weapons might endanger the survival of humanity, but the "more dangerous" threat was the "population explosion." Humanity's ability to defuse the population explosion, he complained, was being hampered by traditional "prejudices" surrounding birth control. These prejudices had become "incorporated into the religious attitude of considerable numbers of people." The solution, according to Chisholm, lay in humanity liberating itself from these supposedly outdated and "irrelevant" customs. When the human race was able to emancipate itself, Chisholm concluded, it would end "the misery being produced even in the highly-developed countries, ... an enormous amount of misery, poverty, and ill health" resulting from "the burden of childbearing on women who do not have methods of reducing the incidence of pregnancy." Thus "the responsible and mature person" had to do his or her share to improve this "threatening situation," and "[s]terilization is, in many types of situations, the most appropriate and effective method of reducing rates of increase in population. Voluntary sterilization, from both the individual and social point of view, is highly reliable, is without aesthetic disadvantages, requires no embarrassing procedures, costs nothing beyond the original operation, and offers no risk to health. Any objections represent only old prejudices based on long past situations and ancient ignorance." Complying with the unprecedented demands of the world in the twentieth century, Chisholm contended, would not only help the planet survive; it would also make individuals happier and healthier mentally and physically.[26]

Chisholm's association with AVS tailed off in the late 1960s as he started to suffer from a series of strokes that forced him to give up his globe-trotting activities. He died on 4 February 1971, but in the meantime his appeals (and those of the AVS) had not fallen on deaf ears. Despite fierce opposition from the Roman Catholic Church, in 1971 the US federal government's Office of Economic Opportunity extended funding for voluntary sterilization services to the nation's 5 million poor women in need of birth control. One year later the entire policy came under intense media criticism when it was revealed that two African-American sisters aged twelve and fourteen had been sterilized in Montgomery, Alabama, under a federally financed program. One study of national sterilization policy disclosed that of 22,175 women who had been sterilized in 1972, 40 per cent were black and 30 per cent received public assistance. The federal government hastily introduced guidelines to curb abuses, and in the meantime the courts moved aggressively to ensure that the only people eligible for sterilization were fully consenting adults.[27]

Similar problems arose overseas when in 1965, through its Agency for International Development, the US government began to provide poor countries with funding to deal with their population problems. Once again controversy plagued the family planning movement when it was revealed that India had been using both financial incentives and outright coercion to persuade countless men and women to undergo sterilization. Revelations about the heavy-handed methods employed to sterilize 7 million Indians during the nation's state of emergency in 1976–77 brought down Prime Minister Indira Gandhi's government in 1977. As readers of novelist Rohinton Mistry's *A Fine Balance* know, these mass sterilization programs in India could hardly be described as voluntary.

What Chisholm would have thought about these programs of forced sterilization is a matter of speculation, although given his endorsement of paying East Indians to be sterilized, it is unlikely he would have objected strenuously. In all probability, he would have turned a blind eye to the more coercive aspects of such policies because in the end he believed that its victims would have enjoyed better mental health after the operation.

No longer stressed by deferred sexual gratification and the burden of raising unwanted children, they would have seen their quality of life so much improved that they would have been happier. What is beyond dispute is that his impassioned support for sterilization as a major component of international family planning played a large role in creating a climate conducive to social experiments such as India's family planning program.

It would be a mistake to say that throughout his career as "doctor to the world," sterilization was the uppermost issue in Chisholm's mind or that population was his sole public health concern. Nor would it be fair to blame him for advocating neo-eugenic ideas that were part of the intellectual stock and trade of so many figures within the global health movement. Chisholm barely lived to see the beginnings of the great revolution in public attitudes toward sexuality and reproduction, an upheaval in social and gender mores that utterly rejected his generation's misogynist and paternalist willingness to advocate programs of birth control that frequently disregarded the borderline between choice and coercion. Like so many of his generation, Chisholm fell prey to the temptation to blur public and private boundaries, to conflate self and society.[28] By the time he died, his views were decidedly out of step with the mounting campaign in favour of women's reproductive right to choose, a movement that would culminate in the US Supreme Court's 1973 ruling *Roe v. Wade*, which struck down as unconstitutional state laws in the United States prohibiting abortion.[29]

Yet that is precisely the point this chaper seeks to make: Chisholm, rather than being "postmodern," was very much a product of elite opinion in his own time, someone whose views on fertility, like Hugh Moore's, were already out of fashion within the population control field by the 1970s. Indeed, there is an elementary consistency that links his opinions expressed at the Dorothea Palmer trial in 1937 and those he voiced in the 1960s when debates over what form of birth control was the best were all the rage. Chisholm's ties to the past were considerably stronger than were his links to the future. If his theories strike current-day historians as progressive and postmodern, it ultimately says more about their ideological assumptions than about Brock Chisholm and the cultural tenor of his own times.

NOTES

1 Allan Irving, *Brock Chisholm: Doctor to the World* (Markham: Fitzhenry and Whiteside, 1998), 95.

2 For a recent and incisive examination of the historical interconnections between the population control and family planning movements, see Donald T. Critchlow, *Intended Consequences: Birth Control, Abortion, and the Federal Government in Modern America* (New York and Oxford: Oxford University Press, 1999).

3 John Rock, *The Time Has Come* (New York: Knopf, 1963), 18. quoted in Lara V. Marks, *Sexual Chemistry: A History of the Contraceptive Pill* (New Haven and London: Yale University Press, 2001), 13.

4 Irving, *Brock Chisholm*, 69.

5 Thomas E. Brown, "Shell-Shock in the Canadian Expeditionary Force, 1914–1918: Canadian Psychiatry in the Great War," in Charles G. Roland, ed., *Health, Disease, and Medicine: Essays in Canadian History* (Toronto: Hannah Institute, 1984), 308–32. See also Ian R. Dowbiggin, *Keeping America Sane: Psychiatry and Eugenics in the United States and Canada, 1880–1940* (Ithaca: Cornell University Press, 1997; paperback edition, 2003), 112–13.

6 Ellen Herman, *The Romance of American Psychology: Political Culture in the Age of Experts* (Berkeley and London: University of California Press, 1996), 55, 85.

7 C.K. Clarke and C.B. Farrar, "One Thousand Cases from the Canadian Army," *Canadian Journal of Mental Hygiene* 1 (1920): 313–17.

8 For more on Clarke and his career in psychiatry, see Dowbiggin, *Keeping America Sane*, especially 130–78. See also Irving, *Brock Chisholm*, 23, 24.

9 For the Hincks quote, see Mark Cardwell, "Dr. Brock Chisholm: Canada's Most Famously Articulate Angry Man," *Medical Post*, 7 April 1998, 52.

10 For the history of Canadian eugenics, see Angus McLaren, *Our Own Master Race: Eugenics in Canada, 1885–1945* (Toronto: McClelland and Stewart, 1990). For the role of psychiatrists in the Canadian eugenics movement, see Dowbiggin, *Keeping America Sane*, 133–90.

11 For Hincks and the eugenics movement in Canada, see Dowbiggin, *Keeping America Sane*, 179–83. Hincks was still advocating sterilization in 1946; see C.M. Hincks, "Sterilize the Unfit," *Maclean's*, 15 February 1946, 39–40.

12 See Angus McLaren and Arlene Tigar McLaren, *The Bedroom and the State: The Changing Practices and Politics of Contraception and Abortion in Canada, 1880–1980* (Toronto: McClelland and Stewart, 1986), 103–19; McLaren, *Our Own Master Race*, 84–6, 113–17.

13 University of Waterloo Library, Dorothea Palmer Collection, WA 17, Brock Chisholm File, N1–N51.

14 "Mothers' Influence Seen as Bane in Army Life By Medical Director," *Toronto Globe and Mail*, 12 February 1944.

15 Herman, *The Romance of American Psychology*, 278.

16 Irving, *Brock Chisholm*, 62.

17 I am grateful to John Farley for this information. He is currently writing a history of Chisholm's years at the WHO.

18 William Vogt, *Road to Survival* (New York: William Sloane, 1948), 42, 146–51, 218, 282–3; cited in Critchlow, *Intended Consequences*, 19.

19 Critchlow, *Intended Consequences*, 14–29.

20 William Ray Vanessendelft, "A History of the Association for Voluntary Sterilization, 1935–1964" (PhD Dissertation, University of Minnesota, 1978). For the links between the AVS and other reform groups in twentieth-century America, see Ian Dowbiggin, "'A Rational Coalition': Euthanasia, Eugenics, and Birth Control in America, 1940–1970," *Journal of Policy History* 14, (2002): 223–60.

21 Edward Innis, general counsel to the American Civil Liberties Union, told the AVS in 1967 that "unless voluntary programs succeed man will almost certainly face authoritarian and repugnant compulsory programs." Seeley G. Mudd Library, Princeton University, Hugh Moore Fund Collection (hereafter cited as HM), series 3, box 15, folder 3. Edward Innis, "World Poverty and the Rights of Man." For Moore's interest in the legalization of euthanasia, see Ian Dowbiggin, *A Merciful End: The Euthanasia Movement in Modern America* (Oxford and New York: Oxford University Press, 2003), 130–2.

22 Social Welfare History Archives, University of Minnesota (hereafter SWHA), EngenderHealth Collection, SWD 15.1, box 14, Chisholm File. Chisholm to Alan Guttmacher, 5 December 1960. Chisholm wrote to Moore that "your work in this field [of population control] is well worth while and [I] hope that it may be extended greatly" (HM, Chisholm to Hugh Moore, 18 December 1959, series 2, box 20, folder 5.

23 Ibid., Chisholm to Hugh Moore, 18 December 1959.

24 Chisholm letter to the editor of *Maclean's*, 26 November 1959; Library and Archives Canada, Brock Chisholm Fonds, MG 30-B56, volume 2, Chisholm, notes to 1962 speech on population.

25 SWHA, SWD 15.1, box 14, Chisholm File, Ruth P. Smith to Chisholm, 13 October 1960.

26 "Dr. Brock Chisholm Warns of Population Peril," *Human Betterment Association of America News*, Spring 1962, 1–2. The full text of Chisholm's speech, titled "World Health and World Population in the Fateful Sixties," and with his own notes and corrections, is in SWHA, SWD 15.1, box 14, Chisholm File.

27 Critchlow, *Intended Consequences*, 144–6.

28 Herman, *The Romance of American Psychology*, 315.

29 David J. Garrow, *Liberty and Sexuality: The Right to Privacy and the Making of Roe v. Wade* (Berkeley and Los Angeles: University of California Press, 1994),

473–599. In the late 1970s women's groups attacked the US Department of Health, Education, and Welfare's sterilization programs because they allegedly involved the sterilization of people incapable of giving their full consent to the operation; see Thomas M. Shapiro, *Population Control Politics: Women, Sterilization, and Reproductive Choice* (Philadelphia: Temple University Press, 1985).

8

Social Disintegration, Problem Pregnancies, Civilian Disasters

Psychiatric Research in Nova Scotia in the 1950s

JUDITH FINGARD AND JOHN RUTHERFORD

During the era of rapid social change in Canada that followed the end of World War II, interest in exploring the intricacies of the human mind rose in prominence in the nation's research agenda. Even Maritime Canadians, who often felt themselves at a disadvantage compared to central Canadians, found that new federal programs, talented researchers, and participation in national initiatives opened up new opportunities for research. Mental health research in Nova Scotia during the 1950s concentrated on the social environment. Psychiatric and psychological projects adopted social science approaches to address accessible neurotic conditions rather than unfathomable psychotic disorders at a time when, as American historian Gerald Grob notes, "the obstacles blocking fundamental biological research into the etiology and physiology of the mental illnesses were formidable."[1]

Before World War II, as Barbara Clow suggests in her study of alternative medicine in cancer treatment, "it is not at all clear what constituted reputable, rigorous research."[2] This uncertainty continued after the war, when, at least in the short term, ethical guidelines for research, if they existed at all, were self-imposed; clinical trials might be inadequately regulated; control groups were not in all instances considered mandatory; and funding from questionable sources was accepted. Even carefully conducted research might produce unexpected results or serendipitous findings. Chlorpromazine, for example, introduced in 1951 as the first psychiatric "miracle drug," began its existence in a French laboratory as an antihistamine.[3] Because it represented such an enormous advance over previous schizophrenia treatments, its quite common and frequently severe side effects did not discourage its use. In other cases, such as that of thalidomide, research legitimized a new drug without adequately investigating unsuspected and tragic side effects, the impact of which was aggravated by flawed Canadian regulatory procedures.[4] Moreover, despite repeated research efforts, it was often difficult to explain the therapeutic efficacy of a particular treatment. Electroconvulsive therapy (ECT) was a case in point. Its beneficial effects were entirely empirical and lacked a theoretical underpinning.[5] Research approaches were also embedded in the fabric of the society in which such studies were conducted. As Patricia Jasen's examination of psychosomatic research on female cancer patients in the United States in the 1950s demonstrates, results often reflected prevailing orthodoxies – in this case, the dominance of psychoanalysis – as well as a priori cultural assumptions about gender, race, class, and conventional wisdom.[6]

While society's faith in research to explain the etiology of disease, provide strategies for prevention, and cure the most intractable conditions may have been unrealistic, it turned the research enterprise into what would become a major industry. The purpose of this chapter is to examine the emergence of research in the area of mental health from a regional perspective under the stimulus of these circumstances. First, we will establish the context in which psychiatric research developed in post-war Nova Scotia. We will then examine three projects as illustrative case studies of this research, describing as well the insights they provide into contemporary attitudes and approaches to social stratification, economic circumstance, and gender. The first, largest, and most influential of these, the Stirling County Study in psychiatric epidemiology, was conceived in the late 1940s and continues to this day. The second and third, the clinical Spontaneous Abortion Study and the opportunistic Springhill Mine Disasters Studies, were begun in the 1950s and completed in the early 1960s. We will conclude with a comparison of these projects in terms of their similarities and differences and place them in relation to psychiatric research being conducted in the rest of Canada during this period.

THE SETTING

Developments in the late 1940s were conducive to the growth of research in the field of mental health. Scientific research, which contributed immeasurably to winning the war for the Allies, had already proven its utility in the fields of medicine, intelligence, and weapons development. The war had also produced an appreciation for the importance of stress in the environment in the etiology of mental breakdown, variously identified as "shell shock" and "battle fatigue or exhaustion."[7] The need for society to cope with what researchers would subsequently show to be relatively common maladies provided an impetus for further examination of the factors responsible for anxiety and depression. In the positive environment of reconstruction following the war, governments, universities, and hospitals turned hopefully to research to solve society's ills, one of which was the apparently high peacetime prevalence of mental disorders. At the same time, the negative atmosphere produced by the threat of destruction by nuclear weapons and the political uncertainty of the Cold War added urgency to the need to understand stress-related illnesses. Compounding this urgency was the dawning realization of how little was actually known about the nature and frequency of mental illness in a period when psychiatric institutions were experiencing mounting pressures and when the leading organization in the mental health movement, the Canadian Mental Health Association, was calling for action.

Equal in importance to the changes and challenges of the post-war and Cold War periods was the emergence of the mental health professions. Led by psychiatry, mental health professionals were motivated to try new approaches in therapy and health care delivery. Local practitioners were eager to exploit the benefits of improved techniques in electroconvulsive therapy and to administer the newly developed antipsychotic (mid-1950s), antidepressive (late 1950s) and anxiolytic (early 1960s) drugs. Psychotherapy completed the psychiatrist's armamentarium and was often used in conjunction with these "medical" treatments. Concurrently, local administrators began to reform practices in asylums by opening previously locked wards. They also encouraged a decreased reliance on large, centralized institutions by establishing new venues for delivering care to the mentally ill, such as the community mental health clinic and the psychiatric unit in the general hospital. These developments positioned psychiatry closer to the "mainstream" of medicine, in which illness was routinely treated using physical and chemical interventions in settings near the patient's home or in hospitals housing the full range of medical specialties. The acceptance of a more "medical" (or biological) view of mental illness led naturally to the conviction that an empirical or even an experimental approach to the study of mental disease was appropriate and would yield beneficial results. This idea was reinforced by the university community, with which departments of psychiatry found themselves affiliated, as research was seen as integral to the responsibilities of an academic unit.[8] Affiliation with a university also provided an opportunity to design and conduct research projects involving related disciplines, such as psychology or sociology, or other clinical or even basic science disciplines.

To exploit fully such opportunities, funding to offset the expenses associated with the conduct of research was required. Prior to the war, a number of private American organizations, prominent among them the Rockefeller Foundation and the Carnegie Corporation, had supported research and training in medicine, as well as in many other areas. Canadian institutions, including those in Nova Scotia, had benefited greatly from funding provided through these sources.[9] Following the war, the Canadian federal government, which before the conflict had supported scientific inquiry through the National Research Council for many years, acknowledged the importance of research to find solutions to specifically health-related problems by establishing the system of Federal Health Grants, in particular the Federal Mental Health Grants (1948), thus joining private foundations as a source for research funding. The Mental Health Grants were channelled through the provincial governments and were therefore responsive to local funding priorities which, in the case of Nova Scotia, were weighted heavily toward training and clinical service. Notwithstanding this focus, Clyde Marshall, the province's director of Mental Health Services, was able to observe, in his ninth report to the government (1956), "that the province contributes a high proportion of the funds it receives from Mental Health Grants on research. In fact, it is the second highest of all the Provinces in Canada."[10] Finally, when it suited its national interests, the US government, through various of its agencies, proved amenable to supporting Canadian research efforts.

Thus by the beginning of the 1950s, a number of factors converged to produce an atmosphere in which psychiatric research could flourish. The war had created a recognition of the need for research into psychiatric illness, as well as a faith in the efficacy of this approach to solving mental health–related problems. Within the psychiatric profession, the development of new medical therapies and new philosophies of care delivery attracted a group of enthusiastic practitioners willing to embrace research as a part of their professional lives. Finally, expanded opportunities for funding made it easier to initiate and pursue research projects. From this supportive milieu, three major studies emerged in Nova Scotia.

THE CASES

The Stirling County Study

The Stirling County Study was conceived in 1948 by Alexander H. Leighton at Cornell University, where he held positions in the Departments of Sociology and Anthropology and in Clinical Psychiatry. An exercise in psychiatric epidemiology, it was designed to explore the distribution of psychiatric disorders in a stable and relatively self-contained community and relate this to social and cultural factors, rather than to investigate a captive population in a psychiatric institution.[11] Thus Leighton was responding to and advancing the post-war conviction that social factors were key determinants of mental health.[12]

The community in which the study was based, "Stirling County," and the largest urban centre located therein, "Bristol," were situated in Nova Scotia.[13] A number of factors, especially the social, ethnic, and economic composition of the population, were responsible for the choice of a Maritime site for this well-planned, carefully constructed, and influential study. The support of the local medical community was important, as was Leighton's acquaintance with Stirling County, which dated from his early childhood. During his summers there, he became friends with Robert O. Jones, whose family lived next door. The two renewed their acquaintance many years later when, in 1940, both were engaged in residency training in psychiatry at Johns Hopkins University in Baltimore. Leighton then mentioned his interest in undertaking a community-based epidemiologic study of psychiatric illness, possibly in Atlantic Canada, an intention he pursued with Jones in 1946 and 1947. By that time, Jones was a professor at Dalhousie University, Halifax, where he successfully established an independent Department of Psychiatry in 1949, and was thus in a position to promote Leighton's project. By 1950 Leighton also had the backing of Clyde Marshall, at the provincial Department of Public Health, whose commitment to research soon led him to provide funding through the Federal Mental Health Grants.[14] Leighton's study was to involve personnel at Cornell, Dalhousie, and Acadia universities (Wolfville, Nova Scotia), with input from Université Laval in Quebec. The team consisted of psychiatrists, psychologists, sociologists, anthropologists, and statisticians, making it a truly interdisciplinary endeavour.[15] The design of the study included the establishment of the Bristol Psychiatric Clinic (later known as the Bristol Mental Health Centre), which opened in 1951.[16]

Following a pilot project conducted between 1948 and 1951, the research team in 1952 undertook the first of four surveys; the others were carried out in 1962, 1970, and 1992. These involved interviews with a sizable sample of the population supplemented by input from general practitioners in the area. The 1952 survey included data derived not only from the health-related, psychological, and pre-tested sociological questionnaires that would be used subsequently (e.g., the Health Opinion Survey and the Family Life Survey) but also from community assessments performed by anthropologists using the key informant approach. These latter studies were aimed at determining the degree of social integration or disintegration, concepts defined by Leighton as contributory factors to the prevalence of mental illness in a given setting. Findings from the 1952 investigation were published in a three-volume study that established a theoretical framework for the project, defined various types of psychiatric disorders, analyzed the community from a number of socially significant perspectives, and then correlated these factors with the extent of breakdown of community structure ("social disintegration") as a contributor to the prevalence of mental illness.[17] Later surveys continued these themes and provided the basis for estimates of incidence as well as prevalence of anxiety and depression in the population, while interviews with general practitioners provided data on psychoses. The project has been continuously funded for over fifty years. Initially it was supported by the Carnegie Corporation of New York and the Milbank Memorial Fund. Later, the US National Institute of Mental Health provided substantial support for the study.[18]

Judging from its longevity and the repeated calls it made upon the people of Stirling County to be participants, it can be inferred that the inhabitants of the area were, and remain, accepting and tolerant of the study and those who conduct it, thus vindicating the conviction that psychiatric research can be successfully pursued in a relatively uncontrolled community setting as well as in an institutional milieu. This acceptance may be due in no small part to the respect shown by Leighton and his co-workers for the feelings and values of those involved and the strenuous efforts exerted to guard their privacy.

The same cannot be said of reaction toward the Bristol Clinic and its staff. Leighton intended that the clinic should provide mental health care services to the community as a quid pro quo for its participation in the Stirling County Study. It was not the first facility of this kind in Nova Scotia, there having been short-lived local mental health centres established by the province in Yarmouth and Sydney in the late 1940s. In addition, Leighton envisaged the clinic as a potential source of data for the study, although it appears that it was never expected to play a major role in this respect. This research potential did, however, allow Clyde Marshall to designate funding to the support of the clinic from the Department of National Health and Welfare through the Canadian Federal Mental Health Grants program, as well as from the Nova Scotia Department of Public Health. The Milbank Memorial Fund and the Carnegie Corporation of New York also contributed to the operational and research costs of the clinic. It was recognized fairly early on that the presence of a mental health clinic in the community might be regarded with at least some skepticism, if not apprehension, because of pre-existing conceptions about the nature of such a facility and the form of disability with which it was designed to deal. Thus Leighton and Alice Longaker remarked that "the clinic may be thought of as a gateway to commitment in a mental hospital, as a place where they hypnotize you, as a place where they give pills for nerves, as some kind of quack outfit."[19] For this reason, the support of local physicians was vital. Initially, relations with the local medical community, which might have been expected to be sympathetic to the clinic's goals, were amicable, and physicians were generally thankful for access to the clinic's services. In time, however, the town's doctors began to grow critical of the clinic's psychiatrists and the way in which care was being delivered, resulting in a rift between the two groups.[20]

Relations between the clinic's staff and the community were at times strained, as well. The clinic was plagued from the outset with difficulty in finding and retaining qualified staff. Disagreements between the staff and members of the community, in particular those associated with the school system, were not uncommon and resulted at least in part from a lack of skill and experience on the part of the staff in dealing with sensitive public issues.[21] Some years later, when the clinic was no longer a project resource, an extraordinarily acrimonious debate over a school issue split the community. The clinic further compromised its public standing and its credibility by taking sides.[22] These factors contributed to a diminished capacity on the part of the clinic to deliver to the community the service that was a part of its mandate. Of particular relevance to this study is the fact that the clinic never did fulfill the second part of the rationale for its existence: that of providing data to advance the aims of the Stirling County Study itself. For a variety of reasons, including a heavy case load, a lack of training and interest in research, and poor record keeping, Leighton was soon forced to conclude that the clinic would not be able to further the research agenda of the study. By the mid fifties, the research function of the clinic was terminated.[23] Only one paper was ever published based on data collected by the clinic.[24] Perhaps ironically, the most lasting monument to the Bristol Psychiatric Clinic was the analysis of its shortcomings produced by Leighton himself.[25]

A complication of conducting research in a community setting is the impossibility of controlling public perceptions of the project. One psychiatrist noted that Stirling County residents thought they were being used as guinea pigs at the clinic because of a perceived emphasis on research rather than treatment.[26] Despite the regularity with which publications appeared and the frequency with which Leighton reiterated his intention of studying the role of the social environment in mental illness, rumours abounded about what were thought to be the *real* objectives of the researchers. From the outset, the Stirling County Study was conceived as an investigation of the socio-economic, rather than the hereditary, factors affecting the development of mental conditions, a protocol which was clearly stated at the inception of the project and which has never been breached.[27] Yet some people came to believe that regardless of its stated purpose, the Stirling County Study was actually designed to investigate inbreeding as a causative factor in mental illness. The explanation for the divergence between perception on the part of the public and intention on the part of the researchers may lie in the research undertaken as part of another, unrelated project known as the South Mountain Study. Funded by the Acadia University Institute, which was established in 1955 "chiefly to sponsor the Fundy clinic,"[28] a new mental health centre inspired by the Bristol Clinic, the South Mountain Study did explore the effects of inbreeding in an isolated community near Wolfville.[29] In retrospect, it is not impossible that the Stirling County and South Mountain research became conflated in the minds of even the better informed members of the public because of the rural setting of both studies and the involvement of former Bristol Clinic personnel in the Fundy clinic. For example, in the mid-1980s, two Acadia University sociologists claimed that the 1950s "Sterling [*sic*] County Studies – which are seriously flawed, not least for their 'blame the victim' orientation – clearly indicated the extent of familial social problems including incest, in regions of the [Annapolis] Valley."[30] The authors incorrectly identified "Sterling [*sic*] County" as the site for the South Mountain Study, which is difficult to explain given their undoubted acquaintance with the Acadia University Institute. During a visit to Acadia University at the time of this controversial research, Leighton was, in fact, asked for his opinion of conditions on South Mountain. Consistent with his philosophy of emphasizing social environmental rather than genetic causation in mental illness, he replied that community development was the way to address the effects of poverty and isolation. But as Leighton and Jane Murphy (formerly Hughes) commented to us, people will cling to their own preconceptions however widely they diverge from the evidence presented to them. Indeed, they remarked that their detractors had rarely bothered to read the three books that provided the enduring framework from which all their subsequent studies derived.[31]

The Stirling County Study reflected the trends and answered the needs of psychiatric research as perceived in the 1950s. First, as an exercise in psychiatric epidemiology, the Study addressed the need for data concerning the prevalence, and later the incidence, of certain types of mental disability in the community. As Leighton observed, it is impossible to plan a service without knowing the extent of the problem.[32] One of its most striking, and for a while controversial, findings was that, if all forms of mental illness were counted, at any given time as much as 20 per cent of a population suffers from mental disorders of sufficient severity as to need psychiatric attention.[33] Second, in the course of this project, Leighton provided a definition of mental illness that suited the framework of the study and that proved consistent with later criteria developed for the Diagnostic and Statistical Manual of Mental Disorders (DSM) III.[34] Third, anticipating developments in the delivery of mental health care, he included a community-based mental health clinic in the design of his study. Though intended in part as a source of data for his research, the Bristol Clinic was a genuine attempt to provide care, counselling, and referrals for the people in the region in which it was located, and it succeeded to a degree in doing so. A recent study suggests that the clinic was a model for the subsequent system of community mental health clinics established according to Clyde Marshall's ambitious plan.[35]

Arguably, a project of the magnitude of the Stirling County Study had the potential to galvanize social psychiatric research in the province and to promote the research agenda of the new Department of Psychiatry. However, despite Leighton's close and continuing relations with local universities (subsequently, in 1975 he was named National Health Scientist at Dalhousie University), the potential for his study to contribute to the department's research productivity was never fully appreciated, exploited, or realized.[36] While there was no animus toward social psychiatry per se, some evidence suggests that Jones, however unreasonably, questioned the extent of government support provided to the Bristol facility in circumstances where local institutions lacked the funding to initiate even modest programs of academic investigation.[37]

In the broader context, it should be noted that the Stirling County Study was not unique. Two other large-scale projects in psychiatric epidemiology being pursued in the 1950s are particularly relevant here, in perhaps unexpected ways. One, the "Lundby" Study in Sweden, like the Stirling Study, is a longitudinal project that continues to the present.[38] The other, the Midtown Manhattan Study in New York City, produced findings on the prevalence of mental illness that confirmed those obtained in Stirling County.[39] Thus the 20 per cent figure, so surprising at the time, was not an attribute peculiar to Nova Scotia but was a finding reflected in other settings as well, a point that Clyde Marshall, mindful of the perception of the province as a "backwater," was able to make with considerable satisfaction.[40] It speaks to Leighton's prominence that he assumed the directorship of the Midtown Manhattan Study upon the death of its founding director, Thomas Rennie, and later collaborated on a publication with the Lundby group as well.[41]

The Spontaneous Abortion Study

The Halifax-based Spontaneous Abortion Study grew out of the close relationship between the Departments of Obstetrics and Gynecology and Psychiatry fostered by Benjamin Atlee, the long-serving head of Obstetrics and Gynecology, and R.O. Jones, the head of Psychiatry.[42] Atlee had an intense interest in psychiatry and was convinced that a patient's psychological makeup was important to her physical well-being.[43] Developments in Psychiatry were favourable for the institution of this study as well. Robert Weil, recently recruited to the Department by Jones, joined the staff in September of 1950. He was engaged in a study of mental illness in the Hutterite community with Joseph Eaton, a sociologist at Wayne (later Wayne State) University (published in 1956 as *Culture and Mental Disorders: A Comparative Study of the Hutterites and Other Populations*). With the blessing of Jones and at the insistence of Atlee, Weil and gynecologist Carl Tupper began pilot studies in the early 1950s into the causes and possible prevention of habitual spontaneous abortion in women who, while wishing to have children, were consistently unable to carry a pregnancy to term. A call for participants in the study was published in 1956.[44] The investigation was designed to be broadly multidisciplinary, and it eventually came to involve obstetricians, psychiatrists, biochemists, anatomical pathologists, and psychologists. The inclusion of psychiatrists in the study arose from Atlee's conviction that emotional factors were important in the etiology of habitual spontaneous abortion.[45]

The study resulted in numerous publications, among them a series of ten numbered papers that appeared between 1956 and 1963 in the *American Journal of Obstetrics and Gynecology*. Four of these papers (the first and third, appearing in 1957, and the ninth and tenth, appearing in 1962 and 1963 respectively) dealt wholly or in part with psychiatric considerations. It was shown that, when properly employed, "psychotherapy has a beneficial effect on this disorder," a conclusion supported by data indicating that women subject to habitual spontaneous abortions could carry a pregnancy to term and deliver a healthy child successfully when counselled by a competent psychotherapist, such as Weil.[46] In the hands of someone without the appropriate training, however, the results could be disastrous. Jones, commenting on one particularly inept practitioner, noted that he was "as good at producing a spontaneous abortion ... as Bob Weil was in stopping it."[47] Although the study was supported throughout by Federal Health Grants, an atmosphere conducive to research had previously been fostered in the Department of Psychiatry by funding from the Rockefeller Foundation.[48]

The Spontaneous Abortion Study was not, in fact, the first instance of collaboration between Psychiatry and Obstetrics and Gynecology. Psychiatrist Ken Hall and social worker Andrew Crook had previously worked in Atlee's prenatal clinic studying the attitudes of women toward childbearing and rearing and then went on to explore "emotional factors relating to performance in natural childbirth." Solomon Hirsch, another psychiatrist, investigated the psychological makeup of unmarried pregnant women.[49] Support for these initiatives is indicative of the general encouragement that psychiatric research received during this period. As a result, Weil and Tupper and their co-workers were able to plan and execute a successful study by seizing upon an opportunity presented by a troubling clinical problem that previous approaches had failed to resolve.

Some of the contemporary attitudes toward women, as well as the societal developments affecting them, could be glimpsed in the context of the study. Women's roles in society were changing in the post-war era, with more women seeking careers outside the traditional home setting. That this shift might in itself produce conflict which could adversely affect women's health was acknowledged in the criteria defining Weil's patient groupings. Although his criteria were couched in language that might not now be considered altogether appropriate, Weil did recognize that women included in his "Independent, frustrated group" of habitual aborters "had often been career women with special interests they had been reluctant to give up for marriage," and that they were married to men "who were very often markedly neurotic," conditions that might contribute to the difficulty they experienced in carrying a pregnancy to term.[50]

It might be argued that the Spontaneous Abortion Study, like the Stirling County Study, was also affected by the milieu in which psychiatric research was conducted in the 1950s. First, the study was initiated on the premise that psychological factors could influence health (not in itself a new idea) and that this premise should be explored in the context of pregnancy. Such a conviction underscored the contemporary faith in research to provide solutions to thorny problems by employing novel approaches, which here included the use of psychotherapy along with other medical interventions. Second, combining psychiatry with obstetrics allied psychiatry with a field of medicine more commonly experienced, and therefore better accepted, by the public. This focus may have had the effect of legitimizing the still suspect field of psychiatry as a tool of conventional medical treatment. Third, the study represented acceptance by psychiatry of its responsibility as an academic department to engage in research.

The Springhill Mine Disasters Studies

The Springhill Mine Disasters Studies were undertaken following each of two mining disasters in Cumberland County, an explosion in the no. 4 mine on 1 November 1956, in which forty-one died, and a "bump" in the no. 2 mine on 23 October 1958, which killed seventy-five men. These terrible events provided the Department of Psychiatry, along with the Departments of Psychology at Dalhousie and Sociology at Acadia University, the opportunity to study the effects of a civil disaster on a one-industry community. Immediately after the 1956 explosion, Andrew Crook, formerly employed by the Department of Psychiatry and by that time the executive director of the Nova Scotia division of the Canadian Mental Health Association (CMHA), arranged for emergency psychological support for the victims of the accident. Robert Weil, other members of the Department of Psychiatry, and Clyde Marshall cooperated with local authorities to establish a service that became known as "psychological first aid."[51] While providing what appears to have been a form of "grief counselling," the service was also used as an opportunity to conduct research into the psychological effects of a disaster on a civilian population. Miners and their families were interviewed using standard psychological techniques. Weil and his colleague Frank Dunsworth published their observations and findings in two papers, one dealing with the effects on the surviving miners and the other focusing mainly on the effects on the town's citizenry.[52]

Following the 1958 "bump," a similar service was established. Once again, this event provided an opportunity for research, the results of which were analyzed far more extensively and were reported in two lengthy published studies, the first appearing in 1960 and the other in 1969.[53] A follow-up study, concerned with longer-term effects, especially relating to unemployment, was undertaken and the unpublished results apparently communicated to the Defence Research Board of the Canadian Department of National Defence in 1961.[54] The papers relating to the 1956 explosion appear to have been produced without benefit of funding. Significantly, funding for the project investigating the 1958 tragedy was provided by the United States National Institute of Mental Health through that country's Disaster Research Group and by the Canadian Defence Research Board.

The study owes much to the expertise and dedication of its protagonists. Weil, with his background in social research and his familiarity in working with social scientists, combined with his training as a clinician, was an ideal person to exploit the opportunity to study the effects of these disasters. The assessment of psychological damage the second of these events left in its wake was continued by Horace D. Beach, a professor of psychology at Dalhousie University, and Robert A. Lucas, a sociologist at Acadia University. Weil remained involved as the leading psychiatric consultant in the assessment of the 1958 disaster, and he continued to pursue his interest in what became known as "disaster research," which culminated in a book chapter in 1973.[55] Beach was commissioned by the Department of Health and Welfare to write a manual for health personnel on how to manage people in disaster situations.[56]

Interest in disaster studies was a reflection of the preoccupation of North American governments with civil defence in the post-war era. For example, Beach's monograph was the thirteenth in the Disaster Studies Series, commissioned by the Disaster Research Group of the National Academy of Sciences–National Research Council in the United States. The US government was so avid for the data the 1958 event might provide that unsolicited funding for the project was offered even as the miners were finally being rescued. It arrived two days after the last survivor was brought to the surface. According to Weil, the Disaster Research Group "was then particularly interested in survival behaviour in shelter & in the post rescue periods."[57] Leonard Denton, the provincial psychologist who administered mental tests to the miners after they recovered from their initial trauma, believes that the American interest in this event related to the possibility of using mines as radiation shelters in the event of nuclear war.[58] Concerned with the limited terms of reference imposed by Washington, Canada's

Defence Research Board (DRB) encouraged the Springhill Research Group to expand upon its initial analysis to include a consideration of "the individual & social reactions of residents of Springhill as they adjust to the October, 1958, mine disaster & the subsequent industrial changes."[59] The DRB provided a grant of $8,920.00 to fund the continued study, which resulted in an unpublished report entitled "Individual and Group Reactions to Disaster and Unemployment: A Follow-up Study."[60] The report suggested, among other things, that the chronic effects of unemployment following in the wake of the 1958 disaster were more debilitating in psychological terms than the event itself. Disaster research resonated strongly in Halifax. Beach and Weil both included in their subsequent analyses of disasters in general the example of the human effects of the Halifax Explosion of 1917, citing the study by Samuel H. Prince, himself a pioneer in the mental health movement. Even Jones was eventually moved to examine his patients' records for evidence of post-explosion trauma, the results of which he communicated in a talk to a local audience.[61]

As with the other two research projects, the Springhill Mine Disasters Studies were influenced by the factors affecting psychiatric research being conducted in the 1950s. The state's interest in studying the effects of the events at Springhill reflected the concerns raised by the Cold War and the belief that research was key to providing answers to anticipated social and psychological problems. As in the Spontaneous Abortion Study and, to some extent, the Stirling County Study, research was coupled with service delivery in which psychotherapy was offered in conjunction with other forms of medical treatment. Finally, because of the wish of governments to obtain data applicable to civil defence, funding to investigate the effects of the 1958 disaster was readily available.

THE COMPARATIVE FRAMEWORK

Since the three major psychiatric studies in Nova Scotia evolved in the same context and were influenced by the same circumstances, it is perhaps not surprising that they share a number of characteristics. First, all three studies were promoted by influential individuals who, while not themselves involved directly with research, were in a position to provide support and encouragement. As the province's most influential psychiatrist, R.O. Jones played a pivotal role in relation to each of these studies. He was a founder and, in 1951, first president of the Canadian Psychiatric Association and president (from 1965 to 1966) of the Canadian Medical Association, the first psychiatrist to hold this position. Though regarded as a pre-eminent clinician and teacher, Jones did not engage in research. He did, however, recognize its importance, sought funding for its support, and recruited researchers to his department. His acquaintance with Leighton and his interest in the Stirling County Study contributed to its being sited in Nova Scotia. His friendship with Atlee, combined with Atlee's obsession with psychiatry, catalyzed the Spontaneous Abortion Study, which in its psychological aspects revolved around Weil, whom Jones had hired. Weil again surfaced in the Springhill Mine Disasters Studies, financial support for which Jones sought from the Defence Research Board.

Clyde Marshall, Nova Scotia's director of Mental Health Services from 1947 to 1970, was also influential in promoting mental health research during this period. He had come to this post after a decade of active and productive research at Yale in the 1930s and was thus sympathetic to the need to support investigation into mental illness and its causes and prevention. As part of his mandate, he was responsible for the distribution of the Federal Mental Health Grants, among others. While the vast majority of the monies under his control was expended for service and training, Marshall ensured that research received its due, and he was particularly sensitive to the needs of the Stirling County Study. Andrew Crook, the provincial leader of the CMHA, indirectly promoted the studies arising from the Springhill mine disasters. It was on Crook's initiative that the emergency psychological service was established following the 1956 explosion.[62] It was Crook who contacted Weil and convinced him of the need to render psychological aid to the stricken community; Weil responded with alacrity, arriving on the scene within a day of the event. Marshall was also involved, though in this case to ensure the effective delivery of service. By December of that year, it was already proposed that the experiences of the miners and their families be the subject of study, an expectation that was fulfilled for this event and, sadly, for the tragedy that struck two years later.

Second, although situated in Canada, all three studies benefited directly or indirectly from support from American agencies, both private and public, as well as from Canadian sources. The Stirling County Study received its inaugural funding from such private institutions as the Milbank Memorial Fund and the Carnegie Corporation of New York.[63] Canadian governmental support was provided by the Department of National Health and Welfare and through the Department of Public Health of Nova Scotia. Later, the US government supported the study through grants from the National Institute of Mental Health.

The Spontaneous Abortion Study was supported throughout its duration by a Canadian Federal Health Grant. However, in a 1953 memorandum concerning an approach to the Rockefeller Foundation, Jones indicated that Rockefeller monies, formerly used for undergraduate and post-graduate training, might, following the establishment of the Federal Mental Health Grants, be used to support research. It was clear from what followed that he intended specifically to pursue projects involving cooperation between his department and the Department of Obstetrics and Gynecology. Thus he noted that "since the financial support of the Rockefeller Foundation was no longer needed for support of the teaching program it was agreed that this could be used to set up a beginning research in this area and a year later, a grant was made to the two departments, to support research in the area of Obstetrics and Psychiatry." The grant to which reference is made was apparently instituted in 1950. The Spontaneous Abortion Study was among those programs whose origins may be traced to the "beginning research" mentioned in the memorandum. By 1953 Jones was able to state, "This study [the Spontaneous Abortion Study] is still in the pilot phase but interesting conclusions are beginning to emerge. This study is supported by a Federal Health Grant." It is clear that by that time, the Rockefeller investment in psychiatric research, though not targeted directly to the support of the Spontaneous Abortion Study, was beginning to pay off.[64] When it suited its agenda, the US government was also eager to support Canadian psychiatric research, as their immediate offer to fund an analysis of the effects of the 1958 Springhill tragedy shows. Jones, sensing that the Canadian defence establishment might share similar interests, was successful in obtaining funding for his colleagues from the Canadian Defence Research Board to expand upon their efforts on behalf of the US National Academy of Sciences–National Research Council–sponsored study. As in the case of the other two projects, American funding might be viewed as having "primed the pump" for research which then received Canadian financial backing.

Finally, these three studies all drew upon the expertise of individuals from a variety of disciplines. While the Stirling County Study was defined as an epidemiologic investigation into the occurrence of mental illness, it was dependent upon the insights of participants drawn from psychology, sociology, anthropology, and statistics in addition to psychiatry. Indeed, Leighton's perspective was informed by his training in anthropology, the influence of which may be seen in his presentation of the data derived from the study. While conducting the Stirling study, he and Jane Murphy were also engaged in anthropological investigations of Yupik-speaking Siberian Eskimos and the Yoruba in Nigeria, and he had earlier conducted research among the Navajo in the American Southwest. Leighton and Murphy's methodological approach should not, however, be confused with that of the Benedict-Mead school of anthropology, as Leighton was insistent upon a detached approach to data gathering.[65] The Spontaneous Abortion Study enlisted perhaps the most diverse group of researchers, involving as it did biochemists, pathologists, psychologists, obstetricians, and psychiatrists. It confirmed the need for emotional support of pregnant women at risk and shaped the approach of later generations of obstetricians.[66] The effects of the mine disasters on the people of Springhill were analyzed by a multidisciplinary team consisting of psychiatrists, psychologists, and sociologists. Participation was a formative experience for Leonard Denton, because it revealed the flawed nature of certain psychological tests when applied to a population under stress; so much so that he never again used the Rorschach.[67]

Although psychiatry, a clinical specialty, provided the common thread that united the studies, the variety of disciplines involved afforded an opportunity to train students in academic research at the graduate level. At Dalhousie University, this training was delivered in the Department of Psychology and the Maritime School of Social Work. Two psychology students wrote master's theses as part of the Spontaneous Abortion Study, and one worked on the follow-up project that was part of the Springhill Mine Disasters Studies.[68] The theses indicate the emphasis on clinical psychology prevalent at the time and are evidence that psychiatry and psychology, two disciplines that did not always see eye to eye in some areas, could collaborate productively in research. The Stirling County Study provided material for numerous master's and doctoral theses, pursued largely, though not exclusively, at American universities (McMillan's master's thesis was completed at Acadia University). In the early stages of the project, two social work students examined attitudes toward mental illness in Stirling County.[69] At the doctoral level, several graduates became noted scholars in Canada, the most influential of whom was Marc-Adélard Tremblay at Université Laval. In Nova Scotia, W.H.D. Vernon, who was head of the Psychology Department at Acadia University when he began his dissertation research with the Stirling project, became administrator of the Bristol Clinic between 1955 and 1957.[70]

Although each of the three studies contributed to graduate training and were similar in many other regards, they did differ in one major respect. The Stirling County Study was firmly grounded in a theoretical construct that informed the conduct of all of its activities.[71] Thus the epidemiological study proceeded from an hypothesis about the importance of the relationship between socio-cultural environment and mental illness. To describe the most extreme community cases, Leighton coined the term "social disintegration" to characterize the cumulative effects of poverty, isolation, and helplessness in producing a breakdown of social structure, the uncertainties of which then predisposed to mental illness. Even the Bristol Psychiatric Clinic, an acknowledged quid pro quo service to the community for its participation in the study, was established as a source of data to complement the findings from the population at large. By contrast, both the Spontaneous Abortion and Springhill Mine Disasters Studies were opportunistic, with no particular premise as a point of departure, other than a conviction that psychiatry can make a difference for those to whom it is made available. Both grew out of clinical services that provided a basis to explore the relationship and efficacy of psychiatry to groups under particular kinds of stress.

It is instructive to contrast mental health research as conducted in Nova Scotia with developments in the rest of the country during this period. The world of mental health care in Canada was a small one. Exchanges between universities, interactions at professional and academic conferences, memberships on association and government committees, and personal acquaintances combined to ensure that information flowed freely from one place to another. For example, the highly influential administrator Charles A. Roberts, who served during this period as the mental health bureaucrat in the Department of National Health and Welfare in Ottawa, had trained with R.O. Jones.[72] Andrew Crook was trained in psychiatric social work at the Mental Hygiene Clinic in Toronto with the mental health movement guru Clarence Hincks.[73] In the area of research, James and Libuse Tyhurst came to Nova Scotia in 1950 to be participants in the Stirling County Study and were also appointed to the Department of Psychiatry at Dalhousie University. James Tyhurst soon became the first director of the Bristol Clinic (1951–53).[74] Leighton commented that although "an exciting clinical director," Tyhurst sometimes "created waves." Significantly, he published no research with the Stirling County Study.[75] There is considerable confusion concerning Tyhurst's credentials and appointments, including the times and duration of his affiliations with various organizations.[76] It would appear that after, and possibly before, his move to the Allan Memorial Institute in Montreal in the early 1950s, he studied reports of disasters from a theoretical perspective, the outcome of which was a definition of "transition states" found in those affected by major natural and man-made disasters. Funded by the Canadian Defence Research Board, the papers describing his findings were known to the Springhill group, and helped them to categorize certain types of crisis-related behaviour.[77]

At the Allan, Tyhurst became associated with Ewen Cameron, whose approach to research differed markedly from that of the Nova Scotia workers. Cameron's research, and that of others of like mind, has received far more publicity than the more psychotherapeutically informed approaches employed by Leighton, Weil, Beach, and their associates. Cameron attempted to demonstrate the efficacy of radically applied electroconvulsive therapy in his "psychic driving" experiments, which were conducted on mentally ill patients without their permission. He was also funded by the American Central Intelligence Agency to explore the effects of "brainwashing," which included the use of LSD on patients in conjunction with his other "depatterning" techniques.[78] The fascination with LSD extended to Saskatchewan, where Humphry Osmond and Abram Hoffer explored the use of this drug for therapeutic purposes.[79] All of these hospital-based researchers employed an experimental approach, sometimes using patients as unwitting subjects, to explore the limits of the human mind and the ways in which it might be controlled or altered. By contrast, the Nova Scotia research was based on an empirical approach, using psychotherapy for the benefit, directly or indirectly, of those involved. The extremes that these two approaches represent indicates the breadth of topics included under the heading "mental health research" during this period.[80]

A brief examination of the funding provided by the Federal Mental Health Grants between 1948/49 and 1956/57 provides some indication of the range of research supported by these grants.[81] In terms of amounts of dollars granted, Nova Scotia ranked fourth in the country, after Ontario, Quebec, and British Columbia. Of the funding channelled to Nova Scotia, virtually all was dedicated to the Stirling County project through the Bristol Clinic, which was by any estimate the largest psychiatric epidemiological study in Canada. Leighton himself, as director of the project, ranked third in the country in level of support. Indeed, without Leighton, Nova Scotia's impact on the national scene, in terms of funding from this source, would appear to have been negligible. (This conclusion, of course, underscores the shortcoming of relying on a single source for data in an analysis of this kind, since neither the Spontaneous Abortion Study nor the Springhill Mine Disasters Studies are captured here.) William Blatz, the famous child psychologist working in Toronto, received by far the greatest amount of Mental Health Grants support, followed by Ewen Cameron and his group at the Allan Memorial Institute.[82] Perhaps predictably, Abram Hoffer followed Leighton. The very large investment by the government in the experimental research of Cameron and Hoffer is indicative of the high priority that this form of investigation was accorded. However, the Mental Health Grants supported projects ranging from the anatomical (microscopic studies of neurocytology) to the sociological (socio-economic case histories of the elderly); from the biochemical (tissue demand for oxygen in patients with various mental illnesses) to the developmental psychological (factors important to the establishment of mental health in schoolchildren).

During the 1960s the increasing pressures of clinical service and of training gradually replaced research in terms of the demands placed on mental health professionals in Nova Scotia. A survey of psychiatric research in the Maritime provinces submitted to the subcommittee on research of the federal Department of National Health and Welfare in 1962 concluded that "the service needs of understaffed areas squeeze out any chance of research which is always regarded in practice, although frequently not in theory, as of second-order priority."[83] A year later Sol Hirsch reported, "In general, as is so often the case, research appeared to be crowded out by service demands. Where there was a shortage of personnel, service always took first place."[84] At the same time, Jones worried that insufficient research funding "would lead to an even greater emigration of research workers from Nova Scotia."[85] At the university level where interdisciplinary cooperation had been so marked, psychiatry and psychology soon went their separate ways. Sociology, identified by Weil as an essential element in successful collaborative research, failed to capitalize on the opportunity to pursue further health-related research.[86] As a result, the Leighton-Murphy study persists as the sole legacy of an era in which American funding joined Canadian support to produce a defining moment in the field of mental health research in Nova Scotia.

NOTES

This chapter is part of a research project funded by a Hannah Grant-in-Aid provided by Associated Medical Services, Inc. A preliminary version was presented at the annual meeting of the Canadian Society for the History of Medicine, Halifax, 2003.

1 Gerald N. Grob, *From Asylum to Community: Mental Health Policy in Modern America* (Princeton: Princeton University Press, 1991), 62. One such area of laboratory research, neurophysiology, experimented unsuccessfully with psychosurgical techniques on chimpanzees, but failed to stop the resort to lobotomies by North American psychiatrists. See Jack D. Pressman, *Last Resort: Psychosurgery and the Limits of Medicine* (Cambridge, New York: Cambridge University Press, 1998).

2 Barbara Clow, *Negotiating Disease: Power and Cancer Care, 1900–1950* (Montreal and Kingston: McGill-Queen's University Press, 2001), 66.

3 Edward Shorter, *A History of Psychiatry: From the Era of the Asylum to the Age of Prozac* (New York: John Wiley & Sons, 1997), 246–55.

4. Barbara Clow, "The Trouble with Normal: Managing the Thalidomide Tragedy in Canada," paper presented to the Department of History seminar program, Dalhousie University, March 2002.

5 Shorter, *A History of Psychiatry*, 218–24; E.R. Kandel, "Disorders of Mood: Depression, Mania, and Anxiety Disorders," in Eric R. Kandel et al., eds., *Principles of Neural Science* (4th ed., New York: McGraw-Hill, 2000), 1213–14.

6 Patricia Jasen, "Malignant Histories: Psychosomatic Medicine and the Female Cancer Patient in Postwar America," *Canadian Bulletin of Medical History* 20, no. 2 (2003): 265–97.

7 See Terry Copp and Bill McAndrew, *Battle Exhaustion: Soldiers and Psychiatrists in the Canadian Army, 1939–1945* (Montreal and Kingston: McGill-Queen's University Press, 1990).

8 Dalhousie University Archives (hereafter DUA), UA 12 (Faculty of Medicine): 52.1, R.O. Jones, "Memoranda: Re Approach to Rockefeller Foundation," [1953].

9 See DUA, UA 12:51.12, 52.1, Annual Reports, Department of Psychiatry, 1950 and 1954.

10 "Ninth Annual Report of the Director of Mental Health Services for the Year Ending 31 March 1956," *Report of the Department of Public Health, Nova Scotia*, 367.

11 Bruce P. Dohrenwend, "The Stirling County Study: A Research Program on Relations between Sociocultural Factors and Mental Illness," *American Psychologist* 12, no. 2 (1957): 78–85; Jane M. Murphy, "The Stirling County Study: Then and Now," *International Review of Psychiatry* 6 (1994): 329–48.

12 See Grob, *From Asylum to Community*, 100–2.

13 In keeping with the protocol adopted by the two successive directors of the study, Alexander H. Leighton and Jane M. Murphy, and in deference to their wishes as stated in an interview with us on 8 August 2003, we will use throughout the pseudonyms employed by them in their publications.

14 "Fourth Annual Report of the Chief of the Neuropsychiatric Division for the Sixteen Months Ending 31 March 1951," *Report of the Department of Public Health, Nova Scotia*, 253; Alexander H. Leighton and Jane M. Murphy, "The Stirling County Study of Psychiatric Epidemiology," in Patrick Flynn, ed., *Dalhousie's Department of Psychiatry: A Historical Perspective* (Halifax: Department of Psychiatry, Dalhousie University, 1999), 313–17.

15 Alexander H. Leighton, "Psychiatric Disorder and Social Environment: An Outline for a Frame of Reference," *Psychiatry* 18, no. 4 (1955): 367–83; Dorothea C. Leighton, "The Distribution of Psychiatric Symptoms in a Small

Town," *American Journal of Psychiatry* 112, no. 9 (1956): 716–23. The project was formally launched in Nova Scotia at a dinner in Halifax on 23 October 1950. See DUA, UAI2:92.1, Jones to Kerr, 12 Oct. 1950; Leighton and Murphy, "The Stirling County Study of Psychiatric Epidemiology," 314.

16 R.C. Bland et al., "Epidemiology," in Quentin Rae-Grant, ed., *Psychiatry in Canada: 50 Years (1951–2001)* (Ottawa: Canadian Psychiatric Association, 2001), 214.

17 Alexander H. Leighton, *My Name Is Legion: Foundations for a Theory of Man in Relation to Culture, The Stirling County Study of Psychiatric Disorder and Sociocultural Environment*, vol. 1 (New York: Basic Books, 1959); Charles C. Hughes, Marc-Adelard Tremblay, Robert N. Rapoport, and Alexander H. Leighton, *People of Cove and Woodlot: Communities from the Viewpoint of Social Psychiatry, The Stirling County Study of Psychiatric Disorder and Sociocultural Environment*, vol. 2 (New York: Basic Books, 1960); Dorothea C. Leighton, John S. Harding, David B. Macklin, Allister M. Macmillan, and Alexander H. Leighton, *The Character of Danger: Psychiatric Symptoms in Selected Communities, The Stirling County Study of Psychiatric Disorder and Sociocultural Environment*, vol. 3 (New York: Basic Books, 1963).

18 Dohrenwend, "The Stirling County Study"; J.M. Murphy et al., "Depression and Anxiety in Relation to Social Status: A Prospective Epidemiologic Study," *Archives of General Psychiatry* 48 (1991): 223–9; DUA, R.O. Jones Papers (MS-13–14), 26.4, Copy of August 1956 List of Mental Health Grant Research Projects 1948–49 to 1956–57.

19 Alexander H. Leighton and Alice Longaker, "The Psychiatric Clinic as a Community Innovation," in Alexander H. Leighton et al., eds., *Explorations in Social Psychiatry* (New York: Basic Books, 1957), 370.

20 Alexander H. Leighton, *Caring for Mentally Ill People: Psychological and Social Barriers in Historical Context* (Cambridge: Cambridge University Press, 1982), 65; authors' second interview with Leighton and Murphy, 6 August 2003.

21 Leighton, *Caring for Mentally Ill People*, 106–9.

22 Ibid., 83–94, 104–12.

23 Ibid., 64–7.

24 E.J. Cleveland and W.D. Longaker, "Neurotic Patterns in the Family," in Leighton et al., *Explorations in Social Psychiatry*, 167–200; authors' second interview with Leighton and Murphy, 6 August 2003.

25 Leighton, *Caring for Mentally Ill People*.

26 Authors' third interview with Everett Smith, 24 March 2004.

27 Alexander H. Leighton, "A Proposal for Research in the Epidemiology of Psychiatric Disorders," in *Epidemiology of Mental Disorder* (New York: Milbank Memorial Fund, 1950), 128–35; Leighton, "Psychiatric Disorder and Social Envi-

ronment"; Dohrenwend, "The Stirling County Study"; Alexander H. Leighton, "The Stirling County Study: Some Notes on Concepts and Methods," in P.H. Hoch and J. Zubin, eds., *Comparative Epidemiology of the Mental Disorders* (New York: Grune and Stratton Inc., 1961), 24–31.

28 Linda Cann, *A Bold Step Forward: The History of the Fundy Mental Health Centre* (Wolfville: Fundy Mental Health Foundation, 1986), 11.

29 The South Mountain research was undertaken between 1956 and 1960 by people in a variety of disciplines at Acadia and Saint Mary's Universities. The projects were designed, according to a somewhat sensationalized journalistic account, to explain what were characterized as long-time "'mountain problems' of deaf mutism, mental retardation, inbreeding, illiteracy and crime." See David Cruise and Alison Griffiths, *On South Mountain: The Dark Secrets of the Goler Clan* (Toronto: Viking, 1997), 58. The research relating to the South Mountain Study is deposited in the Acadia University Archives, Acc.1982.001, 3.2.1–10.

30 Jim Sacouman and Tony Thomson, "The State vs. the South Mountain: The Annapolis Valley Incest Witch-hunt," *New Maritimes* 3, no. 5 (1985): 5.

31 Authors' first interview with Leighton and Murphy, 4 July 2003. By Leighton's accounting as of July 2003, the Stirling County Study and related studies by his group have resulted in the production of 13 books, 228 articles and book chapters, and 27 dissertations.

32 Authors' fourth interview with Leighton and Murphy, 10 July 2004.

33 D.C. Leighton et al., "Psychiatric Findings of the Stirling County Study," *American Journal of Psychiatry* 119, no. 11 (1963): 1021–6; Jane M. Murphy, "Continuities in Community-based Psychiatric Epidemiology," *Archives of General Psychiatry* 37 (1980): 1215–23. "Prevalence" counts everyone who is ill at a given time, whereas "incidence" counts everyone who becomes ill during a given period of time, regardless of how long the illness persists.

34 Jane M. Murphy et al., "Stability of Prevalence: Depression and Anxiety Disorders," *Archives of General Psychiatry* 41 (1984): 990–7; Alexander H. Leighton and Jane M. Murphy, "Nature of Pathology: The Character of Danger Implicit in Functional Impairment," *Canadian Journal of Psychiatry* 42 (1997): 714–21.

35 Joanna Redden, "The Community Mental Health Movement in Nova Scotia, 1945–69: The Case of the Fundy Mental Health Centre," (MA thesis, Dalhousie University, 2000), chapters 2 and 3. For one of several published versions of Marshall's plan, see Clyde Marshall, "Treatment Close to Home: The Nova Scotia Mental Health Plan," *Mental Hospitals: The Journal of Hospital and Community Psychiatry* 3, no. 6 (1962): 306–18.

36 In fact, Leighton seems to be best remembered in the Department of Psychiatry for his so-called seminar on wheels, which was integrated into the psychiatry

residency training program. See Flynn, *Dalhousie's Department of Psychiatry*, 268, 316.

37 See DUA, R.O. Jones Papers, 78.1. Jones's memorandum of a meeting of CMHA (Nova Scotia division), Scientific Planning Committee, Sub-Committee on Career Opportunities in Mental Health and Clyde Marshall, 14 July 1958. Jones notes that although his department could be severely criticized for not having been aggressive in the matter of research, the provision of opportunities for specific staff to do research, such as the psychologist at the Nova Scotia Hospital, required that money be spent on research infrastructure at that hospital, not on the Stirling County Study.

38 Authors' third interview with Leighton and Murphy, 17 April 2004; Murphy, "The Stirling County Study: Then and Now."

39 Leo Srole, Thomas S. Langner, Stanley T. Michael, Marvin K. Opler, and Thomas A.C. Rennie, *Mental Health in the Metropolis: The Midtown Manhattan Study* (New York: McGraw-Hill Book Company, 1962)

40 J. Fingard tape-recorded interviews with Clyde Marshall in April 1985; on deposit with the Public Archives of Nova Scotia.

41 Leighton wrote the foreword to Srole et al., *Mental Health in the Metropolis*, vii-ix. For his directorship, see ibid., 376; D.C. Leighton, O. Hagnell, A.H. Leighton, J.S. Harding, S.R. Kellert, and R.A. Danley, "Psychiatric Disorders in a Swedish and a Canadian Community: An Exploratory Study," *Social Science and Medicine* 5 (1971): 189–210.

42 DUA, UAI2, 51.1, Jones's "Memoranda: Re Approach to Rockefeller Foundation," [1953].

43 Wendy Mitchinson, "H.B. Atlee on Obstetrics and Gynaecology: A Singular and Representative Voice in 20th-Century Canadian Medicine," *Acadiensis* 32, no. 2 (2003): 3–30.

44 Carl Tupper and R.J. Weil, "The Problem of Spontaneous Abortion," *Nova Scotia Medical Bulletin* 35, no. 8 (1956): 212–13. "'Habitual abortion' is defined as the premature spontaneous termination of at least three consecutive pregnancies"; see Carl Tupper and Robert J. Weil, "The Problem of Habitual Abortion," in J.V. Meigs and S.H. Sturgis, eds., *Progress in Gynecology* (New York and London: Grune and Stratton, 1963), 241.

45 "Interview with R.J. Weil, Spring 1996," in Flynn, *Dalhousie's Department of Psychiatry*, 189.

46 William H. James, "The Problem of Spontaneous Abortion: X, The Efficacy of Psychotherapy," *American Journal of Obstetrics and Gynecology* 85, no. 1 (1963): 38–40.

47 DUA, R.O. Jones Papers, 52.10, Jones to R.A. Cleghorn, 5 June 1981.

48 DUA, UAI2, 51.1, Jones's "Memoranda: Re Approach to Rockefeller Foundation,"

[1953]; "Report of the Treasurer," in *The President's Review from the Rockefeller Foundation, Annual Report* (1954), 73.

49 Flynn, *Dalhousie's Department of Psychiatry*, 63–4, 211, 222–3.

50 R.J. Weil and Carl Tupper, "Spontaneous and Habitual Abortion: An Interdisciplinary Study," *Canadian Psychiatric Association Journal* 4, no. 1 (1959): 1–7. For background on the relationships between pregnant women and their doctors, see Wendy Mitchinson, *Giving Birth in Canada* (Toronto: University of Toronto Press, 2002).

51 *Canada's Mental Health* 4, no. 10 (1956): 3–4.

52 F.A. Dunsworth, "Springhill Disaster (Psychological Findings in the Surviving Miners)," *Nova Scotia Medical Bulletin* 37 (1958): 111–14; R.J. Weil and F.A. Dunsworth, "Psychiatric Aspects of Disaster – A Case History: Some Experiences during the Springhill, N.S. Mining Disaster," *Canadian Psychiatric Association Journal* 3, no. 1 (1958): 11–17.

53 H.D. Beach and R.A. Lucas, *Individual and Group Behavior in a Coal Mine Disaster* (Washington: National Academy of Sciences-National Research Council, 1960); Rex A. Lucas, *Men in Crisis: A Study of a Coal Mine Disaster* (New York and London: Basic Books, 1969).

54 DUA, R.J. Weil Papers (MS-2–750), 3.20, "Individual and Social Reactions to Mine Disaster and Subsequent Industrial Dislocation: Progress Report," submitted to the Defence Research Board on Grant no. 9470–05.

55 Robert J. Weil, "Psychiatric Aspects of Disaster," in Silvano Arieti, ed., *The World Biennial of Psychiatry and Psychotherapy*, vol. 2 (New York: Basic Books, 1973), 112–35.

56 [H.D. Beach], *Management of Human Behaviour in Disaster* (Ottawa: Department of National Health and Welfare, 1967).

57 DUA, R.J. Weil Papers, 3.25, Weil's notes on Springhill Disaster Research, item no.9.

58 Authors' first interview with Leonard R. Denton, 25 May 2004.

59 Weil's notes on Springhill Disaster Research, item no.18.

60 DUA, R.O. Jones Papers, 38.2, Mann (DRB) to Jones, 12 December 1958; ibid., 83.6, Mental Health Project 602–5–40: Training Psychologists at Dalhousie University, Report for 1960–61; DUA, R.J. Weil Papers, 3.20, List of project staff and acknowledgments, Sept. 1961. Our attempt to discover the whereabouts of any copy of the 1961 follow-up study in the Defence Research Board papers at the National Archives (now Library and Archives Canada) was unsuccessful (Kara Quann, National Archives of Canada, to Judith Fingard, 5 November 2002.) The author of a recent popular study of the role of racism in the aftermath of the 1958 Springhill disaster gives the document a date of October 1961; see Melissa Fay Greene, *Last Man Out: The Story of the Springhill Mine Disaster* (Orlando:

Harcourt, Inc., 2003), 327. Leonard Denton, one of the psychologists on the research team recalls no such publication. We did however find three papers that were part of the follow-up study: (1) DUA, R.O. Jones Papers, 90.3, "Psychiatric Findings on Trapped and Nontrapped Miners," and another version of same attributed to Charles Boddie (psychiatric resident) and H.D. Beach entitled "Follow-up Psychiatric Findings on Trapped Miners," in DUA, R.J. Weil Papers, 3.18; (2) DUA, R.J. Weil papers, 3.16, H.D. Beach, "Attitudes and Attitude Change in Minetown" (a version of the Livingstone MA thesis, see note 68); (3) DUA, R.J. Weil papers, 3.18, Horace D. Beach, "Follow-up Psychological Findings on Trapped Miners," included in Beach to Weil, 28 October 1970.

61 S.H. Prince, *Catastrophe and Social Change* (New York: Columbia University Press, 1920); DUA, R.O. Jones Papers, 24.8 and 94.8, R.O. Jones, "The Halifax Explosions," paper presented at the Second Annual Conference on Disaster: The Medical Response, Halifax, 1981. Jones also included in his paper the 1945 magazine explosion.

62 Crook's report to the CMHA (NS Division), 8 Nov. 1956, on the role of the CMHA in the Springhill Mine Disaster, *Canada's Mental Health* 4, no. 10 (1956), 3–4.

63 For funding by Milbank, see Grob, *From Asylum to Community*, chapter 7.

64 DUA, UAI2, 52.1, Jones's "Memoranda: Re Approach to Rockefeller Foundation," [1953].

65 Authors' first interview with Leighton and Murphy, 4 July 2003.

66 Authors' interview with Carl Tupper, 23 September 2004. Current research on that small proportion of women with unexplained recurrent miscarriages indicates that supportive clinical care is successful in enabling them to deliver a live baby. As British research professor of obstetrics and gynecology Lesley Regan reports to women from the largest miscarriage clinic in the world, "I cannot give you a scientific explanation for this, but I do recognize that tender loving care in early pregnancy improves the outcome for women who have experienced repeated, unexplained miscarriages." See Lesley Regan, *Miscarriage: What Every Woman Needs to Know – A Positive Approach* (2nd ed., London: Orion Books, 2001) 294.

67 Authors' first interview with Leonard R. Denton, 25 May 2004.

68 John S. Bishop, "A Psychological Study of Spontaneous Abortion" (MA thesis, Dalhousie University, 1957); D.S. Hart, "Psychological Changes in Pregnant Habitual Aborters during Psychotherapy" (MA thesis, Dalhousie University, 1960); Elizabeth R. Livingstone, "Effects of Disaster and Unemployment on Attitudes" (MA thesis, Dalhousie University, 1961).

69 E. Stanley Matheson, "Attitudes toward Mental Illness in Stirling County" (Diploma in Social Work thesis, Maritime School of Social Work, 1951); Ethel

Trainor, "Attitudes of Relatives toward Mental Illness in Stirling County," (MSW thesis, Maritime School of Social Work, 1951).

70 Cited in Leighton, *My Name Is Legion*, 434, 437; Marc-Adélard Tremblay, "The Acadians of Portsmouth: A Study in Culture Change" (PhD thesis, Cornell University, 1954); William Henry Dalton Vernon, "A Psychological Study of Thirty Residents of a Small Town" (PhD thesis, Cornell University, 1957).

71 Leighton, "A Proposal for Research in the Epidemiology of Psychiatric Disorders"; Leighton, "The Stirling County Study: Some Notes on Concepts and Methods"; Leighton, "Psychiatric Disorder and Social Environment"; Dohrenwend, "The Stirling County Study"; A.H. Leighton, "The Initial Frame of Reference of the Stirling County Study: Main Questions Asked and Reasons for Them," in J. Barrett and R. Rose, eds., *Mental Disorders in the Community: Progress and Challenges* (New York: Guilford Press, 1986), 111–27.

72 C.A. Roberts, *From Fishing Cove to Faculty Council ... and Beyond* (Calgary: Pondhead Publishers, 1995).

73 Authors' first interview with Andrew J. Crook, 2 October 2003.

74 DUA, UAI2: 51.12, Annual Report, Department of Psychiatry, 1950; Leighton, *My Name Is Legion*, 434.

75 Authors' second interview with Leighton and Murphy, 6 August 2003.

76 Christopher Hyde, *Abuse of Trust: The Career of Dr. James Tyhurst* (Vancouver and Toronto: Douglas & McIntyre, 1991).

77 J.S. Tyhurst, "The Role of Transition States – Including Disaster – in Mental Illness" (paper presented at the Symposium on Preventive and Social Psychiatry, Walter Reed Army Institute of Research and the National Research Council, Washington, DC, 1957); Tyhurst, "Individual Reactions to Community Disaster: The Natural History of Psychiatric Phenomena," *American Journal of Psychiatry* 107, no. 10 (1951): 764–9; Tyhurst, "Psychological and Social Aspects of Civilian Disaster," *Canadian Medical Association Journal* 76 (1957): 385–93.

78 Anne Collins, *In the Sleep Room: The Story of the CIA Brainwashing Experiments in Canada* (Toronto: Lester & Orpen Dennys, 1988).

79 Erika Dyck, "Prairie Psychiatry Pioneers: Mental Health Research in Saskatchewan, 1951–1971," in this volume.

80 See R.A. Cleghorn, "The Development of Psychiatric Research in Canada up to 1964," *Canadian Journal of Psychiatry* 29, no. 3 (1984): 189–97.

81 DUA, R.O. Jones Papers, 26.4, August 1956 List of Mental Health Grant Research Projects, 1948–49 to 1956–57. For a comparison to the funding supplied by the American National Institute of Mental Health during the period 1947 to 1951, see Grob, *From Asylum to Community*, 66–7.

82 For information on how Blatz used his grants, see Joselyn Motyer Raymond, *The Nursery World of Dr Blatz* (Toronto: University of Toronto Press, 1991), 207–12.

83 DUA, R.O. Jones Papers, 78.6, "Psychiatric Research in the Maritime Provinces," A Report to the Subcommittee on Research, Department of National Health and Welfare, Ottawa, 1962. This comment reflects a comment made by Aldwyn Stokes, Department of Psychiatry, University of Toronto, in 1950; see Roger Baskett, "The Life of the Toronto Psychiatric Hospital," in Edward Shorter, ed., TPH: *History and Memories of the Toronto Psychiatric Hospital, 1925–1966* (Toronto and Dayton: Wall & Emerson, 1996), 126.

84 DUA, R.O. Jones Papers, 80.9, "Survey of Psychiatric Research in Canada," A Report of Subcommittee on Research to the Advisory Committee on Mental Health, 1963.

85 Ibid., 51.17, R.O. Jones, "Trends in Psychiatric Care in Nova Scotia," 1963.

86 DUA, R.J. Weil Papers, 1.23, Weil to Williams (National Academy of Sciences), 26 Aug. 1959. The close cooperation between the disciplines can be gleaned from the 1950s issues of the *Maritime Psychological Association Bulletin*.

9

Prairie Psychedelics
Mental Health Research
in Saskatchewan, 1951–1967

ERIKA DYCK

Research is both an intellectual and a moral problem. It is one thing to have good ideas and quite another to fight them through year after year with small funds in a remote place, in the face of a profession whose views range from open hostility to ordinary indifference.[1]

In the early 1950s a group of clinical researchers in Saskatchewan began making waves in psychiatry for medical experimentation with psychedelic drugs.[2] Psychiatrists Humphry Osmond and Abram Hoffer had found that hallucinogenic drugs such as d-lysergic acid diethylamide (LSD), among others, produced powerful "mind-manifesting" or psychedelic experiences, which they believed provided insight into the biochemical functions of the human mind. One aspect of their studies suggested that the chemically induced experiences simulated disorders such as schizophrenia by producing a "model psychosis." Another dimension of the LSD studies explored the drugs' ability to create a spiritual or transcendental experience with therapeutic benefits. The profound responses to the drugs often gave individuals personal insight into their behaviour, which then acted as a significant tool in psychotherapy. Combining biochemical and psychosocial approaches to therapy, research with psychedelic drugs challenged these psychiatrists to re-evaluate their clinical approaches to understanding and treating mental disorders. Moreover, medical experimentation with LSD emphasized the therapeutic significance of subjective experiences, while many contemporary studies with psychopharmaceuticals focused on applying drugs to target discrete symptoms.

In historical examinations of post-1945 Western psychiatry, theories that did not garner sufficient professional support have often been lost or overlooked. While there are a few historical examinations of LSD trials in psychiatry,[3] some historians have argued that the shift from psychoanalytical to psychopharmacological therapies has overshadowed the importance of other theories produced at this time. Mark Micale, for example, studied medical historian Henri F. Ellenberger, author of *The Discovery of the Unconscious* (1970), and argued that because Ellenberger's approach to the history of psychiatry did not follow directly from either psychoanalysis or psychopharmacology, his place in the history of the discipline has been largely disregarded. Micale, nonetheless, showed how Ellenberger made an unparalleled historical contribution through his voluminous publications, which charted a radically different view of the history of psychiatry based on eclectic influences.[4]

With similar attention to marginalized practices, Jack Pressman explored psychosurgery in the United States and demonstrated that, although the use of lobotomies in psychiatry was quickly eclipsed by psychopharmacology, its contribution to psychiatry had a tremendous influence on the future of biomedical explanations of human behaviour.[5] Furthermore, Pressman's examination drew attention to the importance of personalities, resources, and professional organizations in the development of a professional consensus regarding particular clinical approaches. By examining the internal politics in the profession and their effects on practice, he illustrated a number of non-scientific factors involved in the dissemination of medical knowledge within psychiatry, thus arguing against a presumption of technological determinism. His study encouraged historians to move away from the wholesale demonization of "failed" therapies and instead to begin unravelling the complex set of relationships and priorities within twentieth-century psychiatry that contributed to its "modern" biomedical paradigm.[6]

Social historians of medicine have also begun examining the interface between culture and medicine by investigating the ways in which non-scientific factors shape clinical research and its reception.[7] These studies, similar to Pressman's examination of psychosurgery, further undermine assumptions about medical progress confined within a closed scientific arena. For example, Virginia Berridge and Betsy Thom investigated Britain's establishment of treatment centres for alcoholics in the post–World War II period. The resultant creation of clinics seemed to demonstrate a medical acceptance of alcoholism as a disease; however, advancing the disease paradigm also ensured coverage under Britain's National Health Service. These authors drew attention to the profound socio-political implications that shaped public and medical attitudes towards alcoholism.[8]

In the case of LSD experimentation in Saskatchewan, a number of non-medical factors affected its development. The most significant dynamic that has continued to shape historical accounts of psychedelic drugs emerges from LSD's reputation for dangerousness. Some of the earliest historical accounts of LSD experimentation focused on its use in military experiments. In the 1970s John Marks uncovered a series of CIA-sponsored projects involving LSD trials with prisoners, military personnel, and CIA officers.[9] His study reinforced the connection between the inherent dangers of the drug and the distorted agenda of its investigators. In the Canadian context, a number of legal challenges in the 1980s further drew attention to CIA-funded research concerning LSD trials in Montreal.[10] The public attention garnered by psychiatrist Ewen Cameron's experiments at the Allan Memorial Institute raised awareness about experimental psychopharmacological research in Canada, as well as the vulnerability of patients in mental health institutions. These examinations of LSD also underscored the link between unprofessional activities and LSD experimentation.

By exploring the medical and non-medical dynamics behind psychedelic psychiatry, this chapter reconsiders the role that LSD played in the history of psychopharmacology. Furthermore, it examines the impact of political pressures in post-1945 Saskatchewan that encouraged local researchers to distinguish their approaches from other North American practices. Prairie psychedelic psychiatry was highly politicized long before Timothy Leary, Ken Kesey, or the Beatles popularized the search for inner freedoms, allegedly encapsulated in recreational "acid." Despite evidence that some investigators employed dubious ethical standards in post-war medical experimentation, this case study also demonstrates that not all LSD trials fell into this category. Instead, LSD experimentation in Saskatchewan engaged its investigators in lively professional debates about the modernization of psychiatry and the growing fascination with psychopharmacological treatments.

LSD arrived on the medical scene in the 1950s, alongside thousands of biochemical studies.[11] Many of these inquiries revealed a high level of enthusiasm that chemical substances would revolutionize psychiatry by offering novel insights into mental illnesses which would eventually lead to the identification of their causes. Proof of the biological origins of "madness" would put an end to the long-standing questioning of its place in society. If drugs could provide researchers with conclusive proof of a "madness entity," it would not only resolve these age-old anxieties about

the existence of mental disorders but would also offer salvation to a category of patients who often suffered under the dual burdens of medical
hopelessness and social stigmatization.

One of North America's earliest psychopharmacologists, Thomas Ban,
argued that in the 1950s drug research was responsible for "dragging psychiatry into the modern world."[12] Psychopharmacological developments in
this decade were rewarded with two Nobel Prizes, one to Daniel Bovet for
work on antihistamines and another to James Black for his identification of
histamine receptors. In fact, in an historical examination of psychopharmacology, David Healy argued that nearly all the antidepressants (including
selective serotonin reuptake inhibitors) and antipsychotics, developed out of
the psychopharmacological research that took place in the 1950s.[13] These
contemporaneous developments inspired confidence in the medical con-
tention that psychopharmacological research and treatment would not only
modernize psychiatry but would also pave the way for reforms in mental
health care in the post-war period.

Henri Laborit's discovery of chlorpromazine (thorazine/largactil) in 1952
marked a turning point in the acceptance of psychopharmaceuticals in
mental health treatments.[14] Over the next three decades this antipsychotic
medication ostensibly became responsible for emptying asylums throughout
North America and Europe. Chlorpromazine purportedly reduced psychiatric symptoms in patients to the extent that they could function in the community without institutional care.[15] The consequent dismantling of psychiatric institutions had a revolutionary effect on mental health care, and
although deinstitutionalization introduced new challenges to patients and
psychiatrists, the increased reliance on psychopharmaceuticals in psychiatry
demonstrated the enormous capacity for drugs to change the course of
mental health care in the post-war period.[16]

Experimentation with LSD began in earnest in the 1950s amidst this optimism that drug research, including that with LSD, would improve psychiatric treatment options. Indeed, some trials involved the same investigators
as those who participated in research with chlorpromazine.[17] Several clinicians welcomed LSD into this experimental clinical environment, confident
that biochemical research offered discrete tools necessary for understanding the mysteries of the mind, and many scientists believed that investigations with LSD would advance the medical understanding of mental
disorders. Access to LSD attracted medical researchers with a variety of
approaches to drug experimentation. Some tested its physiological effects
on animals; others used human subjects to report on the drug's capacity to
bring the unconscious to the conscious; and others still engaged in self-

experimentation with the drug. Given its range of applications, LSD also appealed to mental health researchers across paradigmatic approaches. For psychoanalysts, the drug released memories or revealed the unconscious; for psychotherapists, it brought patients to new levels of self-awareness in a short time; and for psychopharmacologists, LSD reactions supported contentions that mental disorders had chemical origins. For approximately the next fifteen years, clinical research with LSD proceeded with relatively few impediments.

While chlorpromazine had a profound influence on mental health care reforms in the post-war period, this case study of psychopharmacological experimentation illustrates that there is ample evidence to suggest that results from LSD trials also played a key role in influencing mental health care policy in Saskatchewan. LSD studies conducted in that province were instrumental in expanding a particular kind of psychiatric discourse in mental health reforms, one that relied on a combination of biochemical, psychological, and social explanations for disorder. Psychedelic therapies relied on a biochemical model of mental illness that fundamentally rested on a scientific observation of experience. By combining a rigidly scientific study of biochemistry with a more subjective analysis of experience, psychiatrists Abram Hoffer and Humphry Osmond presented their psychedelic approach as a new theory in psychiatry. They merged philosophical traditions with emerging biomedical promises. Despite some resemblance to both psychoanalysis and psychopharmacology, the psychedelic therapy relied on a different etiological understanding of mental disorders with an alternative approach to treatment. Hoffer and Osmond distinguished their approach from psychoanalysts, whom they regarded as dogmatic therapists largely concerned with treating middle-class patients. Similarly, they did not entirely see themselves as psychopharmacologists, who they felt were obsessed with the collection of data without consideration for the deeper meanings of experience. Armed with their own delicate mixture of influences, Hoffer and Osmond promoted an explanation of mental disorders that tempered psychopharmacology and psychoanalysis with a new approach that incorporated the use of psychedelics as a means for binding disparate theoretical influences.

The prairie psychedelic psychiatrists felt that, traditionally, individuals with mental disorders and their family members suffered disproportionately, when compared to individuals with physical illnesses. In an effort to combat the stigma associated with mental disorders, psychedelic psychiatrists used their research with LSD to demonstrate that mental disorders were much like physical disorders and that treatment should be universally accessible without judgment. The Saskatchewan government, elected on a mandate to implement a system of state-funded public health care, was sympathetic to this view of mental illness and embarked on health care reforms that considered mental health care to be an integral part of its vision for publicly funded health services.

SASKATCHEWAN'S SOCIO-POLITICAL CONTEXT

Prior to 1945, national surveys ranked Saskatchewan's psychiatric facilities as substandard. Separate inquiries conducted by Clarence Hincks and Henry E. Sigerist identified overcrowding in hospitals and a severe lack of health care professionals as serious detriments to the provision of proper care in the province.[18] Historically, the region's inhospitable climate, lack of urban amenities, undiversified economy, and sparsely populated rural areas made attracting professionals to the region extremely difficult.[19] The prolonged economic and climatic devastation faced by prairie residents during the Depression of the 1930s compounded the difficulties in constructing new facilities and hiring sufficient staff. The election of North America's first socialist government occurred in Saskatchewan in 1944; this development, in combination with improved regional economic conditions, created an opportunity for Saskatchewan residents to address the serious deficiencies in local health care services. The newly elected Co-operative Commonwealth Federation (CCF) outlined an agenda of health care reform in the province that included provisions for mental health care.

The resultant allure of a socialist political environment, particularly one committed to health care reform, attracted people from all over the world to Saskatchewan. Contemporary observers suggested that the CCF's electoral landslide, followed by successive re-elections, piqued the curiosity of intellectuals, artists, and would-be politicians, among others, with an infectious optimism for constructing a socialist political culture.[20] Saskatchewan's traditionally depressed economy and developing cultural institutions received an influx of cosmopolitanism as curious individuals arrived in the region to observe socialism in action, bringing with them their energy, ideas, and experiences. Reflecting on this theme, intellectual James Labounty states: "It was an age of bold experiments. Tommy Douglas' CCF was in power, and intellectuals flocked to the province to see the workings of the first socialist government in North America. The pioneering spirit went beyond art and medicare, though, it dared to explore the brain, the psyche and dimensions that passeth all understanding."[21]

Premier Tommy Douglas's CCF government created a socio-political environment that set new priorities for experimental research and innovation, with health care at the forefront of the political agenda.

The history of medicare in Saskatchewan has been described in many places and need not be repeated here.[22] But the way in which the development of this program transformed the region into an attractive destination for conducting medical experimentation warrants a closer examination. The erosion of the region's professional class during the 1930s, in combination with political support for activist health reforms, created a fertile research environment in the post-war period. Local residents readily embraced new and replenished services into communities that had struggled to retain professionals during the Depression.[23] After World War II the CCF government established connections with other social democratic states and recruited doctors and medical researchers to fill positions in the rapid expansion of a provincial civil service that included health professions.[24] Enticed by research grants, professional autonomy, and an opportunity to participate in the formation of North America's first program of socialized medicine, the once-desperate region recast itself in the post-war period as an exciting, even cosmopolitan, place to be.

Evidence from correspondence, biographies, and oral interviews reveals the significant drawing power of the cultural and political climate in Saskatchewan in this period. A delicate and complicated set of historical and psychological factors gave rise to a new vision for the region that, above all, created opportunities for daring experimentation. One interviewee suggested that there was a high level of innovation and excitement in Saskatchewan that, he indicated, was influenced by the strong socialist orientation, which attracted people who shared this ideological view.[25] Another interviewee described Saskatchewan as "the most exciting place to be"; during the post-war period curious individuals collected in small towns and brought worldly perspectives to these rural communities.[26] The province quickly gained a reputation for innovation, which helped to attract professionals to the historically under-diversified region.

The CCF government fostered this enthusiasm and created career opportunities in the province that were in many ways unparalleled elsewhere in the country. Newly trained professionals could begin their careers in authoritative positions.[27] Once hired, they often enjoyed research freedom, professional status, and job security. Research labs and provincial grants did little to make the winters bearable, but slowly the province appealed to researchers with arguably its greatest asset: space – professional, geographical, and political. Within this context, medical experimentation flourished, and with political support, researchers explored new medical ideas in a relatively flexible research environment.

During this period the medical and psychiatric professions in the province existed in a relatively unbureaucratized state. The situation appealed to professionals from outside the province who were interested in a socially progressive, research-intensive environment. Since Saskat-chewan's mental health facilities required significant attention, the government actively recruited individuals to fill authoritative positions. Many of these recruits, in turn, attracted other researchers to the province for an opportunity to work with dynamic research teams in this unique North American politi-cal context. Many such recruits stayed only briefly in the province, while others settled in the region permanently, but Saskatchewan's political facelift had a positive influence on its capacity to attract energetic researchers. In a letter to the federal Department of Public Health, the Saskatchewan Psychiatric Association commented on the province's success in attracting "hard-working, full-time private psychiatrists."[28] Contempo-rary observers suggested that the resultant collection of intellectuals in mental health research made for an exciting and collegial environment that could not be replicated in regions with an existing professional bureaucracy.

In addition to taking practical steps to recruit professionals, Douglas strove to encourage a change in attitudes concerning mental illness.[29] He deplored the current tradition of placing individuals with mental ill-nesses in custodial institutions. He maintained that overcrowded and understaffed asylums produced terrible conditions for therapy. More-over, where professionals were available, they were often too busy attending to day-to-day administrative duties rather than engaging in medical research that might produce more satisfying alternatives to insti-tutionalization. Douglas subscribed to the idea that a hospital should be a place of last resort, and that care among relatives and within a famil-iar community was almost always preferable to long stays in a hospi-tal.[30] The premier believed that psychiatric services, therefore, should be provided in a comprehensive manner that emphasized preventative med-icine and cooperation in the community. His strategy for accomplishing this objective involved a combination of support for psychiatric research and the initiation of an aggressive public education program. This outlook set the agenda for mental health reforms in the province that emphasized medical research and embraced new approaches to concep-tualizing mental illnesses.

PSYCHEDELIC THERAPY

By the 1950s, Saskatchewan had already gained a reputation for innovation in political experimentation, and as it continued to attract health professionals, it soon developed a strong current of interest in medical experimentation as well. In October 1951 Humphry Osmond arrived in Saskatchewan after responding to an advertisement in *The Lancet* for a deputy director of psychiatry at the provincial Mental Hospital in Weyburn. Osmond was born in Surrey, England, on 1 July 1917. He spent his childhood in London and earned a medical degree from the University of London in 1942. During World War II he served as a British navy surgeon and then returned to London and took a position as the senior registrar in the psychiatric unit at St George's Hospital. There he developed an interest in biochemical theories of mental disorders, but found that this approach did not gain currency in a London psychiatric community heavily influenced by psychoanalytic theories.[31]

At St George's Hospital, Osmond had worked closely with colleague John Smythies and cultivated a keen interest in chemically induced reactions in the human body. Smythies and Osmond, with the aid of organic chemist John Harley-Mason, examined the chemical properties of mescaline, the psychoactive agent in the peyote cactus. Nearly two years of research led them to conclude that mescaline "caused symptoms in normal people that were similar to the symptoms of schizophrenia."[32] Further interrogation suggested that mescaline's chemical structure appeared very similar to adrenaline. These findings led to their supposition that schizophrenia resulted from a biochemical "imbalance." Furthermore, they believed that this imbalance might be caused by a "defect in the metabolism of adrenaline leading to the body's production of a substance chemically akin to mescaline."[33] This tantalizing assertion captivated Osmond's interests for the next two decades and inspired him to embark on a variety of drug experiments. Osmond's and Smythies' colleagues at St George's Hospital were not particularly interested in this biochemical research, but Osmond was intent on continuing. One of his colleagues recalled that Osmond "wanted to get as far away from Britain as he could to continue the work for which he had received no encouragement in a largely psychoanalytic environment."[34] When the opportunity to work in Saskatchewan presented itself, Osmond relocated his family from London, England, to Weyburn, Saskatchewan, and enthusiastically established a research program involving biochemical experimentation.

Shortly after arriving in Saskatchewan, Osmond met Abram Hoffer. Hoffer was also born in 1917, but far from cosmopolitan London. He had grown up in a small farming community named after his father, Israel Hoffer – Hoffer, Saskatchewan.[35] He also took a different path into medicine. Abram Hoffer graduated from the provincial university in Saskatoon with a bachelor of sciences degree in agricultural chemistry in 1937. Three years later he completed a master's degree in agriculture, after which he spent a year at the University of Minnesota conducting research on cereal chemistry. Stimulated by this subject, he continued in this field and in 1944 graduated with a PhD in agriculture with a dissertation that examined B vitamins in cereal chemistry. With a strong background in agricultural chemistry, Hoffer then applied himself to the field of medicine.

He began his medical training in Saskatchewan and then completed his medical doctorate at the University of Toronto in 1949.[36] By this time he had developed a particular interest in psychiatric disorders through his medical training. On 1 July 1950 Hoffer was hired at the Regina General Hospital to work as a half-time psychiatrist in the Munroe Wing, a psychiatric unit.[37] His other half-time position, with the Department of Public Health, obliged him to concentrate on psychiatric research.[38] His combined areas of expertise in chemical studies and medical practice made Hoffer an attractive candidate for establishing a research program, particularly with the contemporary trend toward studies of chemical treatments. In 1952, the provincial director of the Psychiatric Services Branch, D.G. McKerracher, convinced Hoffer to return to Saskatoon and concentrate on research full-time.

Hoffer and Osmond soon joined forces and began collaborating over their mutual research interests in biochemical experimentation. Osmond's curiosity with hallucinogens quickly introduced him to d-lysergic acid diethylamide (LSD), which he discovered produced similar reactions to those observed in normals under the influence of mescaline, although LSD was a much more powerful drug. Initial research with LSD also fitted neatly into the political vision for mental health reforms in the province. Early trials indicated that the drug had the potential to improve mental health care by advancing a theory of mental illness that explained it as the manifestation of metabolic functions. This assertion pointed to the possibility that mental illness was in fact a biological process and thus could be studied and ultimately treated using modern medical technology. It suggested that, like physical illnesses, mental illnesses might one day be observable through the microscope. In addition to the implications for therapy, this supposition offered evidence that mental illnesses did not result from immoral decisions, dysfunctional families, or inappropriate manners and that they deserved medical, rather than social, attention.

Hoffer and Osmond analyzed LSD from biochemical and experiential perspectives to ascertain its use for psychiatry. Osmond's interest in experimenting with psychedelic drugs began with self-experimentation. His own responses led him to believe that through chemically induced experiences one could come to understand the perceptions of patients with schizophrenia. One of his first experiences with mescaline provided him with a firsthand understanding of perceptual disturbances that seemed to match those described by patients with psychotic symptoms. In his report on his first experience, Osmond stated: "One house took my attention. It had a sinister quality, since from behind its drawn shades, people seemed to be looking out and their gaze was unfriendly. We met no people for the first few hundred yards, then we came to a window in which a child was standing and as we drew nearer its face became pig-like. I noticed two passersby, who, as they drew nearer, seemed hump-backed and twisted and their faces were covered ... The wide spaces of the streets were dangerous, the houses threatening, and the sun burned me."[39] Astounded by the drug's capacity to suspend his own sense of logic, reality, and comfort, Osmond continued to monitor his own reactions for their similarity to perceptions of reality as described by schizophrenic patients. He reasoned that such drug-induced experiences provided a valuable analytical method for understanding patients' perspectives and behaviour.

Osmond felt that patients' perceptions of disorder had often been dismissed by other doctors as "tiresome vapourings of paranoid and disgruntled people whose embittered stories would not, we feel, be typical."[40] His self-experimentation with LSD, however, encouraged him to reconsider patients' own depictions of illness. In 1957 psychologist Robert Sommer joined Osmond to study autobiographies of patients with mental disorders. After collecting hundreds of writing samples, they settled on a collection of accounts from patients who had been hospitalized, which represented frank autobiographies and offered descriptions that were overtly focused on illustrating mental illness or institutionalization.[41] The final list of volumes consisted of thirty-seven titles, involving twenty-five male and twelve female authors.[42] A group comprised of lay and professional participants read the material and subsequently constructed an analysis of patients' perceptions. The investigators found a common trend in the samples that illustrated the authors' regular struggles to suppress or ignore sensory data. They also discovered that these authors often revealed a sophisticated understanding of the psychological theories explaining their illnesses, while some patients even offered their own interpretations. Overall, Sommer and Osmond concluded that this kind of study presented mental health professionals with a rich, untapped resource for investigating mental illnesses.[43]

The examination of patients' autobiographies confirmed Osmond's assumptions that reactions to LSD and patients' experiences with psychotic symptoms held tremendous similarities. He and Sommer stated that "the reader receives the impression that each author considers his experiences unique and beyond the realm of comparison. This is a similar attitude to many of those who have taken mescaline or LSD. They do not see how one experience can validly be compared with another."[44] The results of the autobiography study persuaded Osmond to continue exploring the two sets of experiences in tandem. He felt that the remarkable consistencies among the experiences shed light on the progression of illness and, moreover, that a concentration on perceptual disturbances provided psychiatrists with alternative methods for observing the onset of illness.

Osmond's insistence that psychiatrists study the subjective experiences of their patients did not sit well with many of his colleagues. He responded to his critics by contending that the major challenge facing orthodox psychiatry was its unwillingness to investigate phenomena that fell outside established practices. Given the lack of certainties in mental health research, he advised that no possibilities should be discounted when advancing theories or hypotheses in psychiatric research. He critically examined the nature of psychiatric research, concluding that in their desire to more succinctly define psychiatry somewhere between general medicine and philosophy, psychiatrists had sought the development of a professional language of expertise that did not suit the needs of the discipline. Instead, it relied on fact collection or the empirical method, systematic theories, and scientific methodologies that all depended on assembling observable data, and therefore it could not adequately accommodate immeasurable qualities.[45] Yet continued self-experimentation with LSD, together with the conviction that it produced a model psychosis, encouraged Osmond to conclude that psychiatry needed a different professional discourse, one that appreciated subtleties in experience, attitude, and behaviour.

Hoffer and Osmond steadfastly alleged that interpreting experiences required sound scientific methodology; indeed they stated that "specialties whose scientific background is poorly developed or in which science proves difficult to apply lag behind the more fortunate. Psychiatry is one of the laggards. ... Starved of scientific guidance and stimulation, psychiatry fell back on the descriptive study of symptoms, dogma, system building and empiricism which is the fate of medicine without science."[46] Without sufficient scientific analysis that merged subjective and objective data, they argued, the field of psychiatry could not move beyond listing and comparing symptoms. Debates would, they contended, continue unresolved over the core features of illnesses, the particular manifestations of illness in an individual, and the appropriate course of treatment. Such an uncoordinated approach to mental illness, they argued, delayed the development of effective cures by concentrating professional energies on the illness rather than its cause.

They believed that the lack of a satisfactory discourse on classification and treatment of illness left the field in stasis.[47] The discipline of psychiatry refused to explore ideas that strayed beyond observable measurement, and thus the profession had curtailed its ability to discover effective cures for mental disorders. General medicine, by comparison, accepted the x-ray machine, electronic devices, and modern biochemical methods that allowed it to produce new therapies, often despite the corresponding medical expertise to explain how such stimuli affected the human body. Hoffer pointed out the irony in psychiatrists using tools of medicine to control symptoms, especially tranquilizers, but refusing to embrace biochemical therapies for curing disorders.[48] Indeed, he argued that tranquilizers only created a different kind of psychosis that obstructed more effective cures, thus illustrating the compounded problems psychiatry faced in its reluctance to embrace biomedical cures for mental illness. Moreover, his views demonstrated consternation with the professional desire to develop drug treatments that controlled symptoms, rather than direct research towards the etiological developments of disorders.

For both Hoffer and Osmond, experimentation with psychedelic drugs offered insight into the causation of mental disorder based on a combination of empirical and experiential observations.[49] The resultant psychedelic therapy challenged researchers to reconceptualize mental illness in terms of an individual's experiences and self-awareness, thus abandoning rigid systems of symptom classification based on interpretations from an observer, in favour of interdisciplinary collaboration involving the patient. Their approach to classification promoted a different kind of medical discourse for advancing clinical assessments based on connections among individuals' experiences, beliefs, and behaviours.

Observations made by volunteers who experimented with LSD in the clinical context, many of whom were psychiatrists themselves, encouraged researchers to look more closely at how insight from LSD experiences might benefit patients. If, indeed, LSD reactions mimicked psychosis, then provisions for care could also be improved after identifying the stimuli in a patient's environment that caused negative feelings or reactions.[50] Furthermore, as mental health care professionals gained an appreciation for distortions in thinking, feeling, and behaving, communication barriers between staff and patients might be reduced. Insight gained from these LSD trials contributed to the mounting optimism concerning progressive developments in reforming accommodation for patients suffering from mental illnesses.

Other observations from these trials led to a belief that LSD and other psychedelic drugs were additionally capable of producing a "transcendental feeling of being united with the world."[51] LSD, for example, produced a "mind-manifesting" experience that led to personal insight, transcendence, or spiritual enlightenment; therefore the psychedelic experience itself had therapeutic potential. Osmond assumed a lead role in the development of this approach to therapy, and several psychiatrists examining LSD observed its "psychedelic" qualities. An interim report on the therapeutic use of LSD from University of Regina psychologist Duncan Blewett described this aspect of LSD research in detail. Excerpts from his report list the common LSD reactions:

1 A feeling of being at one with the Universe.
2 Experience of being able to see oneself objectively or a feeling that one has two identities.
3 Change in usual concept of self with concomitant change in perceived body.
4 Changes in perception of space and time.
5 Enhancement in the sensory fields.
6 Changes in thinking and understanding so the subject feels he develops a profound understanding in the field of philosophy or religion.
7 A wider range of emotions with rapid fluctuation.
8 Increased sensitivity to the feelings of others.
9 Psychotic changes – These include illusions, hallucinations, paranoid delusions of reference, influence, persecution and grandeur, thought disorder, perceptual distortion, severe anxiety.[52]

From this catalogue of experiences, Blewett, Osmond, and others reasoned that LSD was useful in creating a psychedelic effect where subjects learned new values or gained important insights about themselves and their surroundings. This premise formed the basis of psychedelic therapy. Employing LSD in a therapeutic context required an appreciation for subjective experiences as a critical component in identifying and healing mental disorders. This approach, however, did not fit neatly into the emerging psychopharmacological paradigm that emphasized the use of drugs for controlling symptoms.

Supporters of psychedelic therapy argued that mental health research focused too much on collecting data about symptoms and that a more qualitative approach was necessary for appreciating experiences. On this subject, Humphry Osmond stated: "Our preoccupation with behaviour because it is measurable, has had us assume that what can be measured must be valuable, and vice versa ... An emphasis on the measurable and the reductive has resulted in the limitation of interest by psychiatrists and psychologists to aspects of experience that fit in with this concept."[53] Osmond thus reasoned that in order for psychiatrists to incorporate psychedelic therapy with any success, the profession needed to entertain new directions in research that gave sophisticated attention to the delicate combinations of spirituality and science. A psychedelic reaction, or a state of oneness with the universe, was often the goal of psychedelic psychotherapy, but patient records indicated that this state of awareness was rarely achieved. Nonetheless, patients undergoing psychedelic therapy had a range of experiences that often resulted in personal insights which, at least initially, assisted in their recoveries.[54]

Patients undergoing psychedelic therapy received a briefing from the attending psychiatrist before taking the drug, signed a consent form, and participated in a session that lasted approximately eight hours, with nurses and clinicians present. The principal investigator encouraged patients under the influence of LSD to discuss the reasons why they had sought therapy. During this time one member of the research team, often a nurse, made a transcript of the session. At the conclusion of the session, the psychiatrist encouraged the patient to submit a report of his or her experience within a couple of days. Although few patients had psychedelic experiences, many reported profound reactions that gave them insight into their behaviour, relationships, or addictions, which they felt could not be achieved without the aid of LSD. After the drug started taking effect, investigators probed patients with questions about their behaviour, life experiences, and relationships, as part of the psychotherapeutic experience. Reports from such sessions indicated that the drug assisted in the recollection, and often reconciliation, of past experiences. Investigators believed that LSD significantly enhanced the psychotherapy process by allowing participants to arrive at profound personal insight in a single session.[55]

The most frequently treated cases involved patients suffering from alcoholism. Patient records and follow-up reports, where available, indicated a high rate of personal insight among alcoholics treated with a combination of LSD and psychotherapy. Patients in this category routinely reported periods of sobriety following the LSD treatment session, used in conjunction with Alcoholics Anonymous.[56] Transcripts from these cases suggested that these patients experienced highly personal reactions that led them to appreciate the seriousness of their dependence on alcohol and its impact on their families, their employers, and their own health. Experiences, however, differed greatly among individuals. Some patients had pleasant reactions that, combined with psychotherapy, led them to appreciate the nature of their disorder. For example, one patient remarked that he had always felt alone and sought comfort in alcohol. During his LSD therapy he had visual hallucinations depicting his life surrounded by family and friends, and he began to feel the strain that alcohol put on these relationships.[57] Others had painful emotional reactions that exposed horrific images and feelings. In both cases, patients felt either coaxed or frightened into sobriety by the experience of the drug reaction. Yet others still had mild reactions with no appreciable change in behaviour or, worse, had terrifying experiences with no therapeutic value.[58] Prospects for sobriety loosely corresponded with the intensity of the LSD reaction; those with religious or terrifying experiences appeared to fare better than those with mild responses.

Although Hoffer and Osmond immediately identified the significance of the subject's experience in affecting the outcome of the treatment, they similarly recognized that their study needed to be well grounded in a biological approach. Their biochemical research on schizophrenia supplied some of the theoretical background for explaining the results of their trials with alcoholics. Accordingly, they elaborated a biochemical disease concept based on their earlier studies which demonstrated an increased rate of adrenaline production in patients with schizophrenia.[59] Related research on chronic alcoholics indicated that alcoholics exhibited comparable levels of adrenaline production, particularly during episodes of delirium tremens. Hoffer and Osmond thus pronounced a biochemical link between mental illness and addiction that placed both diseases under the authority of psychiatrists, within the medical arena, and beyond moral reproach.

The integrated psychedelic psychiatry earned professional support and satisfied local political goals. The research possibilities generated by Hoffer and Osmond's theories attracted other individuals to the province, where they eagerly contributed to the expansion of biochemical studies. The psychiatric research program also fulfilled two important objectives outlined by the CCF government in Saskatchewan: the biochemical experimentation advanced a theory of mental illness that satisfied a vision for a research-intensive program that would eventually transform the image of mental health care in the province, and the allure of the research program attracted researchers to the region and helped to address the critical shortages in health care professionals.

Despite local support, psychiatrists throughout North American increasingly questioned Hoffer and Osmond's claims. By the mid-1960s, LSD emerged in the popular press as an extremely dangerous drug and one that was insidiously associated with a youth-led cultural revolution. By 1961 Osmond had relocated with his family to Princeton University in New Jersey, but he maintained regular contact with Hoffer, and they attempted to counter claims made by their critics that LSD research was a wasted exercise. Despite their repeated attempts, the popular image of the dangerousness of the drug prevailed and cast a dark shadow over Hoffer's and Osmond's research program in Saskatchewan.

At the outset, however, LSD experimentation in the region appealed to several psychiatrists and government officials alike as a legitimate scientific endeavour that could lead to major breakthroughs in mental health treatments. Their commitment to integrating empathy into psychiatric research and practice demonstrated a professional concern for patients and ethical medical experimentation. In post-war Saskatchewan, LSD experimentation received significant support as a viable medical technology. As the investigations progressed, many believed that LSD studies offered demonstrable proof that mental illnesses existed biologically and that their care should be equal to that available for physical ailments – that is to say, without discrimination or stigmatization. The stimulation of theories about mental health captivated interests in this region, which was politically committed to reshaping attitudes towards health. Consequently, support for LSD experimentation was part of a regional commitment to health reforms.

Before leaving his post at Weyburn, Osmond wrote a letter to Premier Tommy Douglas describing his faith in the psychiatric research. He stated "The research is making really encouraging progress. [Ten years ago] it seemed wholly improbable that our idea would last more than a year or so. It is now becoming the centre of more and more attention and gradually confirmation is seeping in ... I could not have done it alone ... I'm not sure what the social implications will be of a measurable, visible, biochemical schizophrenia but it is, I think, (and one can always be a bit premature) very close round the corner."[60] Hoffer similarly congratulated the provincial government for its foresight in supporting an untested theory. He claimed "The support from our own Provincial Government cannot be esti-mated in dollars and cents. There is no other province in Canada which could have provided better soil for such a program. The contribution has been in the form of providing opportunity, providing the co-operation of their professional people and in diverting a substantial proportion of the Mental Health Grant toward research."[61] Taken together, these comments from Osmond and Hoffer indicated that they shared a belief that psychedelic research would reform mental health care. In addition, they applauded the CCF government's courage in supporting measures that made Saskatchewan a fertile region for medical experimentation. Post-war Saskatchewan pre-sented itself as a jurisdiction committed to sweeping reforms, and conse-quently, the biochemical research initiated by Hoffer and Osmond assumed a regional quality.

Saskatchewan's political culture provided an ideological sanctuary for LSD experimentation, which meant that psychiatrists such as Hoffer and Osmond were not actively working to define themselves *against* an exist-ing order. Yet despite their concerted efforts to distinguish themselves from traditional psychiatrists, they did not identify with contemporary critics of psychiatry. Their approach to LSD experimentation did not form part of the anti-psychiatry discourse, as it did in the case of R.D. Laing's LSD experi-ments in Glasgow, for example. Laing identified himself against the pro-fessional establishment and worked diligently to create a supportive research environment as a necessary precursor for advancing scientific the-ories.[62] In Saskatchewan, Hoffer and Osmond *were* the establishment. The overwhelming difference in these two cases was the regional context in which they operated or the sites of their "working utopias," the place where, sociologist Nick Crossley claims, "imaginative projections achieve some degree of concrete realisation."[63]

NOTES

I want to thank David Wright and James Moran for creating this edited volume and the two anonymous reviewers who generously provided comments on this chapter. An earlier version was presented at the Canadian Society for the History of Medicine meeting in Winnipeg (2004), and I am grateful also for the feedback I received at that conference. This project has received funding from McMaster University and a Social Sciences and Humanities Research Council grant. Lastly, I wish to thank all of the individuals – psychiatrists, patients, politicians, and others – who have shared with me their memories and impressions of Saskatchewan and the LSD experiments.

1 Saskatchewan Archives Board (hereafter SAB), A207, XI. 8. (1952–1966), Humphry Osmond, "Models of Madness," *New Scientist* 12 (no date): 778.

2 The term "psychedelic" was coined by Dr Humphry Osmond in 1957 in Osmond, "A Review of the Clinical Effects of Psychotomimetic Agents," *Annals of the New York Academy of Sciences* 66 (1957): 418–34.

3 For examples of historical examinations of LSD in psychiatry, see Stephen Snelders, "LSD and the Dualism between Medical and Social Theories of Mental Illness," in Marijke Gijswijt-Hofstra and Roy Porter, eds., *Cultures of Psychiatry and Mental Health Care in Postwar Britain and the Netherlands* (Amsterdam and Atlanta, GA: Editions Rodopi B.V., 1998), 103–20; Stephen Snelders and Charles Kaplan, "LSD in Dutch Psychiatry: Changing Socio-Political Settings and Medical Sets," *Medical History* 46, 2 (2002): 221–40; Steven Novak, "LSD before Leary: Sidney Cohen's Critique of 1950s Psychedelic Research," *Isis* 88, 1 (1997): 87–110; Bram Enning, "The Success of Jan Bastiaan," (forthcoming PhD dissertation, University of Maastricht); and Patrick Barber, "Chemical Revolutionaries – Saskatchewan's Psychedelic Drug Experiments and the Theories of Drs. Abram Hoffer, Humphry Osmond and Duncan Blewett" (MA thesis, University of Regina, 2005).

4 Mark Micale, "Henri F. Ellenberger: The History of Psychiatry as the History of the Unconscious," in Mark S. Micale and Roy Porter, eds., *Discovering the History of Psychiatry* (Oxford: Oxford University Press, 1994), 117.

5 See also Joel Braslow, *Mental Ills and Bodily Cures: Psychiatric Treatment in the First Half of the Century* (Berkeley: University of California Press, 1997).

6 Jack Pressman, *Last Resort: Psychosurgery and the Limits of Medicine* (Cambridge: Harvard University Press, 1998), 3–4.

7 Examples of works in the history of medicine that investigate the socio-political dynamic in the reception of science include E.M. Tansey, "'They Used to Call It Psychiatry': Aspects of the Development and Impact of Psychopharmacology," in Gijswijt-Hofstra and Roy Porter, *Cultures of Psychiatry and Mental Health Care in Postwar Britain and the Netherlands*, 79–102; Roger Cooter and Stephen Pumfrey, "Separate Spheres and Public Places: Reflections on the History of Science Popularisation and Science in Popular Culture," *History of Science* 32, 3 (1994): 237–67; Harry Marks, "Trust and Mistrust in the Marketplace: Statistics and Clinical Research, 1945–1960," *History of Science* 38, 3 (2000): 343–55; John Abraham, *Science, Politics and the Pharmaceutical Industry: Controversy and Bias in Drug Regulation* (London: University College Press, 1995); Virginia

Berridge, "History and Twentieth-Century Drug Policy: Telling True Stories?" *Medical History* 47, 4 (2003): 518–24; and John C. Burnham, *Bad Habits: Drinking, Smoking, Taking Drugs, Gambling, Sexual Misbehavior, and Swearing in American History* (New York: New York University Press, 1993).

8 Betsy Thom and Virginia Berridge, "'Special Units for Common Problems': The Birth of Alcohol Treatments in England," *Social History of Medicine* 8, 1 (1995): 91.

9 During the Cold War, American government officials reasoned that homosexual behaviour was symptomatic of communist affiliation, suggesting that a secretive lifestyle was unique to communists. See Gary Kinsman, "'Character Weaknesses' and 'Fruit Machines': Towards an Analysis of the Anti-homosexual Security Campaign in the Canadian Civil Service," *Labour* 35 (1995): 133–61.

10 For a description of his experiments, see D.E. Cameron, "Psychic Driving," *American Journal of Psychiatry* 112, 7 (1956): 502–9; and D. Ewen Cameron, J.G. Lohrenze, and K.A. Handcock, "The Depatterning Treatment of Schizophrenia," *Comprehensive Psychiatry* 3 (1962): 65. For an explanation of the subsequent legal inquiries, see Anne Collins, *In the Sleep Room: The Story of the CIA Brainwashing Experiments in Canada* (Toronto: Lester and Orpen Dennys, 1988); J.D.M. Griffin, "Cameron's Search for a Cure," *Canadian Bulletin of Mental Health* 8 (1991): 121–6; and Harvey Weinstein, *Psychiatry and the CIA: Victims of Mind Control* (Washington, DC: American Psychiatric Press, 1990).

11 LSD was discovered by Albert Hofmann in 1938; his first reported experience with the drug occurred in 1943, and the drug became widely available for medical research by the end of the 1940s. See Albert Hofmann, *LSD, My Problem Child* (New York: McGraw-Hill, 1980).

12 Tom Ban as quoted in Tansey, "'They Used to Call It Psychiatry,'" 79.

13 David Healy, *The Creation of Psychopharmacology* (Cambridge: Harvard University Press, 2002), 77–8.

14 David Healy, *The Anti-Depressant Era* (Cambridge: Harvard University Press, 1997), 43–5.

15 For examples of literature on deinstitutionalization, see Simon Goodwin, *Comparative Mental Health Policy: From Institutional to Community Care* (London: Sage Publications, 1997); Wolf Wolfensberger, Bengt Nirje, et al., eds., *The Principle of Normalization in Human Services* (Toronto: National Institute on Mental Retardation, 1972); Kathleen Jones, *Asylums and After: A Revised History of the Mental Health Services: From the Early 18th Century to the 1990s* (London: Athlone Press, 1993); and Gerald Grob, *From Asylum to Community: Mental Health Policy in Modern America* (Princeton: Princeton University Press, 1991).

16 The thalidomide crisis of 1962, however, drew attention to fears that medical "wonder drugs" were not necessarily safe. Birth deformities in children whose

mothers took thalidomide raised serious concerns about the consequences of promoting pharmaceuticals.

17 For example, see K.F. Killam, "Studies of LSD and Chlorpromazine," *Psychiatric Research Reports* 6 (1956): 35; H.A. Abramson and A. Rolo, "Lysergic Acid Diethylamide (LSD-25) Antagonists: Chlorpromazine," *Journal of Neuropsychiatry* 1 (1960): 307–10; and D.B. Sankar, D.V. Siva, E. Gold, and E. Phipps, "Effects of BOL, LSD and Chlorpromazine on Serotonin Levels," *Federation Proceedings [American Physiological Society]* 20 (1961): 344.

18 C.M. Hincks, *Mental Hygiene Survey of Saskatchewan* (Regina: Thomas A. McConnica, King's Printer, 1945), 8; and H.E. Sigerist, *Saskatchewan Health Services Survey Commission* (Regina: King's Printer, 1944). See also Jacalyn Duffin and Leslie A. Falk, "Sigerist in Saskatchewan: The Quest for Balance in Social and Technical Medicine," *Bulletin for the History of Medicine* 70 (1996): 658–83.

19 Arguably, this concept is ahistorical. Census data indicates that since the population boom, fuelled by the promises of free land, Saskatchewan's population has remained virtually unchanged (1911–2002 census data). Closer examination, however, reveals the effects of prolonged brain drain in the province, which perpetuates existing problems with economic diversification and the attraction of professionals. See B.S. Basran, "The Rural Depopulation of the Prairies," in J. A. Fry, ed., *Economy, Class and Social Reality: Issues in Contemporary Canadian Society* (Toronto: Butterworths, 1979). For specific issues concerning attracting doctors to the region, see L. Horlick, *Built Better than They Knew: Saskatchewan's Royal University Hospital, a History, 1955–1992* (Saskatoon: Louis Horlick, 2001).

20 This sentiment is repeatedly borne out by oral interviews. Several individuals recalled in oral interviews an attraction to the region that was explicitly related to its socialist politics and the progressive research environment it fostered.

21 James Labounty, "Dr Yes," *Western Living*, 2001, 43, Archives of the Centre for Addiction and Mental Health, Toronto, Arthur Allen file.

22 For examples of the history of medicare in Saskatchewan, see Duane Mombourquette, "An Inalienable Right: The CCF and Rapid Health Care Reform, 1944–1948," *Saskatchewan History* 3 (1991): 101–16; Howard Shillington, *The Road to Medicare in Canada* (Toronto: Del Graphics Pub., 1972); Edwin Tollefson, *Bitter Medicine: The Saskatchewan Medicare Feud* (Saskatoon: Modern Press, 1964); Aleck Ostry, "Prelude to Medicare: Institutional Change and Continuity in Saskatchewan, 1944–1962," *Prairie Forum* 20, 1 (1995): 87–105; Robin F. Badgley and Samuel Wolfe, *Doctors' Strike: Medical Care and Conflict in Saskatchewan* (Toronto: Macmillan of Canada, 1967); and Malcolm G. Taylor, *Health Insurance and Canadian Public Policy* (Montreal: McGill-Queen's University Press, 1978).

23 Joan Feather, "From Concept to Reality: Formation of the Swift Current Health Region, *Prairie Forum* 16, 1 (1991): 59–79; and Joan Feather, "Impact of the Swift Current Health Region: Experiment or Model?" *Prairie Forum* 16, 2 (1991): 225–45.

24 A.W. Johnson, *Dream No Little Dreams: A Biography of the Douglas Government of Saskatchewan, 1944–1961* (Toronto: University of Toronto Press, 2004).

25 Oral Interview with Arnie Funk, August 2003. This individual was an American graduate student in psychology and had learned about Saskatchewan's plans to establish a publicly funded health system. He came to the province with a desire to observe how the elimination of user fees influenced health outcomes. He received a bursary from the Saskatchewan government and subsequently spent two years pursuing graduate research at the hospital in Moose Jaw.

26 Oral interview with Joyce Munn, July 2003.

27 D.J. Buchan, *Greenhouse to Medical Centre: Saskatoon's Medical School, 1926–1978* (Saskatoon: College of Medicine, University of Saskatchewan, 1983), 169–70.

28 SAB, R45 75(9–1), Psychiatric Services, Miscellaneous, M.D. Rejskind, president, Saskatchewan Psychiatric Association, to Hon. Gordon B. Grant, minister of public health, 16 November 1966.

29 Douglas had some personal experience in this area. Firstly, he lived in and represented the constituency of Weyburn, where the largest provincial mental health facility was located. Secondly, as a master's student, he had written a thesis titled "The Problems of the Subnormal Family" (MA thesis, McMaster University, 1933).

30 Douglas, "The Problems of the Subnormal Family."

31 Elaine Woo, "Obituaries: Humphry Osmond, 86; Coined Term 'Psychedelic,'" *Los Angeles Times*, 22 February 2004, B-18.

32 Excerpt from John Smythies' autobiography, unpublished (2004). I am grateful to Dr Smythies for sharing his work with me.

33 Ibid. Smythies states that this was the first biochemical theory of schizophrenia.

34 Abram Hoffer, "Humphry Osmond Obituary: Doctor Who Helped Discover the Hallucinogenic Cause of Schizophrenia," *Guardian Weekly*, 4–10 March 2004, 23.

35 For further information on the municipality of Hoffer, Saskatchewan, see Clara Hoffer and Fannie Kahan, *Land of Hope* (Saskatoon: Modern Press, 1960). As Hoffer and Kahan make clear, Abram's father came to Saskatchewan as part of a Jewish agricultural relocation program. Hoffer senior was sent to Saskatchewan to establish an agricultural community that would absorb Jewish immigrants. Although the program was not very successful, it is likely that Abram developed an interest in agriculture in this context.

36 At this time the University of Saskatchewan did not have a full medical program available and medical students were therefore obliged to complete their degrees elsewhere.

37 SAB, A207, Correspondence, McKerracher, A. Hoffer to D.G. McKerracher, 20 April 1950, 1.

38 Ibid., A. Hoffer to D.G. McKerracher, 23 April 1952, 1.

39 Humphry Osmond, "On Being Mad," *Saskatchewan Psychiatric Services Journal* 1 (1952): 4. See also Humphry Osmond and John Smythies, "Schizophrenia: A New Approach," *Journal of Mental Science* 98 (1952): 309–15.

40 Robert Sommer and Humphry Osmond, "Autobiographies of Former Mental Patients," *Journal of Mental Science* 107 (1960): 648.

41 Ibid., 650.

42 Ibid., 652. They used the patients' descriptions or diagnoses to categorize them according to type of illness, which gave them an over-representation of alcoholics and paranoids with relatively fewer non-paranoid schizophrenics.

43 Ibid., 660.

44 Ibid., 658.

45 Humphry Osmond, "Inspiration and Method in Schizophrenia Research," *Diseases of the Nervous System* 4 (1955): 1–4.

46 Humphry Osmond and Abram Hoffer, "A Small Research in Schizophrenia," *The Canadian Medical Association Journal* 80 (1959): 91.

47 See Humphry Osmond and Abram Hoffer, "On Critics and Research," *Psychosomatic Medicine* 21 (1959): 311–20

48 See Abram Hoffer and Humphry Osmond, *The Hallucinogens* (Academic Press: New York, 1967) and Provincial Archives of Ontario, RG 10-163-0-461, box 13, A. Hoffer, *Manual For Treating Schizophrenia and Other Conditions Using Megavitamin Therapy* (New York: American Schizophrenia Foundation and University Books, c. 1967), 27.

49 Miriam Siegler and Humphry Osmond, *Models of Madness, Models of Medicine* (New York: MacMillan, 1974).

50 For examples of their studies particularly related to design concepts, see Humphry Osmond, "Function as the Basis of Psychiatric Design," *Mental Hospitals,* May 1957, 23–9; Archives of the Centre for Addiction and Mental Health, Toronto, Arthur Allen papers, Kyoshi Izumi, "An Analysis for the Design of Hospital Quarters for the Neuropsychiatric Patient," 8; Kyoshi Izumi, "The Yorkton Psychiatric Centre," *Mental Hospitals,* May 1957, 87; and Robert Sommer, "The Physical Environment of the Ward," *Hospitals* 40 (1966): 71–4.

51 SAB, A207, box 37, 233–A, LSD, Gustav R. Schmiege, "The Current Status of LSD as a Therapeutic Tool" (unpublished article), 5.

52 University of Regina Archives, RG 88–29. Duncan Blewett Papers. Writings of Duncan Blewett, "Interim Report on the Therapeutic Use of LSD" (1958), 4–5.

53 Humphry Osmond as quoted ibid., 8.

54 SAB, A207, A.II. "Hallucinogens," "Patient Files" [anonymous; names removed by author]. Records from Saskatchewan's Psychiatric Research branch suggested that some psychiatrists used LSD in psychotherapy for disorders that included "homosexuality," obsessive-compulsive disorder, depression, and, most commonly, alcoholism.

55 Most patients treated in this manner had already established relationships with their psychiatrists.

56 Cure rates varied. Reports indicate anywhere between 30 to 80 per cent rate of sobriety in cases involving LSD and chronic alcoholism. Follow-up periods also varied between approximately six months and two years.

57 This patient remained sober for over forty years.

58 Observations from author's review of over two hundred patient files: SAB, A207, A.II.5 to A.II.12, Hallucinogens, Patients, 1956–66.

59 Abram Hoffer, "A Program for the Treatment of Alcoholism: LSD, Malvaria, and Nicotinic Acid," in Harold Abramson, ed., The Use of LSD in Psychotherapy and Alcoholism (New York, 1967), 343–406.

60 SAB, Regina R-33.1, XVI, 573a, Humphry Osmond to T.C. Douglas, 14 July 1960, 2.

61 SAB, A207 XVIII, 2.b, Abram Hoffer, "Funding for Saskatchewan Psychiatric Research," May 1955, 1. National Health Grants and Rockefeller Foundation grants provided the remaining funding for their research program.

62 Nick Crossley, "Working Utopias and Social Movements: An Investigation Using Case Study Materials from Radical Mental Health Movements in Britain," Sociology 33, 4 (1999): 809–30.

63 Ibid., 810.

Selected Bibliography

Abraham, John. *Science, Politics and the Pharmaceutical Industry: Controversy and Bias in Drug Regulation*. London: University College London Press, 1995.

Andrews, Jonathan, and Anne Digby, eds. *Sex and Seclusion, Class and Custody: Perspectives on Class and Gender in the History of British and Irish Psychiatry.* Amsterdam: Rodolpi, 2004.

Arieti, Silvano, ed. *The World Biennial of Psychiatry and Psychotherapy.* 2nd ed. New York: Basic Books, 1973.

Atkinson, Dorothy, Mark Jackson, and Jan Walmsley, eds. *Forgotten Lives: Exploring the History of Learning Disability*. Kidderminster: British Institute of Learning Disabilities, 1997.

Baehre, Rainer. "'The Ill-Regulated Mind': A Study in the Making of Psychiatry in Ontario, 1830–1921." PhD dissertation, York University, 1985.

– "Imperial Authority and Colonial Officialdom of Upper Canada in the 1830s: The State, Crime, Lunacy and Everyday Social Order." In Louis Knafla Louis and Susan Binnie, eds., *Law, Society and the State: Essays in Modern Legal History.* Toronto: University of Toronto Press, 1995.

Barrett, J., and R. Rose, eds. *Mental Disorders in the Community: Progress and Challenges.* New York: Guilford Press, 1986.

Bartlett, Peter. "Structures of Confinement in 19th-Century Asylums: A Comparative Study Using England and Ontario." *International Journal of Law and Psychiatry* 23 (2000): 1–13.

Bartlett, Peter, and David Wright, eds. *Outside the Walls of the Asylum: The History of Care in the Community, 1750–2000.* London: The Athlone Press, 1999.

Berrios, German. *A History of Mental Symptoms: Descriptive Psychopathology since the Nineteenth Century.* Cambridge: Cambridge University Press, 1996.
- "J.C. Prichard and the Concept of 'Moral Insanity.'" *History of Psychiatry* 10, no. 1 (1999): 111–26.
Berrios, German, and Hugh Freeman., eds. *150 Years of British Psychiatry, 1841–1991.* London: Gaskell, 1991.
Berrios, German, and Roy Porter, eds. *A History of Clinical Psychiatry: The Origin and History of Psychiatric Disorders.* London: The Athlone Press, 1996.
Braslow, Joel. *Mental Ills and Bodily Cures: Psychiatric Treatment in the First Half of the Century.* Berkeley: University of California Press, 1997.
Brookes, Barbara, and Jane Thomson, eds. *"Unfortunate Folk": Essays on the History of Mental Health Treatment, 1863–1992.* Dunedin, NZ: University of Otago Press, 2001.
Brown, Thomas E. "'Living with God's Afflicted': A History of the Provincial Lunatic Asylum at Toronto, 1830–1911." PhD thesis, Queen's University, 1980.
- "Workman, Joseph." In *Dictionary of Canadian Biography*, vol. 12.
Bynum, W.F., Roy Porter, and Michael Shepherd., eds. *The Anatomy of Madness: Essays in the History of Psychiatry.* 3 vols. London: Tavistock, 1985–87.
Cellard, André. "La curatelle et l'histoire de la maladie mentale au Québec," *Histoire sociale/Social History* 19 (1986): 443–50.
- *Histoire de la folie au Québec, de 1600 à 1850: Le désordre.* Québec: Boréal, 1991.
Cherry, Steven. *Mental Health Care in Modern England: The Norfolk Lunatic Asylum, St Andrew's Hospital, 1810–1998.* London: Boydell & Brewer, 2003.
Chesler, Phyllis. *Women and Madness.* New York: Avon Books, 1973.
Chunn, Dorothy E., and Robert Menzies. "Out of Mind, Out of Law: The Regulation of 'Criminally Insane' Women inside British Columbia's Public Mental Hospitals, 1888–1973." *Canadian Journal of Women and the Law* 10 (1998): 306–37.
Cleghorn, R.A. "The Development of Psychiatric Research in Canada up to 1964." *Canadian Journal of Psychiatry* 29, no. 3 (1984): 189–97.
Coleborne, Catharine, and Dolly MacKinnon, eds. *"Madness" in Australia: Histories, Heritage and the Asylum.* St Lucia: University of Queensland Press, 2003.
Collins, Anne. *In the Sleep Room: The Story of the CIA Brainwashing Experiments in Canada.* Toronto: Lester and Orpen Dennys, 1988.
Copp, Terry, and Bill McAndrew. *Battle Exhaustion: Soldiers and Psychiatrists in the Canadian Army, 1939–1945.* Montreal and Kingston: McGill-Queen's University Press, 1990.
Crossley, Nick. "Working Utopias and Social Movements: An Investigation Using Case Study Materials from Radical Mental Health Movements in Britain." *Sociology* 33 (1999): 809–30.

Davies, Megan J. "The Patient's World: British Columbia's Mental Health Facilities, 1920–1935." MA thesis, University of Waterloo, 1987.

Digby, Anne. *Madness, Morality and Medicine: A Study of the York Retreat, 1792–1914.* Cambridge: Cambridge University Press, 1985.

Dowbiggin, Ian. *Keeping America Sane: Psychiatry and Eugenics in the United States and Canada, 1880–1940.* Ithaca: Cornell University Press, 1997, 2003.

– "'Keeping This Young Country Sane': C.K. Clarke, Immigration Restriction, and Canadian Psychiatry, 1890–1925." *Canadian Historical Review* 76 (1995): 598–627.

– *A Merciful End: The Euthanasia Movement in Modern America.* Oxford and New York: Oxford University Press, 2003.

– "'A Rational Coalition': Euthanasia, Eugenics, and Birth Control in America, 1940–1970." *Journal of Policy History* 14 (2002): 223–60.

Dwyer, Ellen. *Homes for the Mad: Life inside Two Nineteenth-Century Asylums.* New Brunswick, NJ, and London: Rutgers University Press, 1982.

Ernst, Waltraud. *Mad Tales from the Raj: The European Insane in British India, 1800–1858.* London: Routledge, 1991.

Finnane, Mark. "Asylums, Families and the State." *History Workshop Journal* 20 (1985): 134–48.

– *Insanity and the Insane in Post-Famine Ireland.* London: Croom Helm, 1981.

Flynn, Patrick, ed. *Dalhousie's Department of Psychiatry: A Historical Perspective.* Halifax: Department of Psychiatry, Dalhousie University, 1999.

Foucault, Michel. *Folie et déraison: Histoire de la folie à l'âge clas*sique. Paris: Plon, 1961. Trans. Richard Howard as *Madness and Civilization: A History of Insanity in the Age of Reason.* New York: Pantheon, 1965.

Fox, Richard W. *So Far Disordered in Mind: Insanity in California, 1870–1930.* Berkeley: University of California Press, 1978.

Freeman, Hugh, and German Berrios, eds. *150 Years of British Psychiatry, 1841–1991.* Vol. 2, *The Aftermath.* London: The Athlone Press, 1996.

Friedland, Martin L. *The Case of Valentine Shortis: A True Story of Crime and Politics in Canada.* Toronto: University of Toronto Press, 1986.

Geller, Jeffrey L., and Maxine Harris, eds. *Women of the Asylum: Voices from Behind the Walls, 1840–1945.* New York: Anchor Doubleday 1994.

Gijswijt-Hofstra, Marijke, and Roy Porter, eds. *Cultures of Psychiatry and Mental Health Care in Postwar Britain and the Netherlands.* Amsterdam: Rodolpi, 1998.

Goffman, Erving. *Asylums: Essays on the Social Situation of Mental Patients and Other Inmates.* New York: Anchor Books, 1961.

Goldberg, Ann. *Sex, Religion and the Making of Modern Madness.* Oxford: Oxford University Press, 1999.

Goldstein, Janet. *Console and Classify: The French Psychiatric Profession in the Nineteenth Century.* Cambridge: Cambridge University Press, 1987.

Goldstein, Michael S. "The Sociology of Mental Health and Illness." *Annual Review of Sociology* 5 (1979): 381–409.

Goodwin, Simon. *Comparative Mental Health Policy: From Institutional to Community Care.* London: Sage Publications, 1997.

Goulet, Denis, and André Paradis. *Trois siècles d'histoire médicale au Québec.* Montréal: VLB éditeur, 1992.

Goulet, George R.D. *The Trial of Louis Riel: Justice and Mercy Denied: A Critical, Legal and Political Analysis.* Calgary: Tellwell, 1999.

Greenland, Cyril. "The Life and Death of Louis Riel. Part II: Surrender, Trial, Appeal and Execution." *Canadian Psychiatric Association Journal* 10 (1965): 253–65.

Grenier, Guy. *Les monstres, les fous et les autres: La folie criminelle au Québec.* Montréal: Éditions Trait d'union, 1999.

Griffin, J.D.M. "Cameron's Search for a Cure." *Canadian Bulletin of Mental Health* 8 (1991): 121–6.

Grob, Gerald. *From Asylum to Community: Mental Health Policy in Modern America.* Princeton: Princeton University Press, 1991.

– *The Mad among Us: A History of the Care of America's Mentally Ill.* Cambridge: Harvard University Press, 1994

– *Mental Institutions in America: Social Policy to 1875.* New York: Free Press, 1973.

Hacking, Ian. *Rewriting the Soul: Multiple Personality and the Sciences of Memory.* Princeton: Princeton University Press, 1995.

Harris, Ruth. *Murders and Madness: Medicine, Law, and Society in the Fin de Siècle.* Oxford: Clarendon Press, 1989.

Hatfield, Agnes B., and Harriet P. Lefley, eds. *Families of the Mentally Ill: Coping and Adaptation.* New York: The Guildford Press, 1987.

Healy, David. *The Anti-Depressant Era.* Cambridge: Harvard University Press, 1997.

– *The Creation of Psychopharmacology.* Cambridge: Harvard University Press, 2002.

Herman, Ellen. *The Romance of American Psychology: Political Culture in the Age of Experts.* Berkeley and London: University of California Press, 1996.

Hoff, Paul. "Emil Kraepelin and Forensic Psychiatry." *International Journal of Law and Psychiatry* 21 (1998): 343–53.

Hofmann, Albert. *LSD, My Problem Child.* New York: McGraw-Hill, 1980.

Horden, Peregrine, and Richard Smith, eds. *The Locus of Care: Families, Communities, Institutions, and the Provision of Welfare since Antiquity.* London: Routledge 1998.

Hudson, Edna, ed. *The Provincial Asylum in Toronto.* Toronto: Toronto Regional Architectural Conservancy, 2000.

Hurd, Henry M. *The Institutional Care of the Insane in the United States and Canada*. Baltimore: Johns Hopkins University Press, 1916–17.

Irving, Allan. *Brock Chisholm: Doctor to the World*. Markham: Fitzhenry and Whiteside, 1998.

Jackson, Mark. "'It Begins with the Goose and Ends with the Goose': Medical, Legal, and Lay Understandings of Imbecility in Ingram v Wyatt, 1824–1832." *Social History of Medicine* 11 (1998): 361–80.

Jasen, Patricia. "Malignant Histories: Psychosomatic Medicine and the Female Cancer Patient in Postwar America." *Canadian Bulletin of Medical History* 20 (2003): 265–97.

Johnston, Christine. *Father of Canadian Psychiatry*. Victoria: Ogden Press, 2000.

Jones, Kathleen. *Asylums and After: A Revised History of the Mental Health Services*. London: The Athlone Press, 1993.

– *A History of the Mental Health Services*. London: Routledge and Kegan Paul, 1972.

Keating, Peter. *La science du mal: L'institution de la psychiatrie au Québec, 1800–1914*. Québec: Boréal, 1993.

Kelm, Mary-Ellen. *Colonizing Bodies: Aboriginal Health and Healing in British Columbia, 1900–50*. Vancouver: UBC Press, 1998.

– "Women and Families in the Asylum Practice of Charles Edward Doherty at the Provincial Hospital for the Insane, 1905–1915." MA thesis, Simon Fraser University, 1990.

– "Women, Families and the Provincial Hospital for the Insane, British Columbia, 1905–1915." *Journal of Family History* 19 (1994): 177–93.

Kirk-Montgomery, Allison. "Courting Madness: Insanity and Testimony in the Criminal Justice System of Victorian Ontario." PhD thesis, University of Toronto, 2001.

Labrum, Bronwyn. "Looking Beyond the Asylum: Gender and the Process of Committal in Auckland, 1870–1910." *New Zealand Journal of History* 26 (1992): 125–45.

Leighton, Alexander H. *Caring for Mentally Ill People: Psychological and Social Barriers in Historical Context*. Cambridge: Cambridge University Press, 1982.

Leighton, Alexander H., and Jane M. Murphy. "Nature of Pathology: The Character of Danger Implicit in Functional Impairment." *Canadian Journal of Psychiatry* 42 (1997): 714–21.

Leighton, Alexander H., et al., eds. *Explorations in Social Psychiatry*. New York: Basic Books, 1957.

Leighton, D.C., et al. "Psychiatric Findings of the Stirling County Study." *American Journal of Psychiatry* 119 (1963): 1021–6.

McCandless, Peter. *Moonlight, Magnolias, and Madness: Insanity in South Caro-

line from the Colonial Period to the Progressives Era. Chapel Hill and London: University of North Carolina Press, 1996.

Marsh, Diane T. *Families and Mental Retardation: New Directions in Professional Practice*. New York: Praeger, 1992.

Melling, Joseph, and Bill Forsythe, eds. *Insanity, Institutions and Society: A Social History of Madness in Comparative Perspective*. London: Routledge, 1999.

Menzies, Robert. "Historical Profiles of Criminal Insanity." *International Journal of Law and Psychiatry* 25 (2002): 379–404.

– "'I Do Not Care for a Lunatic's Role': Modes of Regulation and Resistance inside the Colquitz Mental Home, British Columbia, 1919–33." *Canadian Bulletin of Medical History* 16 (1999): 181–213.

Menzies, Robert, and Dorothy E. Chunn. "The Gender Politics of Criminal Insanity: 'Order-in-Council' Women in British Columbia, 1888–1950." *Histoire sociale/Social History* 31 (1999): 241–79.

Micale, Mark, and Roy Porter, eds. *Discovering the History of Psychiatry*. Oxford: Oxford University Press, 1994.

Michael, Pamela. *Care and Treatment of the Mentally Ill in North Wales, 1800–2000*. Cardiff: University of Wales Press, 2003.

Mills, James H. *Madness, Cannabis and Colonialism: The "Native Only" Lunatic Asylums of British India, 1857–1900*. London: Palgrave MacMillan, 2000.

Miron, Janet. "'As in a Menagerie': The Custodial Institution as Spectacle in the Nineteenth Century." PhD dissertation, York University, 2004.

Mitchinson, Wendy. *Giving Birth in Canada*. Toronto: University of Toronto Press, 2002.

– *The Nature of Their Bodies: Women and Their Doctors in Victorian Canada*. Toronto: University of Toronto Press, 1991.

– "Reasons for Committal to a Mid-Nineteenth-Century Ontario Insane Asylum: The Case of Toronto." In *Essays in the History of Canadian Medicine*, ed. Wendy Mitchinson and Janice Dickin McGinnis. Toronto: McClelland and Stewart, 1988.

Mohr, James. "The Origins of Forensic Psychiatry in the United States and the Great Nineteenth-Century Crisis over the Adjudication of Wills." *Journal of the American Academy of Psychiatry and the Law* 25 (1997): 273–84.

Montigny, Edward-André. "'Foisted Upon the Government': Institutions and the Impact of Public Policy upon the Aged: The Elderly Patients of Rockwood Asylum, 1866–1906." *Journal of Social History* 28 (1995): 819–36.

Moran, James E. "Asylum in the Community: Managing the Insane in Antebellum America." *History of Psychiatry* 9, no. 2 (1998): 217–40.

– *Committed to the State Asylum: Insanity and Society in Nineteenth-Century Quebec and Ontario*. Montreal and Kingston: McGill-Queen's University Press, 2000.

Morton, Desmond, ed. *The Queen v Louis Riel*. Toronto: University of Toronto Press, 1974.

Murphy, Jane M. "Continuities in Community-based Psychiatric Epidemiology." *Archives of General Psychiatry* 37 (1980): 1215–23.

– "The Stirling County Study: Then and Now." *International Review of Psychiatry* 6 (1994): 329–48.

Murphy, Jane M., et al. "Depression and Anxiety in Relation to Social Status: a Prospective Epidemiologic Study." *Archives of General Psychiatry* 48 (1991): 223–9.

– "Stability of Prevalence: Depression and Anxiety Disorders." *Archives of General Psychiatry* 41 (1984): 990–7.

Noll, Steven, and James Trent, eds. *Mental Retardation in America: A Historical Reader*. New York: New York University Press, 2004.

Nootens, Thierry. "Fous, prodigues et ivrognes: Internormativité, et déviance à Montréal au 19ᵉ siècle." PhD thesis, Université de Québec à Montréal, 2003.

Novak, Steven. "LSD before Leary: Sidney Cohen's Critique of 1950s Psychedelic Research." *Isis* 88 (1997): 87–110.

Nye, Robert. *Crime, Madness, and Politics in Modern France: The Medical Concept of National Decline*. Princeton: Princeton University Press, 1984.

Oppenheim, Janet. *Shattered Nerves: Doctors, Patients, and Depression in Victorian England*. New York: Oxford University Press, 1991.

Peterson, Dale. *A Mad People's History of Madness*. Pittsburgh: University of Pittsburgh Press, 1982.

Plotkin, Mariano, ed. *Argentina on the Couch: Psychiatry, State, and Society, 1880 to Present*. Albuquerque: University of New Mexico Press, 2003.

Porter, Roy. *Madness: A Brief History*. Oxford: Oxford University Press, 2003.

– "The Patient's View: Doing Medical History from Below." *Theory and Society* 14 (1985): 175–98.

– *A Social History of Madness*. New York: E.P. Dutton, 1989.

Porter, Roy, and Andrew Wears, eds. *Problems and Methods in the History of Medicine*. London: Croom Helm, 1987.

Porter, Roy, and David Wright, eds. *The Confinement of the Insane: International Perspectives, 1800–1965*. Cambridge: Cambridge University Press, 2003.

Pressman, Jack D. *Last Resort: Psychosurgery and the Limits of Medicine*. Cambridge, New York: Cambridge University Press, 1998.

Prestwich, Patricia E. "Family Strategies and Medical Power: 'Voluntary' Committal in a Parisian Asylum, 1876–1914." *Journal of Social History* 27 (1994): 799–818.

Rae-Grant, Quentin, ed. *Psychiatry in Canada: 50 Years (1951–2001)*. Ottawa, Canadian Psychiatric Association, 2001.

Reaume, Geoffrey. *Remembrance of Patients Past: Patient Life at the Toronto Hospital for the Insane, 1870–1940*. Toronto: Oxford University Press, 2000.

Redden, Joanna. "The Community Mental Health Movement in Nova Scotia, 1945–69: The Case of the Fundy Mental Health Centre." MA thesis, Dalhousie University, 2000.

Ripa, Yannick. *Women and Madness: The Incarceration of Women in Nineteenth-Century France*. Trans. Catherine du Peloux Menagé. Cambridge: Polity Press, 1990.

Robinson, Daniel. *Wild Beasts and Idle Humours: The Insanity Defence from Antiquity to the Present*. Cambridge: Harvard University Press, 1996.

Rosenberg, Charles. *The Trial of the Assassin Guiteau: Psychiatry and the Law in the Gilded Age*. Chicago: University of Chicago Press, 1968.

Rosenberg, Charles, and Janet Golden, eds. *Framing Disease: Studies in Cultural History*. New Brunswick, NJ: Rutgers University Press, 1992.

Rothman, David. *The Discovery of the Asylum: Social Order and Disorder in the New Republic*. Boston: Little Brown, 1971.

Sadowsky, Jonathan. *Imperial Bedlam: Institutions of Madness in Southwest Nigeria*. Berkeley: University of California Press, 1999.

Scheff, Thomas J., ed. *Mental Illness and Social Processes*. New York: Harper and Row, 1967.

Scull, Andrew. *The Most Solitary of Afflictions: Madness and Society in Britain, 1700–1900*. New Haven: Yale University Press, 1993.

– *Museums of Madness: The Social Organization of Insanity in Nineteenth-Century England*. London: Allen Lane, 1979.

– ed. *Madhouses, Mad-Doctors, and Madmen: The Social History of Psychiatry in the Victorian Era*. Philadelphia: University of Pennsylvania Press, 1981.

– ed. *Social Order/Mental Disorder: Anglo-American Psychiatry in Historical Perspective*. Berkeley: University of California Press, 1989.

Scull, Andrew, Charlotte MacKenzie, and Nicholas Hervey. *Masters of Bedlam: The Transformation of the Mad-Doctoring Trade*. Princeton: Princeton University Press, 1996.

Sedgwick, Peter. *Psycho Politics: Laing, Foucault, Goffman, Szasz, and the Future of Mass Psychiatry*. New York: Harper and Row, 1982.

Shorter, Edward. *From Paralysis to Fatigue: A History of Psychosomatic Illness in the Modern Era*. New York: Free Press, 1992.

– *A History of Psychiatry: From the Era of the Asylum to the Age of Prozac*. New York: John Wiley & Sons, 1997.

– ed. *TPH: History and Memories of the Toronto Psychiatric Hospital, 1925–1966*. Toronto and Dayton: Wall & Emerson, 1996.

Shortt, S.E.D. *Victorian Lunacy: Richard M. Bucke and the Practice of Late Nine-teenth-Century Psychiatry.* Cambridge: Cambridge University Press, 1986.

Showalter, Elaine. *The Female Malady: Women, Madness and English Culture, 1830–1980.* New York: Pantheon, 1985.

Smith, C.J., and J.A. Giggs, eds. *Location and Stigma: Contemporary Perspectives on Mental Health and Mental Health Care.* Boston: Unwin Hyman, 1988.

Smith, Roger. *Trial by Medicine: Insanity and Responsibility in Victorian Trials.* Edinburgh: Edinburgh University Press, 1981.

Snelders, Stephen, and Charles Kaplan. "LSD in Dutch Psychiatry: Changing Socio-Political Settings and Medical Sets." *Medical History* 46 (2002): 221–40.

Srole, Leo, Thomas S. Langner, Stanley T. Michael, Marvin K. Opler, and Thomas A.C. Rennie. *Mental Health in the Metropolis: The Midtown Manhattan Study.* New York: McGraw-Hill Book Co., 1962.

Stalwick, Henry. "A History of Asylum Administration in Pre-Confederation Canada." PhD thesis, University of London, 1969.

Terbenche, Danielle. "'Curative' and 'Custodial': Benefits of Patient Treatment at the Asylum for the Insane, Kingston, 1878–1906." *Canadian Historical Review* 86 (2005): 29–52.

Thifault, Marie-Claude. "L'enfermement asilaire des femmes au Québec: 1873–1921." PhD thesis, Université d'Ottawa, 2003.

Tomes, Nancy. *The Art of Asylum-Keeping: Thomas Story Kirkbride and the Origins of American Psychiatry.* Philadelphia: University of Pennsylvania Press, 1994.

– *A Generous Confidence: Thomas Story Kirkbride and the Art of Asylum-Keeping, 1840–1883.* Cambridge: Cambridge University Press, 1985.

Vanessendelft, William Ray. "A History of the Association for Voluntary Steriliza-tion, 1935–1964." PhD dissertation, University of Minnesota, 1978.

Verdun-Jones, Simon N., and Russell Smandych. "Catch-22 in the Nineteenth Century: The Evolution of Therapeutic Confinement for the Criminally Insane in Canada, 1840–1900." *Criminal Justice History* 2 (1981): 85–108.

Walker, Nigel. *Crime and Insanity in England.* Vol. 1, *The Historical Perspective.* Edinburgh: Edinburgh University Press, 1968.

Walton, John. "Lunacy in the Industrial Revolution: A Study of Asylum Admissions in Lancashire, 1848–1850." *Journal of Social History* 13 (1979): 1–22.

Warsh, Cheryl Krasnick. "The First Mrs Rochester: Wrongful Confinement, Social Redundancy and Commitment to the Private Asylum, 1883–1923." *Canadian Historical Association/Société historique du Canada, Historical Papers/Commu-nications historiques,* 1988, 145–67.

– "'In Charge of the Loons': A Portrait of the London, Ontario Asylum for the Insane in the Nineteenth Century." *Ontario History* 74 (1982): 138–84.

- *Moments of Unreason: The Practice of Canadian Psychiatry and the Homewood Retreat, 1883–1923.* Montreal and Kingston: McGill-Queen's University Press, 1989.

Weinstein, Harvey. *Psychiatry and the* CIA: *Victims of Mind Control.* Washington, DC: American Psychiatric Press, 1990.

Wright, David. "Getting Out of the Asylum: Understanding the Confinement of the Insane in the Nineteenth Century." *Social History of Medicine* 10 (1997): 137–55.

Wright, David, and Anne Digby, eds. *From Idiocy to Mental Deficiency: Historical Perspectives on People with Learning Disabilities.* London: Routledge, 1996.

Index

Aberdeen, Ishbel Gordon, Countess of, 34
Aboriginal patients, 13; admission to hospital, 158–9, 160, 173n24; assimilation of, 163–4; certification of, 161; children of, 154, 155; deaths of, 151–2, 165–6, 166, 167; diagnosis, 159, 160; education levels, 154, 155; in Essondale, 149, 152, 161, 162, 163, 164, 165, 166, 167, 168; experiences in mental hospitals, 162, 163–4; families' correspondence with, 163, 165; families of, 163, 165; gender, 154, 155; geographic origins, 155, 157; identification of, 158; and insanity, 149; institutionalization of, 154–6; interventions on behalf of, 165, 166–7; labour of, 162; language knowledge, 151, 162; length of hospitalization, 166, 167; letters to authorities, 150–2; marital status, 154, 155; occupations, 154, 155; outcomes of institutionalization, 166, 167; probationary discharges, 166–7; in psychiatric historical record, 151; racialization by staff, 163; releases of, 166, 167; religion, 154, 155; resistance by, 164, 169; return to village, 150, 151; status Indians among, 154, 155; suicides, 168–9; treatment of, 151, 160, 162; violent acts by, 174–5n33; women, 154, 162, 163–4; from Yukon Territory, 154–5
Aboriginal peoples: assimilation of, 158; concept of identity, 158; contact with Europeans, 156–7, 158; criminalization of culture/practices, 158; diversity in BC, 162; imprisonment rate, 158; intervention with, 158; isolated surveillance of, 158; land, 157–8; in mental health settings, 158; as patients, 13; population, 157; reserves, 157–8; residential schools, 156, 158, 162; social regulation of, 161; state institutional responses to, 13
abortion, 187
Acadia University, 197; Department of Sociology, 204; Institute, 200
adrenaline, 229, 236
agricultural labour: and mental health, 70, 73, 74, 76, 77, 78, 79, 80, 82, 86
Alberta: sterilization laws in, 179–80, 180
alcohol/alcoholism, 64, 130–1, 132, 222–3, 236
Alden, Francis, 124–5
alienists. See asylum doctors; psychiatrists
Allan Memorial Institute, 210, 211, 223
Amherstburg asylum. See Malden Asylum
anglophones: admissions to asylums, 103; in cities, 99–100; institutionalization by, 99–100
antidepressive drugs, 195, 224
antipsychotic drugs, 195, 224
anxiolytic drugs, 195
Ardagh, John, 77
armed forces: mental breakdown in, 178, 182, 185
Association for Voluntary Sterilization (AVS), 181, 185–6
asylum doctors, 7, 120. See also psychiatrists
asylum visiting, 10–11, 19; as anachronistic, 28; anxiety and, 36–7; attendants and, 40; and boundary between normal and